Alexandra J. Rosborough

KETO SLOW COOKER COOKBOOK

250 Keto Quick and Easy Recipes to Prepare Delicious and Healthy Dishes. Discover How Simply It Is to Lose Weight and Stay Healthy

© Copyright 2020 - All rights reserved.

Table of Contents

Introduction

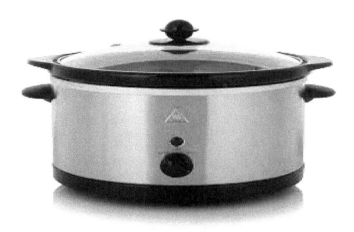

Keto is short for Ketogenic. A Ketogenic diet is a diet with very low carbohydrate intake. By eating little or no carbohydrates, the body has very little of its own glucose or blood sugar to burn. So, it produces "ketones," which are very small molecules that the body can use as an alternative source of fuel. As carbohydrates break down into blood sugar, removing them or limiting them drastically in your diet obligates the body to produce ketones from fat in the liver. Through a ketogenic or keto diet, you are basically changing the fuel for your body. Limiting your blood sugar supply will force the body to burn fat faster. You'll lose weight and be less hungry. The quickest way to produce ketones is through fasting. But fasting is not a daily option. On the other hand, following a keto diet is. You eat well and burn fat at the same time.

What Can I Eat, and What Do I Need to Avoid?

The keto diet offers a varied selection of foods to cook with. Fish, seafood, meat, eggs, cheese, and vegetables are included along with natural fats like butter and olive oil. The important thing is to consume as few carbs as possible on a daily basis. By consuming fewer carbs, you'll burn more fat. This means avoiding starch and sugar. Bread, pasta, potatoes, and rice along with candy, some fruits, sodas, juices, and beer should be avoided. And your food should have a relatively high-fat content with only moderately high protein content. Excess protein can become blood sugar as well.

What Can I Drink?

Water, water, and more water. But you can also drink tea, coffee and even a glass of red wine. No sugar, no sweeteners, and only a small amount of milk or cream are ideal in your coffee and tea.

The Advantages of Cooking with a Slow Cooker

Why should you use a slow cooker as opposed to following the Keto way of life with regular stovetop and oven cooking? There are numerous advantages to using a slow cooker. One great reason alone is that it's economical! You save money and time. The slow cooker uses much less energy than a regular oven, so for people who embrace low energy consumption and consequentially low-cost living, the slow cooker is a great ally to have in the kitchen. It does a wonderful job of tenderizing less expensive cuts of meats helping to trim costs of your food budget, and with less cleaning due to one-pot dinners, you'll even save a little on water consumption and cleaning products.

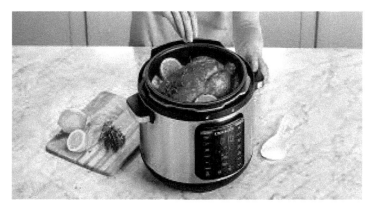

The slow cooker offers a wide variety of one-pot lunches and dinners, including casseroles, chili, soups, stews, and even pizza! Many of these meals can be frozen for use another day, and this avoids wasting leftovers. As to the cooking, the length of time amalgamates all the flavors and seasonings. While a slow cooker may seem more adapted to the winter months with those steaming soups and stews, it's actually great for summer because it doesn't overheat your entire kitchen. And it's literally impossible to burn food or scorch your slow cooker. You'll have a healthier and great tasting meal waiting for you when it's dinnertime. No more takeouts!

Why Should I Follow a Keto Diet or Lifestyle?

The most obvious benefit is weight loss. And while you increase your fat-burning capacity, your insulin levels will be reduced. A keto diet really helps in controlling blood sugar levels. If you suffer from type-2 diabetes, Keto eating may help you in managing your condition, and if you are pre-diabetes, Keto may help you avoid developing the condition. You may see improved levels for some types of cholesterol and improved blood pressure. You'll also have better appetite control. As a result of following a keto diet, you may experience better digestive tract performance with less gas and cramps, less heartburn, and you'll definitely experience fewer sugar cravings.

Will I Suffer on a Keto Diet?

Absolutely not! Most diets tend to be very restrictive, and after a few days, you're literally dying to run to the closest fast-food shack to relieve your discomfort. As you'll learn by preparing and enjoying the many recipes in this book, the food is delicious, filling, and fast and easy to prepare. So, let's get started. Welcome to the mouthwatering world of Keto low-carb dieting!

CHAPTER 1:

The Health Benefits of the Keto Diet

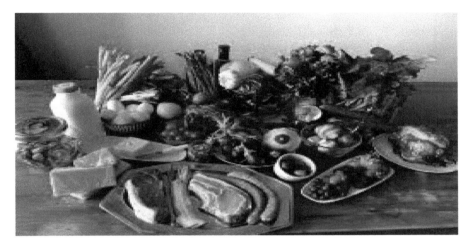

The keto diet allows for an optimal intake of carbohydrates, as well as the optimal use of energy, all of which depend on your way of life. People who are not active or have a sedentary job are much better off with a low carb intake. Those that are more active, especially people who are in contact with sports on a daily basis, can add some more carbs to their diet because they will burn it all off in that same day, and so there will be no carbs left over to turn into fats. Regardless of your lifestyle, everyone benefits from the keto diet in the following ways:

Weight Loss

Far more important than the visual aspect of excess weight is its negative influence on your body. Too much weight affects the efficiency of your body's blood flow, which in turn also affects how much oxygen your heart is able to pump to every part of your system. Too much weight also means that there are layers of fat covering your internal organs, which prevents them from working efficiently. It makes it hard to walk because it puts great pressure on your joints and makes it very difficult to complete even regular daily tasks. A healthy weight allows your body to move freely and your entire internal system to work at its optimal levels.

Cognitive Focus

In order for your brain to function at its best, it needs to have balanced levels of all nutrients and molecules, because a balance allows it to focus on other things, such as working, studying, or creativity. If you eat carbs, the sudden insulin spike that comes with them will force your brain to stop whatever it was doing and to turn its focus on the correct breakdown of glucose molecules. This is why people often feel sleepy and with a foggy mind after high-carb meals. The keto diet keeps the balance strong so that your brain does not have to deal with any sudden surprises.

Blood Sugar Control

If you already have diabetes or are prone to it, then controlling your blood sugar is obviously of the utmost importance. However, even if you are not battling a type of diabetes at the moment, that doesn't mean that you are not in danger of developing it in the future. Most people forget that insulin is a finite resource in your body. You are given a certain amount of it, and it is gradually used up throughout your life. The more often you eat carbs, the more often your body needs to use insulin to break down the glucose, and when it reaches critically low levels of this finite resource, diabetes is formed.

Lower Cholesterol and Blood Pressure

Cholesterol and triglyceride levels maintain or ruin your arterial health. If your arteries are clogged up with cholesterol, they cannot efficiently transfer blood through your system, which in some cases even results in heart attacks. The keto diet keeps all of these levels at an optimal level so that they do not interfere with your body's normal functioning.

CHAPTER 2:

Tips to be Considered When Cooking on Slow Cookers

1. If you are trying a recipe that is not written for the slow cooker, then reduce the amount of liquid in the recipe by at least one-third because no liquid escapes during its cooking process.

   But then, for slow cooker recipes, don't add much liquid as slow cookers are good at retaining moisture. If at all, it seems dry, you can top up the water.

2. Don't open and close the lid many times as the heat will be lost. This will slow the cooking time. Every time you open the lid, about 20 minutes of cooking time is lost.

3. The inner pot of the slow cooker should always be at room temperature. When you are using frozen foods, make sure to thaw them before cooking in the slow cooker.

4. When cooking rice, make sure to clean them well, because the more starch you can remove from the rice, the better will be the end result as it won't be a sticky mess then.

5. Make sure to brown the meat well. The slow cooking method usually results in less color because of the appliance's gentle heat. So to avoid the dish being bland and to make it more flavourful, always brown the meat before adding it to the slow cooker.

6. When cooking in the slow cooker, make sure not to fill them more than two-thirds full and not less than half full. Cooking too much or too little can affect the cooking time, safety, and quality.

7. Avoid lean meats in the slow cooker. The same also holds true while cooking delicate vegetables for a long time, like peas, as these veggies become mushy.

   If it needs to be added, just add it to the end of the cooking time.

   When both veggies and meat need to be cooked at the same time, place the veggies on the bottom and then the meat on top. This is because vegetables cook slower than meat and poultry.

8. Don't add too many spices as they become spicier with time.

9. Prolonged cooking of dairy products can cause them to separate and curdle.

10. Regarding settings, one hour on high power is more or less equal to two hours on low power. Similarly, one hour in the oven at 350 ° F is equal to four hours on high heat.

Myths About the Slow Cooker

1. Though we *shouldn't open the lids frequently*, opening the lid by the end of the cooking period wouldn't do much harm as most of the cooking is already done with.

2. Another myth is that *slow cookers are suitable only for making stews and soups*. Though they are exceptional for making these two types, they are also fitting for making a number of other fares. Anything that does well on low heat and cooking on stovetops and oven will also work well on the slow cooker.

3. *Everything slow cooked will be watered.* Slow cookers retain moisture and don't lose much liquid during the cooking process as they never get a chance to reduce the way it does in the stovetop over direct heat. This may sometimes lead to watered sauces and gravies. But then this can be rectified either by using thickeners or by cooking it open during the last stages of cooking.

4. *You can dump all ingredients and go.* Though it is true to a good extent, they are several things you need to do to prepare yourself for more flavor. You need to brown the meat or sauté the onion before adding them to the slow cooker. Sometimes you need to add delicate ingredients, which can only be added at the end stage, etc.

5. You *can't make pasta in slow cookers* as it would result in a big white mess. Provided you take proper measures, it isn't hard to make good pasta in slow cookers.

CHAPTER 3:

Breakfast Recipes

Nutritious Burrito Bowl

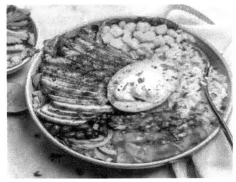

Preparation Time: 18 minutes

Cooking time: 7 hours

Servings: 6

Ingredients:

- 10 oz. chicken breast
- 1 tablespoon chili flakes
- 1 teaspoon salt
- 1 teaspoon onion powder
- 1 teaspoon minced garlic
- ½ cup white beans, canned
- ¼ cup green peas
- 1 cup chicken stock
- ½ avocado, pitted
- 1 teaspoon ground black pepper

Directions:

1. Put the chicken breast in the slow cooker.
2. Sprinkle the chicken breast with chili flakes, salt, onion powder, minced garlic, and ground black pepper. Add the chicken stock.
3. Close the slow cooker lid and cook the dish for 2 hours on HIGH.

4. After this, open the slow cooker lid and add the white beans and green peas.
5. Mix and close the lid. Cook the dish for 5 hours more on LOW.
6. When the time is done, remove the meat, white beans, and green peas from the slow cooker. Transfer the white beans and green peas to the serving bowls.
7. Shred the chicken breast and add it to the serving bowls too.
8. After this, peel the avocado and chop it. Sprinkle the prepared burrito bowls with the chopped avocado. Enjoy!

Nutrition: calories 192, fat 7, carbs 13, protein 11

Quinoa Curry

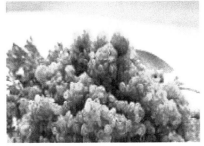

Preparation Time: 20 minutes

Cooking time: 9 hours

Servings: 7

Ingredients:

- 8 oz. potato
- 7 oz. cauliflower
- 1 cup onion, chopped
- 7 oz. chickpea, canned
- 1 cup tomatoes, chopped
- 13 oz. almond milk

- 3 cup chicken stock
- 8 tablespoon quinoa
- 1/3 tablespoon miso
- 1 teaspoon minced garlic
- 2 teaspoon curry paste

Directions:

1. Peel the potatoes and chop them.
2. Put the chopped potatoes, onion, and tomatoes into the slow cooker. Combine the miso, chicken stock, and curry paste together.
3. Whisk the mixture until the ingredients are dissolved in the chicken stock. Pour the chicken stock in the slow cooker too.
4. Separate the cauliflower into the florets.
5. Add the cauliflower florets and the chickpeas to the slow cooker.
6. Add the almond milk, quinoa, and minced garlic. Close the slow cooker lid and cook the dish on LOW for 9 hours.
7. When the dish is cooked, chill it and then mix it gently.
8. Transfer the prepared curry quinoa to the bowls. Enjoy!

Nutrition: calories 262, fat 4, carbs 18, protein 12

Ham Pitta Pockets

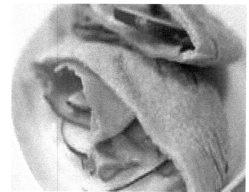

Preparation Time: 14 minutes
Cooking time: 1.5 minutes
Servings: 6
Ingredients:

- 6 pita breads, sliced

- 7 oz. mozzarella, sliced
- 1 teaspoon minced garlic
- 7 oz. ham, sliced
- 1 big tomato, sliced
- 1 tablespoon mayo
- 1 tablespoon heavy cream

Directions:

1. Preheat the slow cooker on HIGH for 30 minutes.
2. Combine the mayo, heavy cream, and minced garlic.
3. Spread the inside of the pita bread with the mayo mixture.
4. After this, fill the pitta bread with the sliced mozzarella, tomato, and ham.
5. Wrap the pita bread in foil and place them in the slow cooker.
6. Close the slow cooker lid and cook the dish for 1.5 hours on HIGH.
7. Then discard the foil and serve the prepared pita pockets immediately. Enjoy!

Nutrition: calories 273, fat 3, carbs 10, protein 10

Breakfast Meatloaf

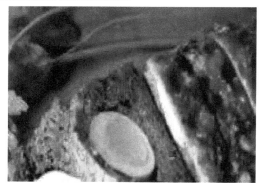

Preparation Time: 18 minutes
Cooking time: 7 hours
Servings: 8
Ingredients:

- 12 oz. ground beef
- 1 teaspoon salt
- 1 teaspoon ground coriander
- 1 tablespoon ground mustard

- ¼ teaspoon ground chili pepper
- 6 oz. white bread
- ½ cup milk
- 1 teaspoon ground black pepper
- 3 tablespoon tomato sauce

Directions:
1. Chop the white bread and combine it with the milk.
2. Stir, then set aside for 3 minutes.
3. Meanwhile, combine the ground beef, salt, ground coriander, ground mustard, ground chili pepper, and ground black pepper.
4. Stir the white bread mixture carefully and add it to the ground beef. Cover the bottom of the slow cooker bowl with foil.
5. Shape the meatloaf and place the uncooked meatloaf in the slow cooker, then spread it with the tomato sauce.
6. Close the slow cooker lid and cook the meatloaf for 7 hours on LOW.
7. Slice the prepared meatloaf and serve. Enjoy!

Nutrition: calories 214, fat 14, carbs 12, protein 9

Breakfast Sweet Pepper Rounds

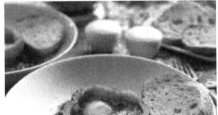

Preparation Time: 10 minutes
Cooking time: 3 hours
Servings: 4
Ingredients:

- 2 red sweet pepper
- 7 oz. ground chicken
- 5 oz. Parmesan
- 1 tablespoon sour cream

- 1 tablespoon flour
- 1 egg
- 2 teaspoon almond milk
- 1 teaspoon salt
- ½ teaspoon ground black pepper
- ¼ teaspoon butter

Directions:
1. Combine the sour cream with the ground chicken, flour, ground black pepper, almond milk, and butter.
2. Beat eggs into the mixture.
3. Remove the seeds from the sweet peppers and slice them roughly.
4. Place the pepper slices in the slow cooker and fill them with the ground chicken mixture.
5. After this, chop Parmesan into the cubes and add it into the sliced peppers.
6. Close the slow cooker lid and cook the dish for 3 hours on HIGH.
7. When the time is done, make sure that the ground chicken is cooked, and the cheese is melted. Enjoy the dish immediately.

Nutrition: calories 261, fat 8, carbs 13, protein 21

Breakfast Cauliflower Hash

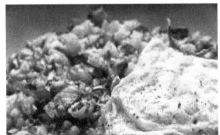

Preparation Time: 17 minutes
Cooking time: 8 hours
Servings: 5
Ingredients:

- 7 eggs
- ¼ cup milk
- 1 teaspoon salt
- 1 teaspoon ground black pepper

- ½ teaspoon ground mustard
- 10 oz. cauliflower
- ¼ teaspoon chili flakes
- 5 oz. breakfast sausages, chopped
- ½ onion, chopped
- 5 oz. Cheddar cheese, shredded

Directions:

1. Wash the cauliflower carefully and separate it into the florets.
2. After this, shred the cauliflower florets.
3. Beat the eggs in a bowl and whisk. Add the milk, salt, ground black pepper, ground mustard, chili flakes, and chopped onion into the whisked egg mixture.
4. Put the shredded cauliflower in the slow cooker. Add the whisked egg mixture. Add the shredded cheese and chopped sausages.
5. Stir the mixture gently and close the slow cooker lid. Cook the dish on LOW for 8 hours. When the cauliflower hash is cooked, remove it from the slow cooker and mix up. Enjoy!

Nutrition: calories 329, fat 16, carbs 10, protein 23

Healthy Low Carb Walnut Zucchini Bread

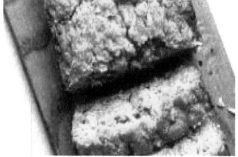

Preparation Time: 17 minutes
Cooking time: 3 hours 10 minutes
Servings: 12
Ingredients:

- 3 eggs
- 1/2 cup walnuts, chopped

- 2 cups zucchini, shredded
- 2 tsp vanilla
- 1/2 cup pyure all-purpose sweetener
- 1/3 cup coconut oil, softened
- 1/2 Tsp baking soda
- 1 1/2 Tsp baking powder
- 2 tsp cinnamon
- 1/3 cup coconut flour
- 1 cup almond flour
- 1/2 Tsp salt

Directions:

1. Mix all the ingredients. Set aside.
2. In another bowl, whisk together eggs, vanilla, sweetener, and oil.
3. Add dry mixture to the wet mixture and fold well.
4. Add walnut and zucchini and fold well.
5. Pour batter into the silicone bread pan.
6. Place the bread pan into the slow cooker on the rack. Cover slow cooker with lid and cook on high for 3 hours.
7. Cut bread loaf into slices and serve.

Nutrition: calories 174, fat 15, carbs 5, protein 7

Savory Creamy Breakfast Casserole

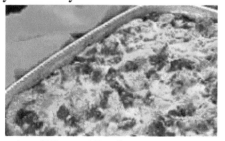

Preparation Time: 17 minutes
Cooking time: 5 hours on low 3 hours on high
Servings: 5
Ingredients:

- 1 tablespoon unsalted butter, Ghee (here), or extra-virgin olive oil
- 10 large eggs, beaten

- 1 cup heavy (whipping) cream
- 1½ cups shredded sharp Cheddar cheese, divided
- ½ cup grated Romano cheese
- ½ teaspoon kosher salt
- ¼ teaspoon freshly ground black pepper
- 8 ounces thick-cut ham, diced
- ¾ head broccoli, cut into small florets
- ½ onion, diced

Directions:
1. Generously coat the inside of the slow cooker insert with the butter.
2. Directly in the insert, whisk together the eggs, heavy cream, ½ cup of Cheddar cheese, Romano cheese, salt, and pepper.
3. Stir in the ham, broccoli, and onion.
4. Sprinkle the remaining 1 cup of Cheddar cheese over the top. Cover and cook for 6 hours on low or 3 hours on high. Serve hot.

Nutrition: calories 465, fat 10, carbs 7, protein 28

Delicious Bacon & Cheese Frittata

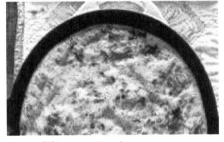

Preparation Time: 15 minutes
Cooking time: 2 hours 30 minutes
Servings: 8
Ingredients:

- 1/2 lb bacon
- 2 tablespoons butter
- 8 oz fresh spinach, packed down
- 10 eggs
- 1/2 cup heavy whipping cream
- 1/2 cup shredded cheese

- Salt and pepper

Directions:
1. Butter or grease the inside of your slow-cooker.
2. Loosely chop the spinach.
3. Cut bacon into half-inch pieces.
4. Beat the eggs with the spices, cream, cheese, and chopped spinach. Then everything will be blended smoothly.
5. Line the bottom of the slow cooker with the bacon.
6. Pour the egg mixture over the bacon.
7. Cover the crockpot and adjust the temperature to high
8. Cook for 2 hours.
9. Serve hot.

Nutrition: calories 392, fat 34, carbs 4, protein 19

Delight Breakfast Meatloaf

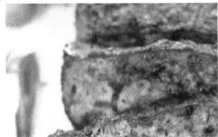

Preparation Time: 10 minutes
Cooking time: 3 hours 10 minutes
Servings: 8
Ingredients:

- 2 lb ground pork
- 2 eggs
- 2 tbsp paprika
- 2 tbsp fresh sage
- 1 tbsp olive oil
- 1 diced onion
- 3 garlic cloves
- 1/4 cup of almond flour

Directions
1. Saute vegetables in the crockpot in the olive oil until brown.

2. Mix together the pork, eggs, sage, paprika, and almond flour thoroughly.

3. Add the cooked onions and garlic.

4. Shape the meat mixture into the shape of a loaf.

5. Put the loaf in the crockpot, cover with the lid, and cook for three hours on low heat.

6. Serve in slices immediately, or save to serve at breakfast later.

Nutrition: calories 406, fat 26, carbs 5, protein 32

Low-Carb Hash Brown Breakfast Casserole

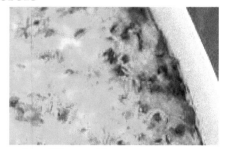

Preparation Time: 10 minutes

Cooking time: 6 hours on low

Servings: 6

Ingredients:

- 1 tablespoon unsalted butter, Ghee (here), or extra-virgin olive oil

- 12 large eggs

- ½ cup heavy (whipping) cream

- 1 head cauliflower, shredded or minced

- 1 onion, diced

- 10 ounces cooked breakfast sausage links, sliced

- 2 cups shredded Cheddar cheese, divided

Directions

1. Generously coat the inside of the slow cooker insert with the butter.

2. In a large bowl, beat the eggs, then whisk in heavy cream, 1 teaspoon of salt, ½ teaspoon of pepper, and the ground mustard.

3. Spread about one-third of the cauliflower in an even layer in the bottom of the cooker.

4. Layer one-third of the onions over the cauliflower, then one-third of the sausage, and top with ½ cup of Cheddar cheese. Season with salt and pepper. Repeat twice more with the remaining ingredients. You should have ½ cup of Cheddar cheese left.

5. Pour the egg mixture evenly over the layered ingredients, then sprinkle the remaining ½ cup Cheddar cheese on top. Cover and cook for 6 hours on low. Serve hot.

Nutrition: calories 523, fat 18, carbs 7, protein 3

Asparagus Smoked Salmon

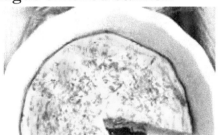

Preparation Time: 15 minutes

Cooking time: 5 hours

Servings: 6

Ingredients:

- 1 tablespoon extra-virgin olive oil

- 6 large eggs

- 1 cup heavy (whipping) cream

- 2 teaspoons chopped fresh dill, plus additional for garnish

- ½ teaspoon kosher salt

- ¼ teaspoon freshly ground black pepper

- 1½ cups shredded Havarti or Monterey Jack cheese

- 12 ounces asparagus, trimmed and sliced

- 6 ounces smoked salmon, flaked

- Generously coat the inside of the slow cooker insert with the olive oil.

- In a large bowl, beat the eggs, then whisk in the heavy cream, dill, salt, and pepper.
- Stir in the cheese and asparagus.

Directions:

1. Gently fold in the salmon and then pour the mixture into the prepared insert. Cover and cook for 6 hours on low or 3 hours on high. Serve warm, garnished with additional fresh dill.

Nutrition: calories 388, fat 19, carbs 10, protein 21

Broccoli Cream Cheese Quiche

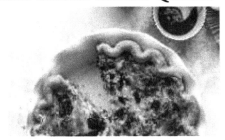

Preparation Time: 10 minutes

Cooking time: 2 hours 30 minutes

Servings: 8

Ingredients:

- 9 eggs
- 2 cups cheese, shredded and divided
- 8 oz cream cheese
- 1/4 Tsp onion powder
- 3 cups broccoli, cut into florets
- 1/4 Tsp pepper
- 3/4 Tsp salt

Directions:

1. Add broccoli into the boiling water and cook for 3 minutes. Drain well and set aside to cool.
2. Add eggs, cream cheese, onion powder, pepper, and salt in a mixing bowl and beat until well combined.
3. Spray slow cooker from inside using cooking spray.
4. Add cooked broccoli into the slow cooker, then sprinkle half cup cheese.

5. Pour egg mixture over broccoli and cheese mixture.
6. Cover slow cooker and cook on high for 2 hours and 15 minutes.
7. Once it done, sprinkle the remaining cheese and cover for 10 minutes or until cheese melted. Serve warm and enjoy.

Nutrition: calories 296, fat 24, carbs 3, protein 16

Delicious Thyme Sausage Squash

Preparation Time: 15 minutes

Cooking time: 6 hours on low

Servings: 4

Ingredients:

- 2 tablespoons extra-virgin olive oil
- 14 ounces smoked chicken sausage, halved lengthwise and thinly sliced crosswise
- ¼ cup chicken broth
- 1 onion, halved and sliced
- ½ medium butternut squash, peeled, seeds and pulp removed and diced
- 1 small green bell pepper, seeded and cut into 1-inch-wide strips
- ½ small red bell pepper, seeded and cut into 1-inch-wide strips
- ½ small yellow bell pepper, seeded and cut into 1-inch-wide strips
- 1 cup shredded Swiss cheese

Directions:

1. In the slow cooker, combine all the ingredients and cook for 6 hours on low.
2. Just before serving, sprinkle the Swiss cheese over the top, cover, and cook for about 3 minutes more to melt the cheese.
3. Make It Paleo Omit the cheese and use a paleo-friendly sausage or diced ham.

Nutrition: calories 502, fat 26, carbs 13, protein 27

Tasty Greek Style Breakfast

Preparation Time: 10 minutes

Cooking time: 5 hours 20 minutes

Servings: 6

Ingredients:

- 8 oz spinach
- 3 cloves chopped garlic
- 12 eggs
- 1/2 cup milk
- 8 oz sliced crimini mushrooms
- 4 oz sun-dried tomatoes
- 1 cup feta cheese
- Salt and pepper

Directions:

1. Butter or grease the inside of your slow cooker.
2. Beat together the eggs, milk, garlic, salt, and pepper separately from the other ingredients.
3. Put in the sun-dried tomatoes, sliced mushrooms, and spinach, stirring well.
4. Put the egg mixture in the slow-cooker.
5. Top it off with the feta cheese. Cover the crockpot and set it on the low setting. Cook for five hours. Serve hot and enjoy!

Nutrition: calories 236, fat 15, carbs 7, protein 18

Mexican Style Breakfast Casserole

Preparation Time: 17 minutes

Cooking time: 2.5 hours on Low, or 4.5 hours on high

Servings: 5

Ingredients:

- 5 eggs
- 6 ounces pork sausage, cooked, drained
- ½ cup 1% milk
- ½ teaspoon garlic powder
- 2 jalapeños, deseeded, finely chopped
- ½ teaspoon ground cumin
- ½ teaspoon ground coriander
- 1 ½ cups chunky salsa
- 1 ½ cup pepper Jack cheese, shredded
- Salt to taste
- Pepper to taste
- ¼ cup fresh cilantro

Directions:

1. Spray the inside of the cooking pot with cooking spray.
2. Whisk together in a bowl, eggs, salt, pepper, and milk.
3. Add garlic powder, cumin, coriander, and sausage and mix well.
4. Pour the mixture into the slow cooker.
5. Close the lid. Set cooker on 'Low' option and timer for 4-5 hours or on 'High' option and timer for 2-3 hours.
6. Place toppings of your choice and serve.

Nutrition: calories 320, fat 24, carbs 5, protein 13

Almond Lemon Blueberry Muffins

Preparation Time: 17 minutes

Cooking time: 2-3 hours on High

Servings: 3

Ingredients:

- 1 cup almond flour
- 1 large egg
- 3 drops Stevia
- ¼ cup fresh blueberries
- ¼ teaspoon lemon zest, grated
- ¼ teaspoon pure lemon extract
- ½ cup heavy whipping cream
- 2 tablespoons butter, melted
- ½ teaspoon baking powder

Directions:

1. Add egg into a bowl. Whisk well
2. Add the rest of the ingredients into the bowl of egg. Whisk well.
3. Pour batter into lined or greased muffin molds. Pour up to ¾ of the cup.

4. Pour 6 ounces of water into the slow cooker. Place an aluminum foil at the bottom of the cooker. Place the muffin molds inside the cooker. Close the lid. Set cooker on 'High' option and timer for 2-3 hours. Let it cool in the cooker for a while. Remove from the cooker. Loosen the edges of the muffins. Invert on to a plate and serve.

Nutrition: calories 223, fat 21, carbs 5, protein 6

Creamy Oregano Chorizo Mushroom

Preparation Time: 10 minutes

Cooking time: 4 hours 30 minutes

Servings: 8

Ingredients:

- 4 bell peppers
- 3 tbsp oregano
- 2 large onions
- 1 lb fresh mushrooms of any kind
- 1 lb cream cheese
- 1 cup milk
- 2 eggs
- 1 lb chorizo style Mexican sausage

Directions:

1. Slice the bell peppers into thick slices.
2. Chop onion into large pieces.
3. Halve or quarter-chop mushrooms, depending on preference.
4. Turn on the slow cooker to high and begin to brown the chorizo, allowing the grease to bubble.
5. Cook onions, peppers, and mushrooms for a few moments in chorizo grease.
6. Combine the creamed cheese, oregano, milk, and eggs until blended smoothly. Pour milk and egg mixture on top of the meat in the crockpot and set to low heat. Cover and let cook for four hours. Serve hot and enjoy!

Nutrition: calories 516, fat 10, carbs 11, protein 22

Healthy Veggie Omelet

Preparation Time: 10 minutes

Cooking time: 1 hour 40 minutes

Servings: 4

Ingredients:

- 6 eggs
- 1 tsp parsley, dried
- 1 tsp garlic powder
- 1 bell pepper, diced
- 1/2 cup onion, sliced
- 1 cup spinach
- 1/2 cup almond milk, unsweetened
- 4 egg whites
- Pepper
- Salt

Directions

1. Spray slow cooker from inside using cooking spray.
2. In a large bowl, whisk together egg whites, eggs, parsley, garlic powder, almond milk, pepper, and salt.
3. Stir in bell peppers, spinach, and onion.
4. Pour egg mixture into the slow cooker.
5. Cover and cook on high for 90 minutes or until egg is set.
6. Cut into the slices and serve.

Nutrition: calories 200, fat 13, carbs 6, protein 13

Parmesan Sausage Mushroom Breakfast

Preparation Time: 15 minutes

Cooking time: On Low for 5 hours

Servings: 4

Ingredients:

- 2 cups cooked ground sausage
- ½ cup chopped onion
- 1 Tbsp. parsley, dried
- 1 tsp garlic powder
- 1 tsp thyme

- 6 crumbled bacon slices, cooked and drained
- 2 cups organic chicken broth
- 1 cup red bell pepper, chopped
- ½ cup Parmesan cheese
- 1 cups heavy white cream
- 2 cups raw mushrooms, sliced
- Pepper
- Salt

Directions:

1. Add all the above ingredients to a large slow cooker.
2. Cook on LOW mode for 4-6 hours. Make sure not to overcook or cook at too high heat, or the cream will separate. Serve hot.

Nutrition: calories 166, fat 15, carbs 3, protein 6

Arugula Cheese Herb Frittata

Preparation Time: 17 minutes
Cooking time: 3 hours 10 minutes
Servings: 6
Ingredients:

- 8 eggs
- 3/4 cup goat cheese, crumbled
- 1/2 cup onion, sliced
- 1 1/2 cups red peppers, roasted and chopped
- 4 cups baby arugula
- 1 tsp oregano, dried
- 1/3 cup almond milk
- Pepper
- Salt

Directions:

1. Spray slow cooker from inside using cooking spray.
2. In a mixing bowl, whisk together eggs, oregano, and almond milk.
3. Season with pepper and salt.
4. Arrange red peppers, onion, arugula, and cheese into the slow cooker.
5. Pour egg mixture into the slow cooker over the vegetables.
6. Cover and cook on low for 3 hours. Serve hot and enjoy.

Nutrition: calories 178, fat 12, carbs 6, protein 11

CHAPTER 4:

Hors d'oeuvres

Pimiento Cheese Dip

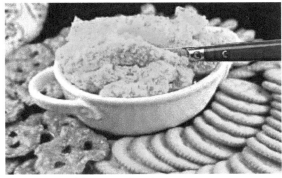

Preparation Time: 10 minutes
Cooking time: 2 hours 15 minutes
Servings: 8
Ingredients:

- 1/2 pound grated Cheddar
- 1/4 pound grated pepper Jack cheese
- 1/2 cup sour cream
- 1/2 cup green olives, sliced
- 2 tablespoons diced pimientos 1 teaspoon hot sauce
- 1/4 teaspoon garlic powder
- 1/4 teaspoon onion powder

Directions:

1. Combine all the ingredients in a Slow Cooker. Cover the pot with its lid and cook on high settings for hours. The dip is best served warm with vegetable sticks or bread sticks.

Nutrition: calories 123, fat 10, carbs 6, protein 16

Zesty Lamb Meatballs

Preparation Time: 15 minutes
Cooking time: 7 hours 15 minutes
Servings: 10
Ingredients:

- 3 pounds ground lamb
- 1 shallot, chopped
- 2 garlic cloves, minced
- 1 tablespoon lemon zest
- 1/4 teaspoon five-spice powder
- 1/2 teaspoon cumin powder
- 1/4 teaspoon chili powder
- 1/2 cup raisins, chopped
- 1 teaspoon dried mint
- Salt and pepper to taste
- 2 cups tomato sauce
- 1 lemon, juiced
- 1 bay leaf
- 1 thyme sprig
- 1 red chili, chopped

Directions:

1. Mix the tomato sauce, lemon juice, bay leaf, thyme sprig, and red chili in your Slow Cooker. Combine the remaining ingredients in a bowl and mix well. Season with salt and pepper and give it a good mix. Form small balls and place them in the sauce. Cover with its lid and cook over low heat for 7 hours. Serve the meatballs warm or chilled.

Nutrition: calories 231, fat 14, carbs 9, protein 18

Spicy Monterey Jack Fondue

Preparation Time: 15 minutes
Cooking time: 4 hours 15 minutes
Servings: 6
Ingredients:

- 1 garlic clove
- 1 cup white wine
- 2 cups grated Monterey Jack cheese
- 1/2 cup grated Parmesan
- 1 red chili, seeded and chopped
- 1 tablespoon cornstarch
- 1/2 cup milk
- 1 pinch nutmeg - 1 pinch salt
- 1 pinch ground black pepper

Directions:

1. Rub the inside of your Slow Cooker's pot with a garlic clove just to infuse it with aroma. Add the white wine into the pot and stir in the cheeses, red chili, cornstarch, and milk. Season with nutmeg, salt, and black pepper and cook on low heat for 4 hours. The fondue is best served warm with bread sticks or vegetables.

Nutrition: calories 278, fat 6, carbs 2, protein 25

Balsamico Pulled Pork

Preparation Time: 10 minutes
Cooking time: 8 hours 15 minutes
Servings: 6
Ingredients:

- 2 pounds boneless pork shoulder
- 2 tablespoons honey
- 1/4 cup balsamic vinegar
- 1/4 cup hoisin sauce
- 1 tablespoon Dijon mustard
- 1/4 cup chicken stock
- 2 garlic cloves, minced
- 2 shallots, sliced
- 2 tablespoons soy sauce

Directions:

1. Combine the honey, vinegar, hoisin sauce, mustard, stock, garlic, shallots, and soy sauce in your Slow Cooker. Add the pork shoulder and roll it in the mixture until evenly coated. Cover the Slow Cooker and cook over low heat for 8 hours. When done, shred the meat into fine pieces and serve warm or chilled.

Nutrition: calories 239, fat 12, carbs 6, protein 21

Pork Ham Dip

Preparation Time: 15 minutes
Cooking time: 6 hours 15 minutes
Servings: 20
Ingredients:

- 2 cups diced ham
- 1 pound ground pork
- 1 shallot, chopped
- 2 garlic cloves, chopped
- 1 teaspoon Dijon mustard
- 1 cup tomato sauce
- 1/2 cup chili sauce
- 1/2 cup cranberry sauce
- Salt and pepper to taste

Directions:

1. Heat a skillet over medium flame and add the ground pork. Cook for 5 minutes, stirring often. Transfer the ground pork to a Slow Cooker and add the remaining ingredients. Adjust the taste with salt and pepper and cook over low heat for 6 hours. Serve the dip warm or chilled.

Nutrition: calories 208, fat 12, carbs 3, protein 15

Cheesy Bacon Dip

Preparation Time: 4 1/4 Hours
Cooking time: 4 1/4 Hours
Servings: 20
Ingredients:

- 1 sweet onions, chopped

- 1 teaspoon Worcestershire sauce
- 1 teaspoon Dijon mustard
- 1 cup cream cheese
- 10 bacon slices, chopped
- 1 cup grated Gruyere
- 1/2 cup whole milk
- Salt and pepper to taste

Directions:

1. Combine all the ingredients in a Slow Cooker. Adjust the taste with salt and pepper and cover with its lid. Cook over low heat for 4 hours. Serve the dip warm or chilled with vegetable sticks, biscuits, or other salty snacks.

Nutrition: calories 342, fat 12, carbs 5, protein 11

Wild Mushroom Dip

Preparation Time: 15 minutes
Cooking time: 4 hours 15 minutes
Servings: 20
Ingredients:

- 1 pound wild mushrooms, chopped
- 1 cup white wine
- 1 cup cream cheese
- 1 cup heavy cream
- 1/2 cup grated Parmesan
- 1 teaspoon dried tarragon
- 1/2 teaspoon dried oregano
- 1/2 teaspoon ground black pepper
- Salt and pepper to taste

Directions:

1. Combine all the ingredients in your Slow Cooker. Adjust the taste with salt and pepper and cook over low heat for 4 hours. Serve the dip warm or chilled.

Nutrition: calories 278, fat 18, carbs 4, protein 22

Bacon Crab Dip

Preparation Time: 15 minutes
Cooking time: 2 hours 15 minutes
Servings: 20
Ingredients:

- 1 pound bacon, diced
- 1 cup cream cheese
- 1/2 cup grated Parmesan cheese
- 1 teaspoon Worcestershire sauce
- 1 teaspoon Dijon mustard
- 1 can crab meat, drained and shredded
- 1 teaspoon hot sauce

Directions:

1. Heat a skillet over medium flame and add the bacon. Sauté for 5 minutes until fat begins to drain out. Transfer the bacon to a Slow Cooker. Stir in the remaining ingredients and cook on high settings for 2 hours. Serve the dip warm or chilled.

Nutrition: calories 380, fat 24, carbs 12, protein 16

Pepperoni Pizza Dip

Preparation Time: 10 minutes
Cooking time: 3 hours 15 minutes
Servings: 10
Ingredients:

- 1 1/2 cups pizza sauce
- 4 pepperoni, sliced
- 2 shallots, chopped
- 2 red bell peppers, diced
- 1/2 cup black olives, pitted and chopped
- 1 cup cream cheese
- 1 cup shredded mozzarella
- 1/2 teaspoon dried basil

Directions:

1. Combine the pizza sauce and the rest of the ingredients in your Slow Cooker. Cover the pot with its lid and cook over low heat for 3 hours.

2. The dip is best served warm with bread sticks or tortilla chips.

Nutrition: calories 180, fat 12, carbs 18, protein 18

Blue Cheese Chicken Wings

Preparation Time: 10 minutes
Cooking time: 7 hours 15 minutes
Servings: 8
Ingredients:

- 4 pounds chicken wings
- 1/2 cup buffalo sauce
- 1/2 cup spicy tomato sauce
- 1 tablespoon tomato paste
- 2 tablespoons apple cider vinegar
- 1 tablespoon Worcestershire sauce
- 1 cup sour cream
- 2 oz. blue cheese, crumbled
- 1 thyme sprig

Directions:

1. Combine the buffalo sauce, tomato sauce, vinegar, Worcestershire sauce, sour cream, blue cheese, and thyme in a Slow Cooker. Add the chicken wings and toss them until evenly coated. Cook over low heat for 7 hours. Serve the chicken wings, preferably warm.

Nutrition: calories 345, fat 18, carbs 7, protein 29

Turkey Meatloaf

Preparation Time: 10 minutes
Cooking time: 6 hours 15 minutes
Servings: 8
Ingredients:

- 1 1/2 pounds ground turkey
- 1 carrot, grated
- 1 sweet potato, grated
- 1 egg
- 1/4 cup breadcrumbs
- 1/4 teaspoon chili powder

- Salt and pepper to taste
- 1 cup shredded mozzarella

Directions:

1. Mix all the ingredients in a bowl and season with salt and pepper as needed. Give it a good mix, then transfer the mixture to your Slow Cooker. Level the mixture well and cover with the pot's lid. Cook over low heat for 6 hours. Serve the meatloaf warm or chilled.

Nutrition: calories 308, fat 6, carbs 2, protein 18

White Bean Hummus

Preparation Time: 15 minutes
Cooking time: 8 hours 15 minutes
Servings: 8
Ingredients:

- 1 pound dried white beans, rinsed
- 2 cups water
- 2 cups chicken stock
- 1 bay leaf
- 1 thyme sprig
- 4 garlic cloves, minced
- Salt and pepper to taste
- 2 tablespoons canola oil
- 2 large sweet onions, sliced

Directions:

1. Combine the white beans, water, stock, bay leaf, and thyme in your Slow Cooker. Add salt and pepper to taste and cook the beans over low heat for 8 hours. When done, drain the beans well (but reserve 1/4 cup of the liquid) and discard the bay leaf and thyme. Transfer the bean to a food processor. Add the reserved liquid and pulse until smooth. Season with salt and pepper and transfer to a bowl. Heat the canola oil in a skillet and add the onions. Cook for 10 minutes over medium flame until the onions begin to caramelize.

2. Top the hummus with caramelized onions and serve.

Nutrition: calories 456, fat 12, carbs 6, protein 11

Tropical Meatballs

Preparation Time: 15 minutes
Cooking time: 7 hours 30 minutes
Servings: 20
Ingredients:

- 1 can pineapple chunks (keep the juices)
- 2 poblano peppers, chopped
- 1/4 cup brown sugar
- 2 tablespoons soy sauce
- 2 tablespoons cornstarch
- 1 tablespoon lemon juice
- 2 pounds ground pork
- 1 pound ground beef
- 4 garlic clove, minced
- 1 teaspoon dried basil
- 1 egg
- 1/4 cup breadcrumbs
- Salt and pepper to taste

Directions:

1. Mix the pineapple, poblano peppers, brown sugar, soy sauce, cornstarch, and lemon juice in a Slow Cooker.
2. Cover and cook over low heat for 7 hours. Serve the meatballs warm or chilled.

Nutrition: calories 421, fat 8, carbs 4, protein 19

Bacon Black Bean Dip

Preparation Time: 15 minutes
Cooking time: 6 hours 10 minutes
Servings: 6
Ingredients:

- 6 bacon slices
- 2 cans black beans, drained
- 2 shallots, sliced
- 1 garlic cloves, chopped
- 1 cup red salsa
- 1/2 cup beef stock
- 1 tablespoon brown sugar
- 1 tablespoon molasses
- 1/2 teaspoon chili powder
- 1 tablespoon apple cider vinegar
- 2 tablespoons Bourbon
- Salt and pepper to taste

Directions:

1. Heat a skillet over medium flame and add the bacon. Cook until crisp, then transfer the bacon and its fat in your Slow Cooker. Stir in the remaining ingredients and cook over low heat for 6 hours. When done, partially mash the beans and serve the dip right away.

Nutrition: calories 321, fat 12, carbs 6, protein 21

Quick Parmesan Bread

Preparation Time: 15 minutes
Cooking time: 1 hour 15 minutes
Servings: 8
Ingredients:

- 4 cups all-purpose flour
- 1/2 teaspoon salt
- 1/2 cup grated Parmesan cheese
- 1 teaspoon baking soda
- 2 cups buttermilk
- 2 tablespoons olive oil

Directions:

1. Mix the flour, salt, parmesan cheese, and baking soda in a bowl. Stir in the buttermilk and olive oil and mix well with a fork. Shape the dough into a loaf and place it in your Slow Cooker. Cover with its lid and cook on high heat for 1 hour. Serve the bread warm or chilled.

Nutrition: calories 378, fat 10, carbs 8, protein 18

Creamy Spinach Dip

Preparation Time: 15 minutes
Cooking time: 2 hours 15 minutes
Servings: 30
Ingredients:

- 1 can crab meat, drained
- 1 pound fresh spinach, chopped
- 2 shallots, chopped
- 2 jalapeno peppers, chopped
- 1 cup grated Parmesan
- 1/2 cup whole milk
- 1 cup sour cream - 1 cup cream cheese
- 1 cup grated Cheddar cheese
- 1 tablespoon sherry vinegar
- 2 garlic cloves, chopped

Directions:

1. Combine all the ingredients in your Slow Cooker. Cover with its lid and cook on high settings for hours.
2. Serve the spinach dip warm or chilled with a vegetable stick or your favorite salty snacks.

Nutrition: calories 388, fat 12, carbs 10, protein 21

Party Mix

Preparation Time: 10 minutes
Cooking time: 1 hour 15 minutes
Servings: 20
Ingredients:

- 4 cups cereals
- 4 cups crunchy cereals
- 2 cups mixed nuts
- 1 cup mixed seeds
- 1/2 cup butter, melted
- 2 tablespoons Worcestershire sauce
- 1 teaspoon hot sauce
- 1 teaspoon salt
- 1/2 teaspoon cumin powder

Directions:

1. Combine all the ingredients in your Slow Cooker and toss around until evenly coated. Cook on high settings for 1 hour. Serve the mix chilled.

Nutrition: calories 180, fat 18, carbs 5, protein 11

Spanish Chorizo Dip

Preparation Time: 10 minutes
Cooking time: 6 hours 15 minutes
Servings: 8
Ingredients:

- 8 chorizo links, diced
- 1 can diced tomatoes
- 1 chili pepper, chopped
- 1 cup cream cheese
- 2 cups grated Cheddar cheese
- 1/4 cup white wine

Directions:

1. Combine all the ingredients in your Slow Cooker. Cook the dip over low heat for 6 hours. Serve the dip warm.

Nutrition: calories 280, fat 18, carbs 9, protein 22

Artichoke Bread Pudding

Preparation Time: 15 minutes
Cooking time: 6 hours 30 minutes
Servings: 10
Ingredients:

- 6 cups bread cubes
- 6 artichoke hearts, drained and chopped
- 1/2 cup grated Parmesan
- 4 eggs
- 1/2 cup sour cream
- 1 cup milk
- 4 oz. spinach, chopped
- 1 tablespoon chopped parsley
- 2 tablespoons olive oil
- Salt and pepper to taste

- 1/2 teaspoon dried oregano
- 1/2 teaspoon dried basil

Directions:

1. Combine the bread cubes, artichoke hearts, and Parmesan in your Slow Cooker. Add the spinach and parsley as well. In a bowl, mix the eggs, sour cream, milk, oregano, and basil, as well as salt and pepper. Pour this mixture over the bread and press the bread slightly to make sure it soaks up all the liquid. Cover the pot with its lid and cook over low heat for 6 hours. The bread can be served both warm and chilled.

Nutrition: calories 411, fat 10, carbs 5, protein 12

Molasses Lime Meatballs

Preparation Time: 17 minutes
Cooking time: 8 hours 15 minutes
Servings: 10
Ingredients:

- 3 pounds ground beef
- 2 garlic cloves, minced
- 1 shallot, chopped
- 1/2 cup oat flour
- 1/2 teaspoon cumin powder
- 1/2 teaspoon chili powder
- 1 egg
- Salt and pepper to taste
- 1/2 cup molasses
- 1/4 cup soy sauce
- 2 tablespoons lime juice
- 1/2 cup beef stock
- 1 tablespoon Worcestershire sauce

Directions:

1. Combine the molasses, soy sauce, lime juice, stock, and Worcestershire sauce in your Slow Cooker. In a bowl, mix the ground beef, garlic, shallot, oat flour, cumin powder, chili powder, egg, salt, and pepper, and mix well. Form small balls

and place them in the sauce. Cover the pot and cook over low heat for 8 hours. Serve the meatballs warm or chilled.

Nutrition: calories 430, fat 16, carbs 8, protein 15

Sausage and Pepper Appetizer

Preparation Time: 15 minutes
Cooking time: 6 hours 10 minutes
Servings: 6
Ingredients:

- 6 fresh pork sausages, skins removed
- 2 tablespoons olive oil
- 1 can fire-roasted tomatoes
- 4 roasted bell peppers, chopped
- 1 poblano pepper, chopped
- 1 shallot, chopped
- 1 cup grated Provolone cheese
- Salt and pepper to taste

Directions:

1. Heat the oil in a skillet and stir in the sausage meat. Cook for 5 minutes, stirring often. Transfer the meat to your Slow Cooker and add the remaining ingredients. Season with salt and pepper and cook over low heat for 6 hours. Serve the dish warm or chilled.

Nutrition: calories 329, fat 12, carbs 9, protein 21

Nacho Sauce

Preparation Time: 15 minutes
Cooking time: 6 hours 15 minutes
Servings: 12
Ingredients:

- 2 pounds ground beef
- 2 tablespoons Mexican seasoning
- 1 teaspoon chili powder
- 1 can diced tomatoes
- 2 shallots, chopped
- 4 garlic cloves, minced
- 1 can sweet corn, drained

- 2 cups grated Cheddar cheese

Directions:
1. Combine all the ingredients in your Slow Cooker. Cook over low heat for 6 hours. This dip is best served warm.

Nutrition: calories 321, fat 16, carbs 4, protein 11

Five-spiced Chicken Wings

Preparation Time: 15 minutes
Cooking time: 7 hours 15 minutes
Servings: 8
Ingredients:

- 1/2 cup plum sauce
- 1/2 cup BBQ sauce
- 2 tablespoons butter
- 1 tablespoon five-spice powder
- 1 teaspoon salt
- 1/2 teaspoon chili powder
- 4 pounds chicken wings

Directions:
1. Combine the plum sauce and BBQ sauce, as well as butter, five-spice, salt, and chili powder in a Slow Cooker. Add the chicken wings and mix well until well coated. Cover and cook over low heat for 7 hours. Serve warm or chilled.

Nutrition: calories 218, fat 12, carbs 6, protein 32

Green Vegetable Dip

Preparation Time: 15 minutes
Cooking time: 2 hours 15 minutes
Servings: 12
Ingredients:

- 10 oz. frozen spinach, thawed and drained
- 1 jar artichoke hearts, drained
- 1 cup chopped parsley
- 1 cup cream cheese
- 1 cup sour cream
- 1/2 cup grated Parmesan cheese
- 1/2 cup feta cheese, crumbled

- 1/2 teaspoon onion powder
- 1/4 teaspoon garlic powder

Directions:
1. Combine all the ingredients in your Slow Cooker and mix gently. Cover with its lid and cook on high settings for hours. Serve the dip warm or chilled with crusty bread, biscuits, or other salty snacks, or even vegetable sticks.

Nutrition: calories 154, fat 12, carbs 9, protein 18

Roasted Bell Peppers Dip

Preparation Time: 15 minutes
Cooking time: 2 hours 15 minutes
Servings: 8
Ingredients:

- 4 roasted red bell peppers, drained
- 2 cans chickpeas, drained
- 1/2 cup water
- 1 shallot, chopped
- 4 garlic cloves, minced
- Salt and pepper to taste
- 2 tablespoons lemon juice
- 2 tablespoons olive oil

Directions:
1. Combine the bell peppers, chickpeas, water, shallot, and garlic in a Slow Cooker. Add salt and pepper as needed and cook on high settings for hours. When done, puree the dip in a blender, adding the lemon juice and olive oil as well. Serve the dip fresh or store it in the fridge in an airtight container for up to 2 days.

Nutrition: calories 342, fat 18, carbs 8, protein 18

Spicy Glazed Pecans

Preparation Time: 15 minutes
Cooking time: 3 hours 15 minutes
Servings: 10
Ingredients:

- 2 pounds pecans

- 1/2 cup butter, melted
- 1 teaspoon chili powder
- 1 teaspoon smoked paprika
- 1 teaspoon dried basil
- 1 teaspoon dried thyme
- 1/4 teaspoon cayenne pepper
- 1/2 teaspoon garlic powder
- 2 tablespoons honey

Directions:

1. Combine all the ingredients in your Slow Cooker. Mix well until all the ingredients are well distributed, and the pecans are evenly glazed. Cook on high settings for hours. Allow them to cool before serving.

Nutrition: calories 321, fat 18, carbs 10, protein 24

Cocktail Meatballs

Preparation Time: 15 minutes
Cooking time: 6 hours 30 minutes
Servings: 10
Ingredients:

- 2 pounds ground pork
- 1 pound ground beef
- 4 garlic cloves, minced
- 1 shallot, chopped
- 1 egg
- 1/4 cup breadcrumbs
- 2 tablespoons chopped parsley
- 1 tablespoon chopped cilantro
- 1/2 teaspoon chili powder
- 2 tablespoons cranberry sauce
- 1 cup BBQ sauce
- 1/2 cup tomato sauce
- 1 teaspoon red wine vinegar
- 1 bay leaf
- Salt and pepper to taste

Directions:

1. Combine the cranberry sauce, BBQ sauce, tomato sauce, and vinegar, as well as bay leaf, salt, and pepper in your Slow Cooker Cover and cook over low heat for 6 hours. Serve the meatballs warm or chilled with cocktail skewers.

Nutrition: calories 211, fat 10, carbs 5, protein 12

Bacon New Potatoes

Preparation Time: 10 minutes
Cooking time: 3 hours 15 minutes
Servings: 6
Ingredients:

- 3 pounds new potatoes, washed and halved
- 12 slices bacon, chopped
- 2 tablespoons white wine
- Salt and pepper to taste
- 1 rosemary sprig

Directions:

1. Place the potatoes, wine, and rosemary in your Slow Cooker. Add salt and pepper to taste and top with chopped bacon. Cook on high settings for hours. Serve the potatoes warm.

Nutrition: calories 298, fat 12, carbs 6, protein 19

Glazed Peanuts

Preparation Time: 10 minutes
Cooking time: 2 hours 15 minutes
Servings: 8
Ingredients:

- 2 pounds raw, whole peanuts
- 1/4 cup brown sugar
- 1/2 teaspoon garlic powder
- 2 tablespoons salt
- 1 tablespoon Cajun seasoning
- 1/2 teaspoon red pepper flakes
- 1/4 cup coconut oil

Directions:

1. Combine all the ingredients in your Slow Cooker. Cover and cook on high settings for hours. Serve chilled.

Nutrition: calories 324, fat 18, carbs 10, protein 24

Beer Bbq Meatballs

Preparation Time: 15 minutes
Cooking time: 7 hours 30 minutes
Servings: 10
Ingredients:

- 2 pounds ground pork
- 1 pound ground beef
- 1 carrot, grated
- 2 shallots, chopped
- 1 egg
- 1/2 cup breadcrumbs
- 1/2 teaspoon cumin powder
- Salt and pepper to taste
- 1 cup dark beer
- 1 cup BBQ sauce
- 1 bay leaf
- 1/2 teaspoon chili powder
- 1 teaspoon apple cider vinegar

Directions:

1. Mix the ground pork and beef in a bowl. Add the carrot, shallots, egg, breadcrumbs, cumin, salt, and pepper, and mix well. Form small meatballs and place them on your chopping board. For the beer sauce, combine the beer, BBQ sauce, bay leaf, chili powder, and vinegar in a Slow Cooker. Place the meatballs in the pot and cover with its lid. Cook over low heat for 7 hours. Serve the meatballs warm or chilled.

Nutrition: calories 375, fat 18, carbs 9, protein 18

Pretzel Party Mix

Preparation Time: 10 minutes
Cooking time: 2 hours 15 minutes
Servings: 10
Ingredients:

- 4 cups pretzels
- 1 cup peanuts
- 1 cup pecans
- 1 cup crispy rice cereals
- 1/4 cup butter, melted
- 1 teaspoon Worcestershire sauce
- 1 teaspoon salt
- 1 teaspoon garlic powder

Directions:

1. Combine the pretzels, peanuts, pecans, and rice cereals in your Slow Cooker. Drizzle with melted butter and Worcestershire sauce and mix well, then sprinkle with salt and garlic powder. Cover and cook on high settings for 2 hours, mixing once during cooking. Allow to cool before serving.

Nutrition: calories 222, fat 18, carbs 8, protein 11

Sausage Dip

Preparation Time: 17 minutes
Cooking time: 6 hours 15 minutes
Servings: 8
Ingredients:

- 1 pound fresh pork sausages
- 1 pound spicy pork sausages
- 1 cup cream cheese
- 1 can diced tomatoes
- 2 poblano peppers, chopped

Directions:

1. Combine all the ingredients in a Slow Cooker. Cook over low heat for 6 hours. Serve warm or chilled.

Nutrition: calories 390, fat 12, carbs 6, protein 11

Spiced Buffalo Wings

Preparation Time: 15 minutes
Cooking time: 8 hours 15 minutes
Servings: 8
Ingredients:

- 4 pounds chicken wings
- 1 cup BBQ sauce
- 1/4 cup butter, melted
- 1 tablespoon Worcestershire sauce
- 1 teaspoon dried oregano
- 1 teaspoon dried basil
- 1 teaspoon onion powder
- 1 teaspoon garlic powder
- 1/2 teaspoon cumin powder
- 1/2 teaspoon cinnamon powder
- 1 teaspoon hot sauce
- 1 teaspoon salt

Directions:

1. Combine all the ingredients in a Slow Cooker. Mix until the wings are evenly coated. Cook over low heat for 8 hours. Serve warm or chilled.

Nutrition: calories 420, fat 10, carbs 8, protein 24

CHAPTER 5:

Chicken

Chicken Pockets

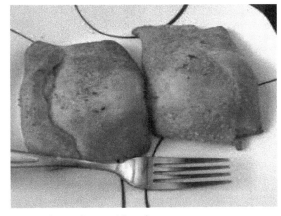

Preparation time: 10 minutes

Cooking time: 4 hours

Servings: 4

Ingredients:

- 4 tablespoons plain yogurt
- 1 oz. fresh cilantro, chopped
- ½ teaspoon dried thyme
- 1-pound chicken fillet, sliced
- 2 tablespoons cream cheese
- 1 red onion, sliced
- 1/3 cup water
- 4 pita bread

Directions
1. Mix plain yogurt with chicken, water, dried thyme, and transfer to the slow cooker.
2. Cook the chicken for 4 hours on High.

3. Then fill the pita bread with cream cheese, onion, cilantro, and chicken.

Nutrition: calories 422, fat 11, carbs 21, protein 40

Jerk Chicken

Preparation time: 15 minutes

Cooking time: 7 hours

Servings: 4

Ingredients

- 1 lemon
- 1-pound chicken breast, skinless, boneless
- 1 tablespoon taco seasoning
- 1 teaspoon garlic powder
- 1 teaspoon ground black pepper
- ½ teaspoon minced ginger
- 1 tablespoon soy sauce
- 1 cup of water

Directions
1. Chop the lemon and put it in the blender.
2. Add taco seasoning, garlic powder, ground black pepper, minced ginger, and soy sauce.
3. Blend the mixture until smooth.
4. After this, cut the chicken breast into the servings and rub with the lemon mixture carefully.

5. Transfer the chicken to the slow cooker, add water, and cook on Low for 7 hours.

Nutrition: calories 150, fat 2, carbs 4, protein 4

Lemon Chicken Thighs

Preparation time: 10 minutes

Cooking time: 7 hours

Servings: 4

Ingredients:

- 4 chicken thighs, skinless, boneless

- 1 lemon, sliced
- 1 teaspoon ground black pepper
- ½ teaspoon ground nutmeg
- 1 teaspoon olive oil
- 1 cup of water

Directions
1. Rub the chicken thighs with ground black pepper, nutmeg, and olive oil.
2. Then transfer the chicken to the slow cooker.
3. Add lemon and water.
4. Close the lid and cook the meal on LOW for 7 hours.

Nutrition: calories 295, fat 12, carbs 1, protein 42

Turkey Breast with Root Vegetables

Preparation time: 25 minutes

Cooking time: 8 hours

Servings: 8

Ingredients:

- 2 cups baby carrots

- 2 fennel bulbs, peeled and sliced
- 1 yellow onion, chopped

- 1 (8-ounce) package button mushrooms
- 1 teaspoon dried thyme
- 1 teaspoon dried rosemary
- 1 teaspoon sea salt
- ¼ teaspoon freshly ground black pepper
- Grated zest of 1 lemon
- 1 (4-to 6-pound) bone-in, skin-on turkey breast

Direction
1. Arrange the baby carrots, fennel, onion, and mushrooms in the bottom of a 4-to-5-quart slow cooker.
2. In a small bowl, combine the thyme, rosemary, salt, pepper, and lemon zest.
3. Rub the turkey breast with the seasoning mixture.
4. Place the turkey, skin-side up, in the slow cooker on top of the vegetables.
5. Cover and cook on low for 8 hours, or until the turkey registers at least 165°F on a food thermometer. Let the turkey stand, covered for 10 minutes before slicing. Remove the turkey skin before serving.

Nutrition: calories 346, fat 2, carbs 6, protein 11

Cranberry Turkey Roast

Preparation time: 15 minutes

Cooking time: 8 hours

Servings: 8

Ingredients:

- 1 (3-pound) bone-in, skin-on turkey breast
- 1 teaspoon sea salt
- ¼ teaspoon freshly ground black pepper
- 2 tablespoons extra-virgin olive oil
- 1 cup apple cider
- 1 (16-ounce) bag fresh cranberries
- Grated zest and juice of 1 orange

- 1 rosemary sprig

Directions

1. Season the turkey breast with salt and pepper.
2. Heat the olive oil in a large skillet over medium heat. Add the turkey, skin-side down, and cook for 5 to 7 minutes, until the skin is browned. Place the turkey, skin-side up, in a 4-quart slow cooker.
3. Add the apple cider to the skillet and bring it to a boil, scraping the brown bits from the bottom of the pan with a spatula or wooden spoon. Pour this into the slow cooker.
4. Add the cranberries, orange zest and juice, and rosemary to the slow cooker.
5. Cover and cook on low for 8 hours, or until the turkey registers at least 165°F on a food thermometer. Let the turkey stand, covered for 10 minutes before you carve and serve with the cranberry mixture.

Nutrition: calories 340, fat 16, carbs 10, protein 35

Turkey Joes

Preparation time: 15 minutes

Cooking time: 6 hours

Servings: 4

Ingredients:

- 1½ pounds lean ground turkey
- ¼ cup tomato paste
- 6 tablespoons ketchup
- 2 tablespoons yellow mustard
- ½ cup water
- ½ small yellow onion, finely chopped
- 2 garlic cloves, minced
- 1 carrot, finely chopped
- 1 teaspoon paprika
- 1 teaspoon ground cumin

- ½ teaspoon sea salt
- ¼ teaspoon freshly ground black pepper
- 4 hamburger or onion buns, split and toasted
- 1 cup shredded Cheddar cheese

Directions

1. Place a large skillet over medium heat. Add the ground turkey and cook, breaking up the meat with a wooden spoon until it is light brown. Drain if necessary.
2. Place the cooked ground turkey, tomato paste, ketchup, mustard, water, onion, garlic, carrot, paprika, cumin, salt, and black pepper in a 3-quart slow cooker. Stir to mix well.
3. Cover and cook on low for 4 to 6 hours or on high for 2 to 3 hours.
4. To serve, spoon about ½ cup of the turkey mixture on the bottom of each bun and top evenly with the cheese. Add the top half of the bun and serve.

Nutrition: calories 544, fat 24, carbs 39, protein 47

Chicken Bowl

Preparation time: 15 minutes

Cooking time: 4 hours

Servings: 6

Ingredients:

- 1-pound chicken breast, skinless, boneless, chopped
- 1 cup sweet corn, frozen
- 1 teaspoon ground paprika
- 1 teaspoon onion powder
- 1 cup tomatoes, chopped
- 1 cup of water
- 1 teaspoon olive oil

Directions

1. Mix chopped chicken breast with ground paprika and onion powder. Transfer it to the slow cooker.
2. Add water and sweet corn. Cook the mixture on High for 4 hours.
3. Then drain the liquid and transfer the mixture to the bowl.
4. Add tomatoes and olive oil. Mix the meal.

Nutrition: calories 122, fat 12, carbs 6, protein 17

Asian Style Chicken

Preparation time: 10 minutes

Cooking time: 8 hours

Servings: 4

Ingredients:

- 1 teaspoon hot sauce
- ¼ cup of soy sauce
- 1 teaspoon sesame oil
- 2 oz. scallions, chopped
- ½ cup of orange juice
- 1 teaspoon ground coriander
- 1-pound chicken breast, skinless, boneless, roughly chopped

Directions

1. Put all ingredients in the slow cooker.
2. Close the lid and cook the meal on Low for 8 hours.
3. Then transfer the chicken and a little amount of the chicken liquid to the bowls.

Nutrition: calories 166, fat 4, carbs 5, protein 25

Oregano Chicken Breast

Preparation time: 10 minutes

Cooking time: 4 hours

Servings: 4

Ingredients:

- 1-pound chicken breast, skinless, boneless, roughly chopped
- 1 tablespoon dried oregano
- 1 bay leaf
- 1 teaspoon peppercorns
- 1 teaspoon salt
- 2 cups of water

Directions

1. Pour water into the slow cooker and add peppercorns and bay leaf.
2. Then sprinkle the chicken with the dried oregano and transfer it to the slow cooker.
3. Close the lid and cook the meal on High for 4 hours.

Nutrition: calories 135, fat 3, carbs 2, protein 24

Thai Chicken

Preparation time: 15 minutes

Cooking time: 4 hours

Servings: 4

Ingredients:

- 12 oz. chicken fillet, sliced
- ½ cup of coconut milk
- 1 teaspoon dried lemongrass
- 1 teaspoon chili powder
- 1 teaspoon tomato paste
- 1 teaspoon ground cardamom
- 1 cup of water

Directions

1. Rub the chicken with chili powder, tomato paste, ground cardamom, and dried lemongrass. Transfer it to the slow cooker.
2. Add water and coconut milk.

3. Close the lid and cook the meal on High for 4 hours.

Nutrition: calories 236, fat 13, carbs 2, protein 25

Chicken Teriyaki

Preparation time: 10 minutes

Cooking time: 4 hours

Servings: 4

Ingredients:

- 1-pound chicken wings

- ½ cup teriyaki sauce
- ½ cup of water
- 1 carrot, chopped
- 1 onion, chopped
- 1 teaspoon butter

Directions

1. Toss butter in the pan and melt it.
2. Add onion and carrot and roast the vegetables for 5 minutes over medium heat.
3. Then transfer them to the slow cooker.
4. Add chicken wings, teriyaki sauce, and water.
5. Close the lid and cook the meal for 4 hours on High.

Nutrition: calories 230, fat 9, carbs 9, protein 35

Stuffed Chicken Breast

Preparation time: 15 minutes

Cooking time: 6 hours

Servings: 4

Ingredients:

- 1-pound chicken breast, skinless, boneless

- 1 tomato, sliced

- 2 oz. mozzarella, sliced
- 1 teaspoon fresh basil
- 1 teaspoon olive oil
- 1 teaspoon salt
- 1 cup of water

Directions

1. Make the horizontal cut in the chicken breast in the shape of the pocket.
2. Then fill it with sliced mozzarella, tomato, and basil.
3. Secure the cut with the help of the toothpicks and sprinkle the chicken with olive oil and salt.
4. Place it in the slow cooker and add water.
5. Cook the chicken on low for 6 hours.

Nutrition: calories 268, fat 12, carbs 8, protein 21

Chicken Pate

Preparation time: 15 minutes

Cooking time: 8 hours

Servings: 6

Ingredients:

- 1 carrot, peeled

- 1 teaspoon salt
- 1-pound chicken liver
- 2 cups of water
- 2 tablespoons coconut oil

Directions

1. Chop the carrot roughly and put it in the slow cooker.
2. Add chicken liver and water.
3. Cook the mixture for 8 hours on Low.
4. Then drain water and transfer the mixture to the blender.
5. Add coconut oil and salt.
6. Blend the mixture until smooth.

7. Store the pate in the fridge for up to 7 days.

Nutrition: calories 190, fat 9, carbs 2, protein 18

Chicken Masala

Preparation time: 10 minutes

Cooking time: 4 hours

Servings: 4

Ingredients:

- 1 teaspoon gram masala
- 1 teaspoon ground ginger
- 1 cup of coconut milk
- 1-pound chicken fillet, sliced
- 1 teaspoon olive oil

Directions
1. Mix coconut milk with ground ginger, gram masala, and olive oil.
2. Add chicken fillet and mix the ingredients.
3. Then transfer them to the slow cooker and cook on High for 4 hours.

Nutrition: calories 358, fat 34, carbs 4, protein 34

Chicken Minestrone

Preparation time: 10 minutes

Cooking time: 3.5 hours

Servings: 4

Ingredients:

- 10 oz. chicken fillet, sliced
- 2 cup of water
- 1 cup tomatoes, chopped
- 1 teaspoon chili powder
- 1 teaspoon ground paprika
- 1 teaspoon ground cumin
- 1 cup Swiss chard, chopped
- ¼ cup red kidney beans, canned

Directions
1. Sprinkle the chicken fillet with chili powder, ground paprika, and ground cumin.
2. Transfer it to the slow cooker.
3. Add tomatoes, water, Swiss chard, and red kidney beans.
4. Close the lid and cook the meal on High for 3.5 hours.

Nutrition: calories 189, fat 5, carbs 10, protein 23

French-Style Chicken

Preparation time: 10 minutes

Cooking time: 7 hours

Servings: 4

Ingredients: 1 can onion soup
- 4 chicken drumsticks
- ½ cup celery stalk, chopped
- 1 teaspoon dried tarragon
- ¼ cup white wine

Directions
1. Put ingredients in the slow cooker and carefully mix them.
2. Then close the lid and cook the chicken on low for 7 hours.

Nutrition: calories 127, fat 3, carbs 5, protein 15

Sweet Chicken Breast

Preparation time: *20 minutes*

Cooking time: *4 hours*

Servings: *4*

Ingredients:

- 2 red onions

- 2 tablespoons of liquid honey
- 1 tablespoon butter
- ½ cup of water
- 1-pound chicken breast, skinless, boneless
- 1 teaspoon curry paste

Directions

1. Rub the chicken breast with curry paste and transfer it to the slow cooker.
2. Slice the onion and add it to the cooker too.
3. Then add water and close the lid.
4. Cook the chicken breast on High for 4 hours.
5. After this, toss the butter in the skillet.
6. Melt it and add chicken.
7. Sprinkle the chicken with liquid honey and roast for 1 minute per side.
8. Slice the chicken breast.

Nutrition: calories 217, fat 24, carbs 14, protein 24

Basil Chicken

Preparation time: 15 minutes

Cooking time: 7 hours

Servings: *4*

Ingredients:

- 2 tablespoons balsamic vinegar
- 1 cup of water
- 1 teaspoon dried basil
- 1 teaspoon dried oregano
- 1-pound chicken fillet, sliced
- 1 teaspoon mustard

Directions

1. Mix chicken fillet with mustard and balsamic vinegar.
2. Add dried basil, oregano, and transfer to the slow cooker.

3. Add water and close the lid.
4. Cook the chicken on low for 7 hours.

Nutrition: calories 222, fat 12, carbs8, protein 33

BBQ Chicken

Preparation time: *15 minutes*

Cooking time: 7 hours

Servings: *2*

Ingredients:

- 1 teaspoon minced garlic
- ½ cup BBQ sauce
- 1 tablespoon avocado oil
- 3 tablespoons lemon juice
- ½ cup of water
- 7 oz. chicken fillet, sliced

Directions

1. Put in the bowl BBQ sauce, minced garlic, avocado oil, and lemon juice.
2. Add chicken fillet and mix the mixture.
3. After this, transfer it to the slow cooker. Add water and close the lid.
4. Cook the chicken on low for 7 hours.

Nutrition: calories 178, fat 21, carbs 15, protein 31

Sugar Chicken

Preparation time: *10 minutes*

Cooking time: *6 hours*

Servings: *6*

Ingredients:

- 1 teaspoon chili flakes
- 6 chicken drumsticks
- 2 tablespoons brown sugar

- 1 tablespoon butter, melted
- 1 tablespoon lemon juice
- 1 teaspoon ground black pepper
- ¼ cup milk

Directions

1. In the bowl, mix chili flakes, brown sugar, butter, lemon juice, and ground black pepper. Then brush every chicken drumstick with the sweet mixture and transfer it to the slow cooker.
2. Add milk and close the lid. Cook the meal on Low for 6 hours.

Nutrition: calories 132, fat 12, carbs 6, protein 11

Chicken and Peppers

Preparation time: *6 hours*

Cooking time: *6 hours*

Servings: *2*

Ingredients:

- 1 pound chicken breasts, skinless, boneless, and cubed
- ¼ cup tomato sauce
- 2 red bell peppers, cut into strips
- 1 teaspoon olive oil
- ½ teaspoon rosemary, dried
- ½ teaspoon coriander, ground
- 1 teaspoon Italian seasoning
- A pinch of cayenne pepper
- 1 cup chicken stock

Directions:

1. In your Slow Cooker, mix the chicken with the peppers, tomato sauce, and the other ingredients, toss, put the lid on and cook on Low for 6 hours. Divide everything between plates and serve.

Nutrition: calories 282, fat 12, fiber 2, carbs 6, protein 18

Chicken Chowder

Preparation time: *6 hours*

Cooking time: *6 hours*

Servings: *4*

Ingredients:

- 3 chicken breasts, skinless and boneless and cubed
- 4 cups chicken stock
- 1 sweet potato, cubed
- 8 ounces canned green chilies, chopped
- 1 yellow onion, chopped
- 15 ounces coconut cream
- 1 teaspoon garlic powder
- 4 bacon strips, cooked and crumbled
- A pinch of salt and black pepper
- 1 tablespoon parsley, chopped

Directions:

1. In your Slow Cooker, mix chicken with stock, sweet potato, green chilies, onion, garlic powder, salt and pepper, stir, cover, and cook on Low for 5 hours and 40 minutes. Add coconut cream and parsley, stir, cover, and cook on Low for 5 minutes more. Ladle chowder into bowls, sprinkle bacon on top, and serve.

Nutrition: calories 232, fat 3, fiber 7, carbs 14, protein 7

Parsley Turkey Breast

Preparation time: 8 *hours*

Cooking time: 8 *hours*

Servings: *4*

Ingredients:

- 3 pounds turkey breast, bone in
- 1 cup black figs
- 3 sweet potatoes, cut into wedges

- ½ cup dried cherries, pitted
- 2 white onions, cut into wedges
- ½ cup dried cranberries
- 1/3 cup water
- 1 teaspoon onion powder
- 1 teaspoon garlic powder
- 1 teaspoon parsley flakes
- 1 teaspoon thyme, dried
- 1 teaspoon sage, dried
- 1 teaspoon paprika, dried
- A pinch of sea salt
- Black pepper to the taste

Directions:

1. Put the turkey breast in your Slow Cooker, add sweet potatoes, figs, cherries, onions, cranberries, water, parsley, garlic and onion powder, thyme, sage, paprika, salt and pepper, toss, cover and cook on Low for 8 hours.

Nutrition: calories 320, fat 5, fiber 4, carbs 12, protein 15

Chili Chicken

Preparation time: *15 minutes*

Cooking time: *7 hours*

Servings: *4*

Ingredients:

- 1 teaspoon chili powder
- 1 tablespoon hot sauce
- 1 tablespoon coconut oil, melted
- ½ teaspoon ground turmeric
- 1 teaspoon garlic, minced
- ½ cup of water
- 1-pound chicken wings

Directions

1. Rub the chicken wings with hot sauce, chili powder, ground turmeric, garlic, and coconut oil.
2. Then pour water into the slow cooker and add prepared chicken wings.
3. Cook the chicken on low for 7 hours.

Nutrition: calories 210, fat 16, carbs 19, protein 33

Orange Chicken

Preparation time: 10 minutes

Cooking time: 8 hours

Servings: 4

Ingredients:

- 1 orange, chopped
- 1 teaspoon ground turmeric
- 1 teaspoon peppercorn
- 1 teaspoon olive oil
- 1 teaspoon salt
- 1 cup of water
- 1-pound chicken breast, skinless, boneless, sliced

Directions

1. Put all ingredients in the slow cooker and gently mix them.
2. Close the lid and cook the meal on Low for 8 hours.
3. When the time is finished, transfer the chicken to the serving bowls and top with orange liquid from the slow cooker.

Nutrition: calories 241, fat 8, carbs 3, protein 23

Bacon Chicken

Preparation time: *10 minutes*

Cooking time: *7 hours*

Servings: *4*

Ingredients:

- 4 bacon slices, cooked
- 4 chicken drumsticks
- ½ cup of water
- ¼ tomato juice
- 1 teaspoon salt
- ½ teaspoon ground black pepper

Directions

1. Sprinkle the chicken drumsticks with salt and ground black pepper.
2. Then wrap every chicken drumstick in the bacon and arrange it in the slow cooker.
3. Add water and tomato juice.
4. Cook the meal on Low for 7 hours.

Nutrition: calories 349, fat 15, carbs 5, protein 32

Bourbon Chicken Cubes

Preparation time: *10 minutes*

Cooking time: *4 hours*

Servings: *4*

Ingredient

- ½ cup bourbon
- 1 teaspoon liquid honey
- 1 tablespoon BBQ sauce
- 1 white onion, diced
- 1 teaspoon garlic powder
- 1-pound chicken fillet, cubed

Directions

1. Put all ingredients in the slow cooker.
2. Mix the mixture until liquid honey is dissolved.
3. Then close the lid and cook the meal on high for 4 hours.

Nutrition: calories 154, fat 12, carbs 6, protein 11

Mexican Chicken

Preparation time: *10 minutes*

Cooking time: 5 *hours*

Servings: *2*

Ingredients:

- Sweet pepper, sliced
- Cayenne pepper
- 1 red onion, sliced
- ½ cup salsa Verde
- 1 cup of water

Directions

1. Pour water into the slow cooker.
2. Add salsa Verde and onion.
3. Then add cayenne pepper and chicken thighs.
4. Cook the mixture on High for 3 hours.
5. After this, add sweet pepper and cook the meal on Low for 3 hours.

Nutrition: calories 327, fat 16, carbs 6, protein 24

Curry Chicken Wings

Preparation time: *15 minutes*

Cooking time: 7 hours

Servings: *4*

Ingredients:

- 1-pound chicken wings

- 1 teaspoon curry paste
- ½ cup heavy cream
- 1 teaspoon minced garlic
- ½ teaspoon ground nutmeg
- ½ cup of water

Directions

1. In the bowl, mix curry paste, heavy cream, minced garlic, and ground nutmeg.
2. Add chicken wings and stir.
3. Then pour water into the slow cooker.
4. Add chicken wings with all remaining curry paste mixture and close the lid.
5. Cook the chicken wings on Low for 7 hours.

Nutrition: calories 154, fat 8, carbs 3, protein 21

Thyme Whole Chicken

Preparation time: *15 minutes*

Cooking time: 9 hours

Servings: *6*

Ingredients:

- 1.5-pound whole chicken
- 1 tablespoon dried thyme
- 1 tablespoon olive oil
- 1 teaspoon salt
- 1 cup of water

Directions

1. Chop the whole chicken roughly and sprinkle with dried thyme, olive oil, and salt.
2. Then transfer it to the slow cooker, add water.
3. Cook the chicken on low for 9 hours.

Nutrition: calories 432, fat 2, carbs 4, protein 18

Fennel and Chicken Sauté

Preparation time: *10 minutes*

Cooking time: *7 hours*

Servings: *4*

Ingredients:

- 1 cup fennel, peeled, chopped
- 10 oz. chicken fillet, chopped
- 1 tablespoon tomato paste
- 1 cup of water
- 1 teaspoon ground black pepper
- 1 teaspoon olive oil
- ½ teaspoon fennel seeds

Directions

1. Heat the olive oil in the skillet.
2. Add fennel seeds and roast them until you get a saturated fennel smell.
3. Transfer the seeds to the slow cooker.
4. Add fennel, chicken fillet, tomato paste, water, and ground black pepper.
5. Close the lid and cook the meal on Low for 7 hours.

Nutrition: calories 100, fat 9, carbs 3, protein 8

Russian Chicken

Preparation time: *10 minutes*

Cooking time: 4 hours

Servings: *4*

Ingredients:

- 2 tablespoons mayonnaise
- 4 chicken thighs, skinless, boneless
- 1 teaspoon minced garlic
- 1 teaspoon ground black pepper
- 1 teaspoon sunflower oil

- 1 teaspoon salt
- ½ cup of water

Directions

1. In the bowl, mix mayonnaise, minced garlic, ground black pepper, salt, and oil.
2. Then add chicken thighs and mix the ingredients well.
3. After this, pour water into the slow cooker. Add chicken thighs mixture.
4. Cook the meal on High for 4 hours.

Nutrition: calories 444, fat 18, carbs 3, protein 32

CHAPTER 6:

Fish and Seafood

Creamy Sea Bass

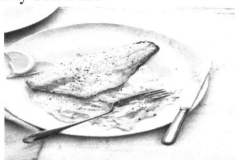

Preparation Time: 15 minutes
Cooking time: 2 hours
Servings: 4
Ingredients:

- 1-pound sea bass fillets, boneless
- 1 teaspoon garlic powder
- ½ teaspoon Italian seasoning
- ½ teaspoon salt
- ¼ cup heavy cream
- 1 tablespoon butter

Directions:

1. In the slow cooker, mix the sea bass with the other ingredients. Close the slow cooker lid and cook for 2 hours on High.

Nutrition: calories 231, fat 14.9, carbs 7.4, protein 24.2

Oregano Crab

Preparation Time: 10 minutes
Cooking time: 40 minutes
Servings:
Ingredients: 1 tablespoon dried oregano

- 2 cups crab meat

- ½ cup spring onions, chopped
- ¾ teaspoon minced garlic
- 1 tablespoon lemon juice
- ½ cup of coconut milk

Directions:

1. In the slow cooker, mix the crab with oregano and the other ingredients and close the lid
2. Cook for 40 minutes on High, divide into bowls, and serve.

Nutrition: calories 151, fat 3, carbs 6, protein 5

Parmesan Salmon

Preparation Time: 10 minutes
Cooking time: 2 hours 30 minutes
Servings: 3
Ingredients:

- 7 oz salmon fillets, boneless
- 1 teaspoon cayenne pepper
- 1 teaspoon chili pepper
- ½ cup coconut cream
- 3 oz Parmesan, grated
- 2 tablespoons lime juice
- 1 teaspoon minced garlic
- ¼ cup fresh chives, chopped

Directions:

1. In the slow cooker, mix the salmon with the coconut cream and the other ingredients and close the lid.

2. Cook on High for 2 hours and 30 minutes and serve.

Nutrition: calories 279, fat 16, fiber 1, carbs 7, protein 18

Balsamic Mussels

Preparation Time: 15 minutes
Cooking time: 2 hours
Servings: 4
Ingredients:

- 1-pound mussels
- 1 tablespoon Balsamic vinegar
- ½ teaspoon stevia extract
- 1 teaspoon lemon zest
- 1 teaspoon lemon juice
- 2 tablespoon sesame oil
- ¼ cup butter
- 4 tablespoons coconut cream

Directions:

1. In the slow cooker, mix the mussels with vinegar, stevia, and the other ingredients.
2. Close the slow cooker lid and cook the catfish for 2 hours on High.
3. Divide into bowls and serve.

Nutrition: calories 279, fat 20, carbs 5, protein 6

Spicy Tuna

Preparation Time: 10 minutes
Cooking time: 1 hour
Servings: 3
Ingredients:

- 12 oz tuna fillet
- 1 tablespoon olive oil
- 1 teaspoon hot paprika
- 1 red chili pepper minced
- ½ teaspoon black pepper
- ½ teaspoon salt
- 1 jalapeno pepper, chopped
- 1/3 cup coconut oil

- 1 garlic clove, chopped

Directions:

1. Put the oil in the slow cooker.
2. Add the fish and the other ingredients and toss gently. Close the lid and cook the oil mixture on High for 1 hour.
3. Divide between plates and serve.

Nutrition: calories 309, fat 12, carbs 1, protein 19

Turmeric Calamari

Preparation Time: 10 minutes
Cooking time: 6 hours
Servings: 5
Ingredients:

- 1-pound calamari rings
- 1 teaspoon turmeric
- 1 teaspoon hot paprika
- 2 tablespoons coconut cream
- ½ teaspoon minced garlic
- 1 tablespoon heavy cream
- ½ teaspoon ground coriander
- ½ teaspoon salt
- ½ teaspoon black pepper

Directions:

1. In the slow cooker, mix the calamari with the turmeric and the other ingredients and close the lid.
2. Cook the seafood for 6 hours on Low.
3. When the time is over, stir the mix and serve.

Nutrition: calories 200, fat 4, carbs 3, protein 14

Thyme Sea bass

Preparation Time: 10 minutes
Cooking time: 4 hours
Servings: 4
Ingredients:

- 11 oz sea bass, trimmed
- 2 tablespoons coconut cream
- 3 oz spring onions, chopped

- 1 teaspoon fennel seeds
- ½ teaspoon dried thyme
- 1 teaspoon olive oil - 1/3 cup water
- 1 teaspoon apple cider vinegar
- ½ teaspoon salt

Directions:
1. In the slow cooker, mix the sea bass with the cream and the other ingredients.
2. Close the lid and cook sea bass for 4 hours on Low.

Nutrition: calories 304, fat 11, carbs 6, protein 1

Shrimp and Zucchini
Preparation Time: 15 minutes
Cooking time: 2 hours
Servings: 6
Ingredients:

- 1-pound shrimp, peeled and deveined
- 2 zucchinis, roughly cubed
- 1 cup cherry tomatoes, halved
- ½ cup Mozzarella cheese, shredded
- 4 tablespoons cream cheese
- 1 tablespoon butter, melted
- 1 teaspoon salt
- 1 tablespoon keto tomato sauce
- ¾ cup of water

Directions:
1. In the slow cooker, mix the shrimp with zucchinis and the other ingredients except for the cheese and toss.
2. Sprinkle the cheese on top, close the lid and cook on High for 2 hours.

Nutrition: calories 223, fat 8, carbs 3, protein 19

Lemon Cod
Preparation Time: 15 minutes
Cooking time: 2 hours
Servings: 4
Ingredients: 20 oz cod fillet

- Juice of 1 lemon

- Zest of 1 lemon, grated
- 2 oz Parmesan, grated
- 1 tablespoon chives, chopped
- 1 teaspoon turmeric powder
- ½ teaspoon salt
- ½ teaspoon ground black pepper
- 1 teaspoon butter
- 1/3 cup organic almond milk

Directions:
1. In the slow cooker, mix the cod with lemon juice, zest, and the other ingredients.
2. Close the lid and cook the sauce for 2 hours on High.
3. Divide between plates and serve.

Nutrition: calories 212, fat 5, carbs 6, protein 30

Cinnamon Mackerel
Preparation Time: 10 minutes
Cooking time: 3 hours
Servings: 4
Ingredients:

- 1 ½ pound mackerel, trimmed
- 1 tablespoon avocado oil
- 1 teaspoon garlic powder
- 1/3 cup coconut milk
- ½ teaspoon salt
- ½ teaspoon basil, dried
- 1 teaspoon cumin, ground
- ¾ teaspoon ground cinnamon

Directions:
1. In the slow cooker, mix the mackerel with the oil and the other ingredients and close the lid.
2. Cook the fish for 3 hours on High.
3. Divide between plates and serve.

Nutrition: calories 228, fat 8, carbs 2, protein 11

Parsley Salmon

Preparation Time: 15 minutes

Cooking time: 2 hours

Servings: 4

Ingredients:

- 10 oz salmon fillet
- 2 tablespoons parsley, chopped
- ½ cup coconut cream
- ½ teaspoon salt
- ½ teaspoon chili flakes
- 1 teaspoon turmeric powder
- 2 oz Parmesan, grated
- 3 tablespoons coconut oil

Directions:

1. In the slow cooker, mix the salmon with the parsley and the other ingredients.
2. Close the lid and cook the meal for 2 hours on High.

Nutrition: calories 283, fat 22, carbs 2, protein 22

Cheesy Tuna

Preparation Time: 10 minutes

Cooking time: 9 hours

Servings: 4

Ingredients:

- 1 cup coconut cream
- 1 tablespoon Ricotta cheese
- 1 teaspoon salt - ½ teaspoon white pepper
- 10 ounces tuna fillet, boneless and cubed
- 1 teaspoon olive oil
- 1 garlic clove, crushed
- 1 teaspoon fennel seeds
- 1/2 cup Cheddar, shredded

Directions:

1. In the slow cooker, mix the tuna with the cream and the other ingredients.
2. Close the lid and cook snapper for 9 hours on Low.

Nutrition: calories 211, fat 4.3, fiber 3.3, carbs 7.8, protein 21

Spiced Shrimp

Preparation Time: 10 minutes

Cooking time: 1 hour

Servings: 2

Ingredients:

- 8 oz shrimp, peeled and deveined
- 1 teaspoon chili powder
- 1 teaspoon nutmeg, ground
- 1 teaspoon coriander, ground
- ½ teaspoon minced garlic
- 1 tablespoon olive oil
- 2 tablespoon coconut cream
- ½ teaspoon salt
- 2 tablespoons water

Directions:

1. In the slow cooker, mix the shrimp with chili powder, nutmeg, and the other ingredients.
2. Close the lid.
3. Cook for 1 hour on High.

Nutrition: calories 200, fat 11, carbs 4, protein 9

Seafood Stew

Preparation Time: 15 minutes

Cooking time: 7 hours

Servings: 4

Ingredients:

- 2 tablespoons olive oil
- 1 cup mussels
- 1 cup salmon fillet, boneless and cubed
- 1 cup shrimp, peeled and deveined
- 3 spring onions, chopped
- ½ green bell pepper, chopped
- 1 garlic clove, diced
- ¾ teaspoon chili flakes
- ¼ teaspoon ground black pepper
- ¼ cup crushed tomatoes
- ½ teaspoon dried thyme

Directions:

1. In the slow cooker, mix the mussels with the salmon and the other ingredients.
2. Stir the mixture and close the lid.
3. Cook the meal for 7 hours on Low.
4. Divide into bowls and serve.

Nutrition: calories 260, fat 15.1, fiber 1.9, carbs 6.2, protein 25.1

Shrimp and Green Beans

Preparation Time: 15 minutes

Cooking time: 3 hours

Servings: 5

Ingredients:

- 1-pound shrimp, peeled and deveined
- ¼ pound green beans, trimmed and halved
- 1 teaspoon salt
- 1 teaspoon chili flakes
- 1 teaspoon paprika
- ½ teaspoon garam masala
- 1 teaspoon coriander, ground
- 1 teaspoon basil, dried
- ¾ cup crushed tomatoes
- 1 tablespoon olive oil
- 3 spring onions, chopped
- 1 green bell pepper, chopped
- 1 cup of water

Directions:

1. In the slow cooker, mix the shrimp with green beans, salt, and the other ingredients.
2. Close the lid and cook for 3 hours on High.
3. Divide into bowls and serve.

Nutrition: calories 202, fat 7, carbs 8, protein 12

Salmon and Spinach Bake

Preparation Time: 10 minutes

Cooking time: 6 hours

Servings: 2

Ingredients:

- 1-pound salmon fillet, chopped
- 1/3 cup spinach, chopped
- ½ cup Cheddar cheese, shredded
- ¾ cup organic coconut milk
- 1 teaspoon butter
- ½ teaspoon ground thyme
- ½ teaspoon salt
- 1/3 cup of water

Directions:

1. In the slow cooker, mix the salmon with spinach and the other ingredients, toss, and close the lid.
2. Cook the salmon bake for 6 hours on Low.

Nutrition: calories 423, fat 16, carbs 3, protein 17

Chili Squid

Preparation Time: 15 minutes

Cooking time: 2 hours

Servings: 4

Ingredients:

- 16 oz squid tubes, trimmed (4 squid tubes)
- 1 cup spring onions, chopped
- 1 teaspoon salt
- ½ teaspoon chili powder
- ½ teaspoon hot paprika
- 1 tablespoon butter
- 1/3 cup heavy cream
- 1 teaspoon ground black pepper
- 1 tablespoon dried dill

Directions:

1. In the slow cooker, mix the squid with spring onions and the other ingredients.

2. Close the slow cooker lid and cook for 2.5 hours on High.

Nutrition: calories 244, fat 8, carbs 7 protein 13

Calamari Rings and Broccoli

Preparation Time: 15 minutes

Cooking time: 4 hours

Servings: 6

Ingredients:

- 1 1/2-pound calamari rings
- 1 cup broccoli florets
- 1 jalapeno pepper, minced
- 1 tablespoon keto tomato sauce
- 1/3 cup heavy cream
- ½ teaspoon salt
- ½ teaspoon chili powder
- 1 teaspoon cumin, ground
- 2 garlic cloves, diced
- 1 tablespoon butter

Directions:

1. In the slow cooker, mix the calamari with broccoli and the other ingredients, toss and close the lid.
2. Cook the meal on Low for 4.5 hours.

Nutrition: calories 210, fat 6.1, carbs 4.7, protein 18.1

Tilapia and Tomatoes

Preparation Time: 15 minutes

Cooking time: 2 hours

Servings: 2

Ingredients:

- 8 oz tilapia fillet (2 servings)
- 1 and ½ cups cherry tomatoes, halved
- 1 tablespoon keto tomato sauce
- 1 tablespoon butter, melted
- 3 tablespoons coconut cream
- ½ teaspoon lemongrass
- ½ teaspoon salt
- ¼ teaspoon chili flakes

Directions:

1. In the slow cooker, mix the tilapia with tomatoes and the other ingredients.
2. Close the slow cooker lid and cook tilapia for 2 hours on High.

Nutrition: calories 308, fat 12.2, carbs 1.9, protein 32.3

Chipotle Salmon Fillets

Preparation Time: 2 Hrs

Cooking time: 2 Hrs

Servings: 2

Ingredients:

- 2 medium salmon fillets, boneless
- A pinch of nutmeg, ground
- A pinch of cloves, ground
- A pinch of ginger powder
- Salt and black pepper to the taste
- 2 tsp sugar
- 1 tsp onion powder
- ¼ tsp chipotle chili powder
- ½ tsp cayenne pepper
- ½ tsp cinnamon, ground
- 1/8 tsp thyme, dried

Directions:

1. Place the salmon fillets in foil wraps. Drizzle ginger, cloves, salt, thyme, cinnamon, black pepper, cayenne, chili powder, onion powder, nutmeg, and coconut sugar on top. Wrap the fish fillet with aluminum foil. Put the cooker's lid on and set the cooking time to 2 hours over low heat. Unwrap the fish and serve warm.

Nutrition: Per Serving: Calories 220, Total Fat 4g, Fiber 2g, Total Carbs 7g, Protein 4g

Cod and Broccoli

Preparation Time: 3 Hrs

Cooking time: 3 Hrs

Servings: 2

Ingredients:

- 1 pound cod fillets, boneless
- 1 cup broccoli florets
- ½ cup veggie stock
- 2 tablespoons tomato paste
- 2 garlic cloves, minced
- 1 red onion, minced
- ½ teaspoon rosemary, dried
- A pinch of salt and black pepper
- 1 tablespoon chives, chopped

Directions:

1. In your Slow Cooker, mix the cod with the broccoli, stock, tomato paste, and the other ingredients, toss, put the lid on and cook on Low for 3 hours. Divide the mix between plates and serve.

Nutrition: calories 200, fat 13, fiber 3, carbs 6, protein 11

Thai Style Flounder

Preparation Time: 6 Hrs

Cooking time: 6 Hrs

Servings: 6

Ingredients:

- 24 oz flounder, peeled, cleaned
- 1 lemon, sliced
- 1 teaspoon ground ginger
- ½ teaspoon cayenne pepper
- ½ teaspoon chili powder
- 1 teaspoon salt
- 1 teaspoon ground turmeric
- 1 tablespoon sesame oil
- 1 cup of water

Directions:

1. Chop the flounder roughly and put it in the Slow Cooker. Add water and all remaining ingredients. Close the lid and cook the fish on low for 6 hours.

Nutrition: Calories: 278 Protein: 7.9g Carbs: 23g Fat: 3.9g

Tuna and Cabbage Mix

Preparation Time: 10 minutes

Cooking time: 3 hours

Servings: 4

Ingredients:

- 2 oz cabbage, shredded
- 11 oz tuna, drained, chopped
- 2 tablespoons keto tomato sauce
- 1/3 cup water
- 1 teaspoon salt
- 1 tablespoon butter
- 1 teaspoon turmeric powder

Directions:

1. In the slow cooker, mix the cabbage with the tuna and the other ingredients, and close the lid.
2. Cook cabbage for 3 hours on High.
3. Divide into bowls and serve.

Nutrition: calories 227, fat 8, carbs 3, protein 15

Mozzarella Fish

Preparation Time: 10 minutes

Cooking time: 2 hours

Servings: 4

Ingredients:

- 1-pound salmon fillet
- ½ cup heavy cream
- ½ cup Mozzarella, shredded
- ½ teaspoon turmeric powder
- 1 teaspoon butter
- ½ teaspoon ground black pepper

Directions:

1. Put the salmon fillet in the slow cooker.
2. Add the rest of the ingredients except the cheese.
3. Top the mix with the Mozzarella, and close the lid.
4. Cook fish gratin for 2 hours on High.

Nutrition: calories 241, fat 14, carbs 3, protein 24

Marinara Shrimp

Preparation Time: 10 minutes

Cooking time: 1 hour

Servings: 2

Ingredients:

- 10 oz shrimp, peeled and deveined
- 3 tablespoons keto marinara sauce
- 2 tablespoons coconut flour
- 1 tablespoon coconut cream

Directions:

1. In the slow cooker, mix the shrimp with the other ingredients and close the lid.
2. Cook the fish for 1 hour on High.

Nutrition: calories 212, fat 4, carbs 7, protein 26

Butter Salmon and Avocado

Preparation Time: 10 minutes

Cooking time: 1 hour 30 minutes

Servings: 1

Ingredients:

- 6 oz salmon fillet
- 1/3 cup butter
- 2 avocados, peeled, pitted, and cubed
- 1 teaspoon garam masala
- 1 teaspoon coriander, ground
- 1 teaspoon lemon juice
- 1 teaspoon apple cider vinegar
- ¼ teaspoon salt

Directions:

1. In the slow cooker, mix the salmon with the butter and the other ingredients and close the lid.
2. Cook salmon for 1.5 hours on High.

Nutrition: calories 370, fat 11, carbs 1, protein 12

Mustard Shrimp

Preparation Time: 10 minutes

Cooking time: 2 hours

Servings: 2

Ingredients:

- 1-pound shrimp, peeled and deveined
- 2 tablespoons Dijon mustard
- ½ cup of coconut water
- 1 teaspoon turmeric powder
- ½ teaspoon salt - 1 teaspoon olive oil

Directions:

1. In the slow cooker, mix the shrimp with the mustard and the other ingredients.
2. Close the lid. Cook the fish on Low for 2 hours.

Nutrition: calories 172, fat 4, carbs 1, protein 32

Salmon and Asparagus

Preparation Time: 15 minutes

Cooking time: 3 hours 30 minutes

Servings: 4

Ingredients:

- 1-pound salmon fillet, boneless
- ¼ pound asparagus, trimmed and halved
- 1 cup coconut cream
- 1 teaspoon dried basil
- ½ teaspoon salt
- 1 teaspoon dried parsley
- Cooking spray

Directions:

1. In the slow cooker, mix the salmon with the asparagus, cream, and the other ingredients and close the lid.

2. Cook the fish loaf for 3.5 hours on Low.

Nutrition: calories 204, fat 9, carbs 6, protein 23

Avocado and Shrimp

Preparation Time: 15 minutes

Cooking time: 2 hours

Servings: 2

Ingredients:

- 1 avocado, peeled, pitted, and cubed
- 8 oz shrimps, raw, peeled
- 1 teaspoon basil, dried
- 1 teaspoon coriander, ground
- 1 teaspoon butter, softened
- ½ teaspoon minced garlic
- ½ teaspoon chili flakes
- 1/3 cup water
- ½ teaspoon onion powder

Directions:

1. In the slow cooker, mix the shrimp with avocado, basil, and the other ingredients and toss.
2. Close the lid and cook the meal on High for 2 hours.

Nutrition: calories 279, fat 13, carbs 12, protein 12

Tilapia and Radish Bites

Preparation Time: 15 minutes

Cooking time: 2 hours 30 minutes

Servings: 2

Ingredients:

- 1 ½ cups radishes, halved
- 1 teaspoon sweet paprika
- ½ teaspoon dried rosemary
- ¼ teaspoon ground black pepper
- ½ teaspoon salt
- 9 oz tilapia fillet, boneless and cubed
- 2 oz Cheddar cheese, sliced
- ¼ cup veggie stock

Directions:

1. In the slow cooker, mix the radishes with the fish and the other ingredients and toss.
2. Close the lid and cook the fish for 2.5 hours on High.

Nutrition: calories 251, fat 8, fiber 1, carbs 1, protein 6

Balsamic Scallops

Preparation Time: 10 minutes

Cooking time: 2 hours

Servings: 4

Ingredients:

- 8 scallops
- 1 tablespoon balsamic vinegar
- 1 teaspoon hot paprika
- ½ teaspoon salt
- 2 tablespoons olive oil
- ½ teaspoon dried rosemary

Directions:

1. In the slow cooker, mix the scallops with the vinegar and the other ingredients, toss and close the lid.
2. Cook bacon scallops for 2 hours on High.

Nutrition: calories 215, fat 6, carbs 1, protein 7

Lemon Crab Legs

Preparation Time: 10 minutes

Cooking time: 3 hours

Servings: 4

Ingredients:

- 12 oz King crab legs
- 1/3 cup butter
- Juice of 1 lemon
- Zest of 1 lemon, grated
- 1 tablespoon yellow curry paste
- ¼ cup of water
- 1 teaspoon minced garlic
- ½ teaspoon salt

Directions:

1. In the slow cooker, mix the crab with the butter and the other ingredients.
2. Close the lid and cook the crab legs for 3 hours on Low.

Nutrition: calories 165, fat 7.8, fiber 0, carbs 4.2, protein 5.6

Cod Patties

Preparation Time: 20 minutes

Cooking time: 1 hour

Servings: 3

Ingredients:

- 8 oz cod fillets, boneless, finely chopped
- 1 egg, beaten
- 1 teaspoon cilantro, dried
- 1 teaspoon Italian seasoning
- ¼ cup fresh basil, blended
- ½ teaspoon salt
- ¼ teaspoon chili powder
- 1/3 cup coconut milk
- 1 tablespoon butter
- 1 tablespoon almond flour

Directions:

1. In the mixing bowl, mix up together the cod with cilantro, seasoning, flour, basil, salt, and chili powder, stir and shape medium patties out of this mix.
2. Toss the butter in the skillet and bring it to boil.
3. Add the patties and cook for 1 minute over medium-high heat.
4. Transfer the patties to the slow cooker and add coconut milk.
5. Close the lid and cook patties for 1 hour on High.

Nutrition: calories 301, fat 21, carbs 5, protein 19

CHAPTER 7:

Meat Recipes

Pepperoncini Beef

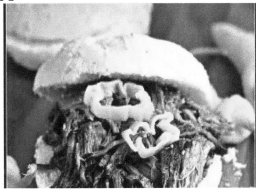

Preparation Time: 10 minutes
Cooking time: 10 hours
Servings: 6
Ingredients:

- 1-pound beef chuck roast
- 18 oz pepperoncini pepper
- 1 cup chicken stock
- 1 teaspoon salt
- 1 teaspoon ground black pepper
- 1 teaspoon paprika
- 1 onion, diced

Directions:

1. Pour the chicken stock into the slow cooker. Add the beef chuck roast and sprinkle with the ground black pepper, salt, paprika, and diced onion. Close the lid and cook for 4 hours on HIGH.
2. Cook for 6 hours.

Nutrition: calories 254, fat 10, carbs 35, protein 9

Curry Lamb

Preparation Time: 14 minutes
Cooking time: 13 hours
Servings: 6
Ingredients:

- 2 tablespoons curry paste
- 1-pound lamb
- 2 tomatoes
- 3 tablespoons pomegranate sauce or juice
- 1 teaspoon salt
- 1 tablespoon apple cider vinegar
- 1 teaspoon nutmeg
- 1 teaspoon cilantro
- 4 tablespoons beef broth
- 1 cup water
- 1 tablespoon butter
- ¼ cup coriander leaves, chopped

Directions:

1. Combine the curry paste with the beef broth and stir the paste until it is dissolved. Slice the tomatoes.
2. Butter the slow cooker bowl and make the layer of the tomatoes in the bottom of the bowl. Combine the pomegranate sauce, salt, apple cider vinegar, nutmeg, cilantro, and chopped coriander leaves together.
3. Then chop the lamb roughly and sprinkle with the pomegranate sauce. Mix using your fingertips. Put the meat on top of the sliced tomatoes.
4. Add water and close the lid. Cook the meat on LOW for 13 hours. Serve the cooked lamb with the lime wedges. Enjoy!

Nutrition: calories 235, fat 15, carbs 4, protein 19

Honey Pulled Pork

Preparation Time: 10 minutes
Cooking time: 7 hours
Servings: 4
Ingredients:

- 4 teaspoons minced garlic
- 1 teaspoon salt
- 1 teaspoon ground black pepper
- 1 teaspoon cilantro
- ¼ cup honey
- 1-pound pork fillet
- 2 cups water
- 1 teaspoon ground chili pepper

Directions:

1. Put the pork fillet in the slow cooker. Sprinkle it with salt, ground black pepper, cilantro, and ground chili pepper. Add the water and close the lid. Cook on HIGH for 5 hours.
2. Then strain the water and shred the pork. Return the pork to the slow cooker and add minced garlic and honey. Stir the shredded meat with a fork.
3. Close the lid and cook on LOW for 2 hours more. Serve it and enjoy!

Nutrition: calories 376, fat 20, carbs 20, protein 29

Delightful Pulled Pork Nachos

Preparation Time: 25 minutes
Cooking time: 5 hours
Servings: 12
Ingredients:

- 7 oz corn tortilla
- 2 tablespoons mayonnaise
- 3 red onions
- 1 cup tomato, chopped
- ½ cup fresh parsley
- 1 garlic clove, peeled
- 1-pound pork shoulder
- 3 tablespoons mustard
- 1 tablespoon ketchup
- 1 teaspoon cayenne pepper
- 1 teaspoon salt
- 2 teaspoons ground black pepper
- 9 oz Cheddar cheese, shredded
- 1 teaspoon dried mint
- 2 cup water

Directions:

1. Peel the onions and slice them. Put 1 tablespoon of onion in the slow cooker.
2. Add the pork shoulder. Sprinkle the meat with the mustard, ketchup, cayenne pepper, salt, ground black pepper, and dried mint. Add the water, then close the lid and cook it for 5 hours on HIGH. Remove the pork shoulder from the slow cooker and shred it.
3. Place a corn tortilla in a skillet and add the shredded meat. Then sprinkle it with a small amount of the chopped tomatoes and onions.
4. Cover it with another corn tortillas. Then sprinkle the mixture with a small amount of cheese. Repeat the layers until you use the entire ingredient.
5. Sprinkle the last layer with cheese and mayonnaise. Chop the garlic and fresh parsley and sprinkle on top as well.
6. Put the dish in the oven and cook it at 350 degrees F for 10 minutes. Enjoy!

Nutrition: calories 204, fat 10, carbs 14, protein 14

Garlic Beef Mash

Preparation Time: 15 minutes
Cooking time: 12 hours
Servings: 4
Ingredients:

- 1-pound beef

- 1 cup garlic cloves, peeled
- 4 cups beef broth
- 1 tablespoon salt
- 1 teaspoon ground black pepper
- 1 teaspoon paprika
- 1 cup onion, roasted
- 3 oz butter

Directions:

1. Put the beef in the slow cooker and add the water. Add salt, ground black pepper, paprika, and peeled garlic cloves.
2. Close the slow cooker lid and cook the meat for 12 hours on LOW. Then strain the water and mash the beef with a fork. Add butter and roasted onion and mix well.
3. Place it in a bowl and serve or keep in the fridge for 1 hour to use the mash as a spread. Enjoy!

Nutrition: calories 462, fat 24, carbs 36, protein 28

Beef Strips in Bread Crumbs

Preparation Time: 17 minutes

Cooking time: 4 hours

Servings: 6

Ingredients:

- ½ teaspoon onion powder
- 1 teaspoon garlic powder
- 1 cup bread crumbs
- 2 large eggs
- ¼ cup sour cream
- 1 tablespoon salt
- 1 teaspoon turmeric
- 1 teaspoon olive oil
- 10 oz beef fillet
- 1 tablespoon balsamic vinegar

Directions:

1. Cut the beef fillet into strips and sprinkle them with the onion powder and garlic

powder. Add salt, turmeric, and balsamic vinegar. Then beat the egg in a separate bowl.
2. Add sour cream and stir well. Dip the beef strips in the egg mixture, and after this, coat them in the bread crumbs. Spray the inside of the slow cooker bowl with the olive oil. Put the beef strips in the slow cooker and close the lid.
3. Cook the dish on HIGH for 4 hours. Stir frequently. Serve the prepared beef strips immediately. Enjoy!

Nutrition: calories 123, fat 6.2, carbs 5, protein 12

Pork and Barley Soup

Preparation Time: 16 minutes

Cooking time: 8 hours

Servings: 9

Ingredients:

- 1 cup barley
- 7 cups water
- 3 oz pickled cucumbers
- 9 oz pork, chopped
- 1 teaspoon paprika
- 1 teaspoon cilantro
- 1 tablespoon ground black pepper
- 1 tomato, chopped
- 1 carrot, peeled
- 1 tablespoon salt
- 1 sweet pepper, chopped
- 1 teaspoon sour cream

Directions:

1. Chop the pickled cucumbers and carrot, then put them in the slow cooker.
2. Add chopped pork, barley, tomatoes, and sweet pepper. After this, add the paprika, cilantro, water, ground black pepper, salt, and sour cream. Mix the soup gently and close the lid.

3. Cook the soup on LOW for 8 hours. Ladle the cooked soup in the bowls. Let it chill gently. Serve!

Nutrition: calories 152, fat 3, carbs 20, protein 11

Hungarian Tender Beef

Preparation Time: 15 minutes
Cooking time: 10 hours
Servings: 4
Ingredients:

- ½ cup tomato puree
- 1-pound beef
- ½ cup garlic clove
- 1 white onion
- ¼ teaspoon caraway seeds
- 1 teaspoon curry powder
- 1 teaspoon chili flakes
- 3 tablespoons sour cream
- 1 teaspoon cilantro
- ½ teaspoon ground nutmeg
- 3 cups water

Directions:

1. Rub the beef with the caraway seeds, curry powder, chili flakes, sour cream, cilantro, and ground nutmeg. Make small cuts in the beef.
2. Peel the garlic cloves and cut them into halves. Fill the beef cuts with the garlic halved. Then rub the meat with the tomato puree and put it in the slow cooker.
3. Chop the onion roughly and sprinkle over the meat. Close the lid and cook for 10 hours on LOW. Stir the meat frequently during cooking. Slice the meat into the serving pieces and transfer them to the plates. Serve it!

Nutrition: calories 217, fat 7.9, carbs 12, protein 26

Stuffed Lamb with Onions

Preparation Time: 15 minutes
Cooking time: 6 hours
Servings: 9
Ingredients:

- 3-pounds lamb fillet
- 5 medium onions
- 3 garlic cloves
- 1 carrot
- 1 tablespoon ground black pepper
- 1 tablespoon olive oil
- ¼ cup sour cream
- 1 tablespoon salt
- 1 teaspoon rosemary

Directions:

1. Peel the onions and slice them. Then peel the garlic cloves and mince them. Combine the sliced onions with the minced garlic.
2. Make a "pocket" in the lamb fillet and fill it with the onion mixture. Peel the carrot and chop it, then stuff it into the lamb as well.
3. After this, secure the lamb fillet with toothpicks. Rub the lamb fillet with the ground black pepper, olive oil, sour cream salt, and rosemary.
4. Wrap the prepared meat in the foil and put it in the slow cooker. Cook the meat on HIGH for 6 hours. Then remove the meat from the slow cooker and discard the foil. Serve it!

Nutrition: calories 440, fat 27.7, carbs 8, protein 38

Lamb Meatballs

Preparation Time: 15 minutes
Cooking time: 6 hours
Servings: 8
Ingredients:

- 19 oz minced lamb
- 2 tablespoons minced garlic
- 1 white onion, diced
- 1 egg
- 1 tablespoon flour
- 1 teaspoon olive oil
- 4 tablespoons flour
- 1 teaspoon salt
- 1 teaspoon turmeric
- 1 teaspoon dried basil
- 2 teaspoons paprika

Directions:

1. Put the minced lamb in a big bowl. Beat the egg into the lamb along with the diced onion.
2. After this, add the minced garlic and flour. Sprinkle the meat with salt, turmeric, dried basil, and paprika. Then make small balls from the lamb mixture and coat them in the flour.
3. Spray the slow cooker bowl with the olive oil.
4. Put the prepared lamb meatballs inside and close the lid. Cook the dish on HIGH for 6 hours. Turn the meatballs to another side after 3 hours of cooking.
5. Then remove the prepared meatballs from the slow cooker and dry them with a paper towel. Serve the lamb meatballs warm.

Nutrition: calories 223, fat 13.3, carbs 6.44, protein 19

Lamb Shoulder

Preparation Time: 30 minutes
Cooking time: 10 hours
Servings: 5
Ingredients:

- 12 oz lamb shoulder
- 1 tablespoon fresh rosemary
- 1 cup beer
- 1 teaspoon cilantro
- 1 tablespoon chili pepper
- 1 tablespoon cayenne pepper
- 1 cup water
- 1 garlic clove, peeled
- 1 teaspoon onion powder
- 1 tablespoon marjoram

Directions:

1. Put the lamb shoulder in a bowl and pour the beer over the lamb.
2. Leave the meat for 20 minutes. Meanwhile, combine the fresh rosemary, cilantro, chili pepper, cayenne pepper, onion powder, and marjoram together.
3. Put the mixture in the slow cooker and add water. Close the lid and cook the liquid on LOW for 1 hour. Peel the garlic clove and put it in the slow cooker liquid after 30 minutes of cooking.
4. Then remove the lamb shoulder from the beer and transfer it to the slow cooker. Close the lid and cook the lamb for 10 hours on LOW.
5. When the time is done, the lamb meat should be very tender. Enjoy the dish!

Nutrition: calories 210, fat 13, carbs 5, protein 17

Lamb Stew

Preparation Time: 20 minutes
Cooking time: 5 hours
Servings: 10
Ingredients:

- 1 cup corn kernels

- 4 oz fresh celery root
- 1 tablespoon ground ginger
- 10 oz lamb cubes
- 1 teaspoon onion powder
- 1 teaspoon garlic powder
- 1 tablespoon tomato sauce
- ½ cup tomato puree
- 1 teaspoon olive oil
- 2 tablespoons flour
- 1 eggplant
- 1 carrot, peeled, grated
- 1 teaspoon cayenne pepper
- 2 cup water
- 5 medium potatoes

Directions:

1. Put the lamb in the slow cooker. Sprinkle the meat with the onion powder, garlic powder, and cayenne pepper. Peel the potatoes and chop them.
2. Add the potatoes into the slow cooker. After this, combine the tomato sauce and tomato puree together. Add the flour and stir.
3. Chop the eggplants and add them to the slow cooker.
4. Grate the fresh celery root. Add the celery root into the slow cooker along with the corn kernels, water, tomato mixture, and carrot.
5. Add the grated carrot to the slow cooker and close the lid.
6. Cook the stew on HIGH for 5 hours. Then open the slow cooker lid and stir the mixture with a spatula. Transfer the lamb stew to the bowls. Enjoy!

Nutrition: calories 265, fat 5.9, carbs 42.39, protein 12

Lamb Casserole

Preparation Time: 16 minutes

Cooking time: 9 hours

Servings: 6

Ingredients:

- 1 cup rice
- 4 cups water
- 13 oz lamb fillet
- 1 tablespoon ground paprika
- 1 onion
- 9 oz Cheddar cheese, shredded
- 3 carrots, chopped
- 1 tablespoon olive oil
- 1 teaspoon ground cinnamon
- 1 tablespoon turmeric
- 5 sweet potatoes

Directions:

1. Combine the rice with the olive oil and turmeric and mix. Transfer the rice to the slow cooker. Make a layer of the chopped carrot in the slow cooker bowl.
2. Then peel the onion and slice. Make the layer of the sliced onion in the bowl as well.
3. Then chop the lamb fillet and add it into the slow cooker. Sprinkle the meat with the ground paprika, salt, and ground cinnamon. Slice the sweet potatoes and cover the meat with the vegetables. Add water and sprinkle the casserole with the cheese.
4. Close the slow cooker and cook the dish on LOW for 9 hours. Then transfer the casserole to the bowls carefully. Serve!

Nutrition: calories 436, fat 20, carbs 42, protein 26

Garlic Lamb

Preparation Time: 10 minutes
Cooking time: 10 hours
Servings: 7
Ingredients:

- 2 oz fresh rosemary
- ½ cup fresh cilantro
- ¼ cup coriander leaves
- 2-pounds lamb fillet
- 1 teaspoon salt
- 1 teaspoon black peas
- 1 teaspoon chili flakes
- 1 cup garlic
- 1 teaspoon garlic powder
- 6 cups water

Directions:

1. Wash the fresh rosemary, cilantro, and coriander leaves carefully and chop them roughly.
2. Then line the slow cooker bowl with the chopped greens and put the lamb fillet inside as well. Sprinkle the lamb fillet with the salt, black peas, chili flakes, and garlic powder.
3. Peel the garlic and mince it. Rub the lamb fillet with the minced garlic and add water.
4. Close the slow cooker lid and cook the lamb for 10 hours on LOW.
5. Strain the liquid from the lamb and transfer the lamb fillet to a plate. Slice it and serve. The lamb fillet will be very aromatic and soft.

Nutrition: calories 375, fat 22, carbs 8, protein 33

Rosemary Lamb

Preparation Time: 20 minutes
Cooking time: 7 hours
Servings: 8
Ingredients:

- 4 tablespoons dried rosemary
- 1 cup tomatillos

- 1 tablespoon minced garlic
- 2 oz fresh rosemary
- 1 onion, grated
- 18 oz lamb leg
- 1 teaspoon salt
- 1 cup cream
- ½ teaspoon ground black pepper

Directions:

1. Chop the tomatillos roughly and put them in the blender.
2. Add the minced garlic, dried rosemary, fresh rosemary, salt, pepper, and grated onion. Pulse the mixture until it is smooth. Then pour the cream into the blender and pulse it for 30 seconds.
3. Put the lamb leg in the slow cooker and sprinkle it with the tomatillo-rosemary mixture.
4. Close the lid and cook it for 7 hours on LOW. Serve the cooled lamb immediately. Enjoy!

Nutrition: calories 168, fat 9, carbs 5, protein 14

Lamb and Apricot Tagine

Preparation Time: 10 minutes
Cooking time: 5 hours
Servings: 7
Ingredients:

- 2-pounds lamb fillet
- ½ cup dried apricots
- 3 tablespoon cashew
- 1 jalapeno pepper
- 2 cups red wine
- 1 tablespoon sugar
- 1 teaspoon salt
- 1 teaspoon ground white pepper
- 1 cup water

Directions:

1. Cut the lamb fillets into bite-sized cubes and put them in the slow cooker.

2. Sprinkle the meat with the cashew, salt, and ground white pepper. Chop the jalapeno pepper and dried apricots. Add all the ingredients into the slow cooker.

3. Then add sugar, red wine, and water.

4. Close the lid and cook the lamb tagine for 5 hours on HIGH. Stir the lamb once per cooking. Stir the cooked dish again. Serve it.

Nutrition: calories 416, fat 25, carbs 9, protein 33

Greek Style Lamb with Olives

Preparation Time: 11 minutes

Cooking time: 7 hours

Servings: 5

Ingredients:

- 1 cup Greek yogurt
- 4 oz black olives
- 8 oz lamb
- 1 tablespoon ground black pepper
- 1 chili, chopped
- 1 teaspoon powdered chili
- 1 tablespoon balsamic vinegar
- 1 teaspoon oregano
- ½ cup chicken stock
- 1 tablespoon lemon zest

Directions:

1. Slice the black olives. Put Greek yogurt in the slow cooker and add the sliced black olives and lamb.

2. Sprinkle the mix with the ground black pepper, powdered chili, balsamic vinegar, oregano, and lemon zest. Add chicken stock and chopped chili.

3. Close the lid and cook the lamb for 4 hours on LOW.

4. Then open the lid and stir, shredding the meat with a fork.

5. Close the lid and cook the lamb for 3 hours more on LOW. Serve the prepared meat with all the juice from the slow cooker. Enjoy!

Nutrition: calories 190, fat 10.4, carbs 8, protein 16

Succulents Lamb

Preparation Time: 10 minutes

Cooking time: 9 hours

Servings: 4

Ingredients:

- 3 tablespoons mustard
- 5 tablespoons olive oil
- 3 tablespoons fresh rosemary
- 1 teaspoon ground coriander
- 1 teaspoon dried mint
- 1 teaspoon salt
- 1 teaspoon paprika
- 4 tablespoons maple syrup
- 1-pound lamb fillet
- 2 tablespoon water

Directions:

1. Combine the mustard and olive oil together. Add the fresh rosemary, ground coriander, dried mint, salt, and paprika.

2. Rub the lamb fillet with the mustard mixture and put it in the slow cooker bowl. Add the water and maple syrup and close the slow cooker lid.

3. Cook the lamb on LOW for 9 hours.

4. When the lamb is cooked, sprinkle with the remaining liquid from the slow cooker. Transfer the meat to a plate and slice. Put the lamb slices on plates and serve!

Nutrition: calories 502, fat 36, carbs 14, protein 28

Moroccan Lamb

Preparation Time: 25 minutes

Cooking time: 13 hours

Servings: 8

Ingredients:

- 2-pound lamb shoulder

- 1 teaspoon cumin seeds
- 1 teaspoon ground cumin
- 1 teaspoon ground coriander
- 1 teaspoon celery root
- 1 teaspoon salt
- 1 teaspoon chili flakes
- 4 tablespoons tomato paste
- 3 tablespoons raisins
- 1 tablespoon dried apricots
- 5 cup water
- 1 cup onion, chopped

Directions:

1. Combine the cumin seeds, ground cumin, ground coriander, celery root, salt, and chili flakes in a shallow bowl.
2. After this, rub the lamb shoulder with the spice mixture and then brush with the tomato paste. Leave the meat for 10 minutes to marinate.
3. Put the chopped onion in the slow cooker with the water.
4. Then put the marinated meat in the slow cooker as well and close the lid.
5. Cook the dish on LOW for 13 hours. Remove the meat from the liquid and serve it. Enjoy!

Nutrition: calories 195, fat 9, carbs 4, protein 23

CHAPTER 8:

Pork Recipes

Slow Cooker Pulled Pork Roast

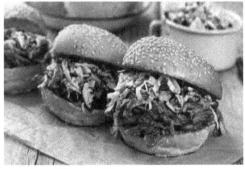

Preparation Time: 15 minutes
Cooking time: 10 hours
Servings: 8
Ingredients

- 1 (3 1/2) pound pork butt roast
- 1 tablespoon chili powder
- 1 tablespoon vegetable oil
- 2 teaspoons pepper
- 2 teaspoons ground cumin
- 2 teaspoons coriander
- 2 teaspoons paprika
- 1 teaspoon allspice
- 1/2 teaspoon salt
- 1/2 cup fancy molasses
- 1/3 cup Heinz® Mustard
- 2 teaspoons cornstarch
- Soft rolls

Directions:
1. Discard all string from the roast and trim away excess fat. In a bowl, put chili powder; mix in garlic, salt, allspice, paprika, coriander, cumin, pepper, chili, and oil to form a paste. Rub all over the whole pork; thoroughly work the spice mixture into the meat. Let the meat marinate for a minimum of 30 minutes or overnight. Remove the roast to a slow cooker.

2. Stir together mustard, molasses, vinegar, and ketchup. Add the mixture onto the roast and cook on low until very soft, or about 8-10 hours.

3. Remove the roast to a big bowl; remove any fat you can see. Separate the meat into long strands with 2 forks. Pour off 1 1/2 cups of the cooking juices and drain into a saucepan. Mix in cornstarch and boil. Cook until bubbly and thick while whisking. Put the shredded meat back into the slow cooker, mix to blend with the leftover cooking juices. Put the meat on soft rolls to enjoy, drizzle the thickened sauce mixture over to taste.

Nutrition: calories 209, fat 18, carbs 7, protein 22

Apple Cider Pulled Pork with Caramelized Onion and Apples

Preparation Time: 10 minutes
Cooking time: 6 hours 20 minutes
Servings: 6
Ingredients

- 3 (12 fluid ounce) bottles hard apple cider
- 1/4 cup brown sugar
- 1 (2 pound) pork tenderloin
- 1 large onion, cut into strips
- 1/2 cup brown sugar

- 1/2 teaspoon ground cinnamon
- 1/2 teaspoon onion powder
- salt and ground black pepper to taste
- 2 large Granny Smith apples - peeled, cored, and sliced
- 6 hard rolls, split

Directions:

1. In a slow cooker, mix together 1/4 cup brown sugar and hard apple cider; stir until dissolved. Add the pork tenderloin.

2. Cook the tenderloin on Low for 6 hours until very soft. Use a fork to shred the pork.

3. During the last 20 minutes of cooking the roast, in a big skillet, melt butter over medium-low heat; cook while mixing the onion for 10 minutes until thoroughly browned.

4. Mix together onion powder, cinnamon, and half a cup of brown sugar; use pepper and salt to season. Mix the sugar mixture and apples into the cooked onion. Put a cover on and cook for another 10 minutes until the sauce is thick and the apples are soft.

5. Put the onion-apple sauce and pork on the rolls using a spoon and enjoy.

Nutrition: calories 221, fat 12, carbs 6, protein 11

Asian Style Country Ribs
Preparation Time: 10 minutes
Cooking time: 9 hours
Servings: 6
Ingredients

- 1/4 cup lightly packed brown sugar
- 1 cup soy sauce
- 1/4 cup sesame oil
- 2 tablespoons olive oil
- 2 tablespoons rice vinegar

Directions:

1. In the crock of a slow cooker, mix together the Sriracha, ginger, garlic, lime

juice, rice vinegar, olive oil, sesame oil, soy sauce, and brown sugar. Put the ribs; place cover and chill. Let the ribs marinate in the refrigerator for 8 hours to overnight.

2. Prior to cooking, allow the marinade to drain and throw. Let cook for 9 hours on Low. Drain the cooked meat, and with 2 forks, pull apart.

Nutrition: calories 553, fat 12, carbs 13, protein 30

Red Beans and Rice
Preparation Time: 20 minutes
Cooking time: 8 hours
Servings: 8
Ingredients

- 8 cloves garlic, chopped
- 1 teaspoon ground black pepper
- 1 teaspoon Creole seasoning, or to taste
- 6 fresh basil leaves, chopped
- 1 ham hock
- 4 cups cooked rice

Directions:

1. In a slow cooker, put water and beans. Heat a skillet on medium-high heat. Brown sausage in skillet; use a slotted spoon to remove sausage from skillet, then put into the slow cooker. Keep drippings. Put garlic, jalapeno pepper, green pepper, and onion into the drippings; mix and cook for 5 minutes till tender. Put everything from the skillet into the slow cooker.

2. Season mixture using creole seasoning and pepper. Add the ham hock and fresh basil leaves. Cover; cook till beans are tender for 8 hours on low. Uncover and put heat on high to cook till it has a creamy texture if the bean mixture is too watery.

Nutrition: calories 324, fat 12, carbs 6, protein 11

Awesome Pulled Pork BBQ

Preparation Time: 15 minutes

Cooking time: 10 hours 15 minutes

Servings: 10

Ingredients

- 1 (5 pound) boneless pork loin roast
- 1 pinch garlic powder, or to taste
- 1 pinch poultry seasoning, or to taste
- salt to taste
- ground black pepper to taste
- 1 large onion, quartered
- 1 apple, cored and quartered
- 3 stalks celery
- 1 (14.5 ounce) can chicken broth

Barbecue Sauce:

- 1/2 cup butter
- 2 cups chopped celery
- 1 1/2 cups chopped onion
- 4 cups ketchup
- 2 cups water
- 2/3 cup cider vinegar
- 1/2 cup brown sugar
- 1/4 cup Worcestershire sauce
- 2 tablespoons prepared mustard
- 1 tablespoon liquid smoke flavoring
- 1 tablespoon garlic powder

Directions:

1. Put the pork into a slow cooker; season with pepper, salt, poultry seasoning, and garlic powder to taste. Add 3 celery stalks, apple, and quartered onion; transfer chicken broth into the slow cooker.

2. Cook for approximately 8 hours till very tender on Low. Transfer pork onto a big platter; discard veggies and juice. Use a fork to shred pork; put back in the slow cooker.

3. As pork is cooking, prep barbecue sauce. Melt butter in a small Dutch oven or big saucepan on medium heat; mix and cook 1 1/2 cups onion and 2 cups celery for about 5 minutes till onion is translucent. Add 1 tbsp. garlic powder, liquid smoke, mustard, Worcestershire sauce, brown sugar, vinegar, water, and ketchup; mix. Lower the heat to low; simmer for approximately 10 minutes till the sauce is thick, occasionally mixing. Transfer barbecue sauce on top of shredded pork.

4. Keep cooking pork for about 2 hours till flavors merge on low heat.

Nutrition: calories 233, fat 12, carbs 18, protein 20

BBQ Pork for Sandwiches

Preparation Time: 17 minutes

Cooking time: 3 hours 10 minutes

Servings: 6

Ingredients

- beef broth
- pork ribs
- barbeque sauce

Direction

1. Cook on high heat for 4 hours until meat can be shredded easily. Transfer the meat and shred with 2 forks. It may seem that it's not successful right away, but it will.

2. Start preheating the oven at 350°F (175°C). Place the shredded pork in a Dutch oven or iron skillet and blend in barbeque sauce. Bake in the prepared oven for 30 minutes until heated thoroughly.

Nutrition: calories 355, fat 18, carbs 15, protein 30

Bacon Wrapped Pork Chops In Zesty Sauce

Preparation Time: 15 minutes

Cooking time: 6 hours 10 minutes

Servings: 6

Ingredients

- 6 (4 ounce) pork chops

- 12 slices bacon
- 1 (12 ounce) bottle tomato-based chili sauce
- 3 tablespoons brown sugar
- 2 tablespoons Dijon mustard
- 1 (8 ounce) can pineapple chunks, drained

Directions:

1. Start preheating the broiler of the oven, then arrange the oven rack approximately 6 inches from the heat.
2. Wrap 2 bacon slices around each pork chop to cover the pork chop entirely, then use toothpicks to secure. Arrange the covered chops on a broiler pan, then broil for 5 minutes on each side until browned.
3. In a bowl, combine Dijon mustard, brown sugar, and chili sauce together. Put the browned pork chops in the bottom of a slow cooker and cover the chops with the chili sauce mixture. Spread the chops with pineapple chunks, then cook in the cooker on Low for 6 hours until they become very tender.

Nutrition: calories 258, fat 22, carbs 16, protein 42

Betty's 3 Bean Hot Dish (a La Minnesota)

Preparation Time: 10 minutes

Cooking time: 1 hour 20 minutes

Servings: 8

Ingredients

- 1/4 pound bacon
- 1 onion, diced
- 1/2 cup ketchup
- 1/2 cup brown sugar
- 1 tablespoon yellow mustard

Directions:

1. In a big skillet, cook bacon over medium-high heat for about 10 minutes with occasional turning until completely brown. Put bacon slices on a paper towel.

When cool enough, crumble. Use a paper towel to wipe out the skillet.

2. In the heated skillet, cook and stir ground beef for 5 to 7 minutes; until it turns brown and crumbly. Drain and remove grease. Add and cook the onion for about 5 minutes until it becomes transparent.
3. In a slow cooker, mix in vinegar, brown sugar, mustard, cooked beef, butter beans, pork and beans, kidney beans, cooked bacon, and ketchup. Stir the mixture until completely combined. Let it cook completely over high heat for 60 minutes until heated through.

Nutrition: calories 369, fat 11, carbs 44, protein 32

Pulled Pork

Preparation Time: 15 minutes

Cooking time: 10 hours

Servings: 6

Ingredients

- 1/4 cup honey
- 2 tablespoons Worcestershire sauce
- 2 tablespoons crushed garlic, or to taste
- 1 teaspoon cayenne pepper
- 1 teaspoon salt
- 3 pounds pork picnic roast
- 3/4 cup water (optional)
- 1 onion, chopped

Directions:

1. In a bowl, stir together salt, cayenne pepper, garlic, Worcestershire sauce, honey, mustard, and beer until the honey dissolves. Add a small amount of the beer marinade to a slow cooker; put in the pork. Pour over the pork with the leftover marinade. Put the cover on and chill overnight, flipping the pork sometimes.
2. In the slow cooker, cook the pork for 8 hours on Low, basting sometimes. If the pork appears dry, add water. Drop onion

around pork and keep cooking for another 2 hours until the pork is very soft.

3. Use 2 forks to pull and shred the pork, disposing any fat pieces. Remove the pork to a serving dish. With a sieve, skim the leftover onion from the slow cooker and put it to the pork.

Nutrition: calories 433, fat 23, carbs 6, protein 42

Casserole in a Slow Cooker

Preparation Time: 15 minutes
Cooking time: 6 hours 5 minutes
Servings: 8
Ingredients

- cooking spray
- 1 (26 ounce) package frozen hash brown potatoes, thawed
- 12 eggs, beaten
- 1 cup milk
- 1 tablespoon ground mustard
- salt and ground black pepper to taste
- 1 (16 ounce) package maple-flavored sausage
- 1 (16 ounce) package shredded Cheddar cheese

Direction

1. Use cooking spray to coat the crock of a slow cooker. Cover the bottom of the slow cooker crock with hash browns.
2. In a bowl, combine black pepper, salt, mustard, milk, and eggs together.
3. Place a large skillet on medium-high heat. Cook sausage while stirring for 5-7 minutes or till browned and crumbly; strain off grease and throw away. Arrange sausage over the hash browns and cover with Cheddar cheese. Transfer the egg mixture over the cheese.
4. Cook for 6-8 hours on low.

Nutrition: calories 432, fat 12, carbs 6, protein 11

Campbell's® Slow Cooked Pulled Pork Sandwiches

Preparation Time: 15 minutes
Cooking time: 8 hours 10 minutes
Servings: 6
Ingredients

- 1 cup ketchup
- 1/4 cup cider vinegar
- 3 tablespoons packed brown sugar
- 12 round sandwich rolls or hamburger rolls, split

Directions:

1. Heat oil on medium-high heat in a 10-in. skillet. Add pork; cook till all sides brown well.
2. Transfer pork from cooker onto cutting board; stand for 10 minutes. Shred pork using 2 forks; put the pork into the cooker.
3. Divide sauce mixture and pork into rolls.

Nutrition: calories 344, fat 31, carbs 8, protein 31

Cantonese Dinner

Preparation Time: 15 minutes
Cooking time: 8 hours 10 minutes
Servings: 5
Ingredients

- 2 pounds pork steak, cut into strips
- 2 tablespoons vegetable oil
- 1 onion, thinly sliced
- 1 (4.5 ounce) can mushrooms, drained
- 1 (8 ounce) can tomato sauce
- 3 tablespoons brown sugar
- 1 1/2 teaspoons distilled white vinegar
- 1 1/2 teaspoons salt
- 2 tablespoons Worcestershire sauce

Directions:

1. Heat oil over medium-high heat in a large, heavy skillet. Brown the pork in oil. Drain off the excess grease.

2. Put Worcestershire sauce, salt, vinegar, brown sugar, tomato sauce, mushrooms, onion, and pork in a slow cooker. Cook on low for 6 to 8 hours or on high for 4 hours.

Nutrition: calories 278, fat 13, carbs 6, protein 11

Carnitas with Pico De Gallo
Preparation Time: 20 minutes
Cooking time: 18 hours 10 minutes
Servings: 10
Ingredients

- 1 tablespoon olive oil
- 6 pounds boneless pork shoulder
- 1 cup ground cumin
- 6 cups water
- 6 tomatoes, chopped
- 1 onion, chopped
- 2 tomatillos, husked and chopped
- 2 jalapeno pepper, seeded and minced
- 1/3 cup lime juice
- 1 tablespoon salt
- 1/4 teaspoon ground black pepper

Directions:

1. Heat olive oil in a big skillet on medium-high heat; sear pork in hot oil for 10 minutes till browned on all sides. Put in a slow cooker with 1 minced jalapeno pepper, garlic, quartered onion, New Mexico chiles, and cumin; put water in, cover; cook for 6-8 hours on high. Lower heat to low; cook for 12-16 hours till pork is easily shredded and tender. When cooked, transfer veggies and pork to a big bowl; use 2 forks to finely shred. Mix enough cooking liquid in to moisten meat to your preference.

2. 2-6 hours before carnitas are ready, prep pico de gallo. Mix 2 minced jalapeno peppers, tomatillos, onion, and tomatoes in a mixing bowl. Season with pepper, salt, and lime juice; stir well. Refrigerate till needed.

Nutrition: calories 635, fat 12, carbs 18, protein 32

Slow Cooker Pork
Preparation Time: 5 minutes
Cooking time: 8 hours
Servings: 8
Ingredients

- 3 pounds pork shoulder
- 2 (1 ounce) packages taco seasoning mix
- chili powder to taste
- crushed red pepper to taste

Direction

1. Put the pork shoulder and taco seasoning into a slow cooker. Put chili powder and/or red pepper flakes, if desired. Put in water until the meat is covered. Put the lid over the pot, then cook for 8 hours on low.

2. Discard pork shoulder from pot, then shred.

Nutrition: calories 328, fat 18, carbs 9, protein 42

Slow Cooker Pork Cacciatore
Preparation Time: 15 minutes
Cooking time: 8 hours 30 minutes
Servings: 4
Ingredients

- 2 tablespoons olive oil
- 1 onion, sliced
- 4 boneless pork chops
- 1 (28 ounce) jar pasta sauce
- 1 (28 ounce) can diced tomatoes
- 1 green bell pepper, seeded and sliced into strips
- 1 (8 ounce) package fresh mushrooms, sliced
- 2 large cloves garlic, minced

- 1 teaspoon Italian seasoning
- 1/2 teaspoon dried basil
- 1/2 cup dry white wine
- 4 slices mozzarella cheese

Directions

1. Brown chops in a large skillet on medium-high. Place into a slow cooker.
2. Cook the onion in oil on medium heat in the same pan until it is browned. Stir in bell pepper and mushrooms, then cook until vegetables are softened. Combine in white wine, diced tomatoes, and pasta sauce. Flavor with garlic, basil, and Italian seasoning. Add onto the pork chops in the slow cooker.
3. Cook for 7-8 hours on Low. Arrange a slice of cheese on each chop and add sauce to cover, then serve.

Nutrition: Calories: 146 Protein: 6.2g Carbs: 41.2g Fat: 5g

Slow Cooker Pork Chops

Preparation Time: 5 minutes

Cooking time: 8 hours

Servings: 4

Ingredients:

- 4 pork chops
- 16 ounces sauerkraut with juice

Directions:

1. Put the chops into the slow cooker's bottom, then pour the sauerkraut on top. Cook about 8 to 9 hours at low or about 4 to 5 hours at high.

Nutrition: calories 178, fat 18, carbs 6, protein 21

Slow Cooker Pork Chops and Sauerkraut

Preparation Time: 10 minutes

Cooking time: 4 hours

Servings: 4

Ingredients

- 1 (27 ounce) can sauerkraut with juice

- 1/2 cup ketchup
- 1/2 cup soy sauce
- 1/4 cup brown sugar
- 1 tablespoon Worcestershire sauce
- 4 pork chops

Directions

1. In a slow cooker, mix ketchup, sauerkraut and juice, soy sauce, Worcestershire sauce, and brown sugar together to form a sauce. Stir in pork chops; toss to cover chops with the sauerkraut sauce.
2. Cook over low heat for around 4 hours till pork is no longer pink in the center. An instant-read thermometer pinned into the center should measure 145 °F (63 °C).

Nutrition: calories 280, fat 12, carbs 6, protein 11

Slow Cooker Pork Chops with Caramelized Onions and Peas

Preparation Time: 10 minutes

Cooking time: 8 hours 22 minutes

Servings: 2

Ingredients

- 2 tablespoons vegetable oil
- 2 pork chops
- 4 large onions, sliced
- 1 clove garlic, crushed
- 2 pinches white sugar
- 3/4 cup hard apple cider
- salt and freshly ground black pepper
- 4 tablespoons frozen baby peas, not thawed
- 1 tablespoon butter

Directions

1. In a skillet, heat oil over medium-high heat and cook pork chops for 7-10 minutes until all sides are brown. Transfer to a slow cooker.
2. In the same skillet, cook onions over medium-low heat for 8-10 minutes until

brown and tender. Add sugar and garlic, stir and cook for 2-3 minutes. Add cider and boil it. Pour over the pork chops in the slow cooker.

3. Cook on Low for 7 1/2 hours until the pork chops are soft. Mix in peas; cook for another 30 minutes until soft.

4. Transfer the pork chops to a serving dish. Add butter to the slow cooker with the sauce, whisk until melted. Pour the sauce over the pork chops.

Nutrition: calories 290, fat 18, carbs 4, protein 20

Slow Cooker Pork Loin Roast with Apple Cranberry Rice

Preparation Time: 15 minutes
Cooking time: 6 hours
Servings: 10
Ingredients

- 2 teaspoons olive oil
- 4 cups cooked rice
- 1 large yellow onion, chopped
- 2 Granny Smith apples, chopped
- 1 1/2 cups dried cranberries
- 1 teaspoon salt
- 1/4 teaspoon ground black pepper, or to taste

Directions:

1. In a big slow cooker, put the pork roast; drizzle olive oil over. Sprinkle herbes de Provence over, use black pepper and salt to season to taste.

2. In a big bowl, combine 1/4 teaspoon black pepper, 1 teaspoon salt, cranberries, apples, onion, and rice. Spoon the rice mixture around and over the pork.

3. Put the cover on and cook for 8-10 hours on Low or for 6 hours on High.

Nutrition: calories 488, fat 19, carbs 10, protein 34

Slow Cooker Pork Tenderloin with Beer and Veggies

Preparation Time: 15 minutes
Cooking time: 4 hours 10 minutes
Servings: 6
Ingredients

- 1 (2 pound) pork tenderloin
- 6 fluid ounces lager-style beer
- 2 cloves garlic
- 1 1/2 teaspoons salt
- 1 teaspoon whole black peppercorns
- 1 teaspoon dried sage

Direction

1. In a slow cooker, mix sage, peppercorns, salt, onion, garlic, mushrooms, carrots, potatoes, vinegar, beer, and pork tenderloin. Place a cover and cook for 4 hours on low.

Nutrition: calories 278, fat 22, carbs 8, protein 18

Slow Cooker Pork With Apricots

Preparation Time: 17 minutes
Cooking time: 6 hours 10 minutes
Servings: 4
Ingredients

- 2 teaspoons olive oil, divided
- 4 (4 ounce) lean boneless pork loin chop
- 1/4 cup chopped fresh cilantro

Directions

1. Heat 1 teaspoon olive oil over medium-high heat in a big non-stick skillet.

2. Season pork chops uniformly with black pepper and 1/4 teaspoon salt; cook for about 2 minutes per side in the hot skillet until browned. Shift chops to a plate, keep drippings in the skillet.

3. In the retained drippings, heat the reserved teaspoon of olive oil; put in onions and add the remaining salt to taste. Sauté onions for about 10 minutes until golden brown.

4. Distribute about 1/2 of the sliced apricots and 1/2 of the cooked onions in the bottom of a slow cooker crock. Place pork chops on top of onions and apricots. Over the pork chops, layer reserved apricots and onions; put in the cinnamon stick, thyme, ginger, and pineapple juice.

5. Cook on low for 6 to 8 hours (or 3 to 4 hours on high) till the pork is fork-tender. Expel the cinnamon stick. Top the mixture with a sprinkling of cilantro.

Nutrition: calories 188, fat 12, carbs 6, protein 11

Slow Cooker Pork with Mushrooms and Barley

Preparation Time: 20 minutes

Cooking time: 8 hours 10 minutes

Servings: 6

Ingredients

- 3 cloves garlic, finely chopped
- 1 teaspoon salt
- 6 pork chops
- 1/2 cup barley
- 8 ounces white mushrooms, sliced
- 1/2 onion, chopped
- 2 (14 ounce) cans chicken broth
- 1/2 cup water
- 2 teaspoons Worcestershire sauce
- 1 bay leaf
- 1 pinch salt and ground black pepper to taste

Direction

1. Rub 1 tsp. salt and chopped garlic into pork chops.

2. Put barley in slow cooker; top using pork chops. Cover using chopped onion and white mushrooms. Add a few grinds of fresh black pepper, salt, bay leaf, Worcestershire sauce, water, and chicken broth.

3. Put the slow cooker on low; cover. Cook for 8 hours.

Nutrition: calories 234, fat 18, carbs 5, protein 28

Slow Cooker Pot Roast with Malbec (Red Wine)

Preparation Time: 10 minutes

Cooking time: 5 hours 10 minutes

Servings: 6

Ingredients

- 2 tablespoons Montreal steak seasoning
- 1 tablespoon salt
- 1 tablespoon dried thyme
- 1 tablespoon dried rosemary
- 1 (2 1/2 pound) beef roast, or more to taste
- 1 (1 ounce) packet dry au jus mix
- 1 (1 ounce) package French onion soup mix
- 1 cup water
- 1 cup Malbec red wine

Direction

1. In a bowl, mix together salt, steak seasoning, rosemary, and thyme. Rub the mixture over the roast.

2. Use a big skillet to cook the roast on medium-high heat for about 10 minutes until browned on all sides.

3. Put the meat in the slow cooker and add onion soup mix and au jus mix. Pour water and Malbec on top of the meat.

4. Let it cook on High for five hours or 8-9 hours on Low.

Nutrition: calories 218, fat 34, carbs 9, protein 34

CHAPTER 9:

Vegetarian & Vegan Recipes

Balsamic Artichoke Summer Dish

Preparation Time: 17 minutes

Cooking time: 3 hours 10 minutes

Servings: 4

Ingredients:

- 6 chopped basil leaves
- ½ cup artichoke hearts, quartered
- ¼ cup halved Kalamata olives
- ¼ cup capers
- 20 diced Roma tomatoes
- 3 tbsps. balsamic vinegar
- 3 tbsps. avocado oil
- ¾ tsp. onion powder
- ¾ tsp. sea salt
- ½ tsp. black pepper
- 2 tbsps. minced garlic

Directions:

1. Combine all the ingredients in the slow cooker and mix well.
2. Cook for 3 hours on high, stirring the mix after every hour.

Nutrition: calories 153, fat 12, carbs 6, protein 23

Thyme Oregano Garlic Mushrooms

Preparation Time: 17 minutes

Cooking time: 3 hours

Servings: 4

Ingredients:

- 24 ounces cremini mushrooms
- 4 minced garlic cloves
- ½ tsp. basil, dried
- ½ tsp. oregano, dried

- ¼ tsp. dried thyme
- 2 bay leaves
- 1 cup vegetable broth
- ¼ cup Half-and-half
- 2 tbsps. unsalted butter
- 2 tbsps. freshly chopped parsley leaves
- Kosher sea salt
- Black pepper

Directions:

1. Combine all the ingredients except the butter, half and half, and fresh parsley in a slow cooker.
2. Cook covered for 3-4 hours on low.
3. 20 minutes prior to the completion of cook time, mix in the butter and half-and-half.
4. Garnish with parsley and serve.

Nutrition: calories 221, fat 12, carbs 6, protein 4

Ricotta Spinach Zucchini Lasagna

Preparation Time: 3½ - 4 hours

Cooking time: 3½ - 4 hours on high

Servings: 8

Ingredients:

- 4 sliced zucchini
- 4 cups of homemade tomato sauce
- 15 ounces ricotta cheese
- 1 large egg
- ¼ cup freshly grated Parmesan cheese
- 1 cup chopped spinach
- Salt

- Pepper
- 16 ounces shredded mozzarella
- 2 tsps. freshly chopped parsley

Directions:

1. Mix together the spinach, egg, ricotta cheese, and half the Parmesan cheese in a bowl.
2. Spread a cup of tomato sauce in a greased slow cooker and spread 5 zucchini slices over it, slightly overlapping.
3. Spread some of the egg mixtures over and sprinkle some Mozzarella.
4. Repeat the layering until all the ingredients are used up, topping with Parmesan cheese and Mozzarella.
5. Cook covered for 3½ - 4 hours on high. Serve garnished with parsley.

Nutrition: calories 231, fat 14, carbs 6, protein 11

Cheesy Spinach Stuffed Mushrooms

Preparation Time: 15 minutes

Cooking time: 6 hours 10 minutes

Servings: 6

Ingredients:

- 2 tablespoons unsalted butter, Ghee or extra-virgin olive oil
- 3 large eggs
- 2 cups shredded Gruyère cheese, divided
- ½ cup chopped walnuts, plus more for garnish
- 1½ pounds cremini or button mushrooms, stems minced, caps left whole
- 2 cups chopped spinach
- ½ onion, minced
- 2 garlic cloves, minced
- 1 tablespoon fresh thyme leaves, plus more for garnish
- ½ teaspoon kosher salt
- ½ teaspoon freshly ground black pepper

Directions:

1. Generously coat the inside of the slow cooker insert with the butter.
2. In a medium bowl, beat the eggs, then stir in 1½ cups of Gruyère cheese, ½ cup of walnuts, the mushroom stems, spinach, onion, garlic, 1 tablespoon of thyme, salt, and pepper. Spoon the mixture into the mushroom caps and place each filled cap in the bottom of the slow cooker in a single layer. Sprinkle the remaining ½ cup of Gruyère cheese over the top. Cover and cook for 6 hours on low. Serve hot, garnished with additional thyme and chopped walnuts.

Nutrition: calories 204, fat 10, carbs 2, protein 22

Rosemary Cheesy Broccoli

Preparation Time: 15 minutes

Cooking time: 5 hours

Servings: 6

Ingredients:

- 8 cups broccoli florets - 1 large onion, chopped - 1 tablespoon fresh rosemary, minced - 1½ cups Swiss cheese, grated
- 1¾ cups homemade tomato sauce
- 1 tbsp. fresh lemon juice
- Sea salt and freshly ground black pepper

Directions:

1. In a large slow cooker, place all ingredients and mix well. Set the slow cooker on Low. Cover and cook for about 5-6 hours. Serve hot.

Nutrition: calories 178, fat 9, carbs 8, protein 18

Garlic Spinach Curry

Preparation Time: 10 minutes

Cooking time: 3 hours 10 minutes

Servings: 6

Ingredients:

- 3 packages (10 ounces) frozen spinach (thawed)

- 1 chopped onion
- 4 minced garlic cloves
- 2 tbsps. curry powder
- 2 tbsps. melted butter
- ½ cup vegetable stock
- ¼ cup heavy cream
- 1 tsp. lemon juice

Directions:

1. Dump all ingredients in a crockpot except the cream and lemon juice.
2. Cook covered for 3-4 hours on low.
3. Mix in the lemon juice and cream 30 minutes prior to the completion of cook time and cook covered. Serve warm.

Nutrition: calories 91, fat 7, carbs 3, protein 4

Parmesan Veggie Casserole

Preparation Time: 17 minutes
Cooking time: 3 hours 10 minutes
Servings: 6
Ingredients:

- 1 tbsp. unsalted butter, melted
- 4 medium zucchinis, peeled and sliced
- 1 green bell pepper, seeded and sliced
- 2 cups finely chopped fresh tomatoes
- 1 thinly sliced white onion
- 1 tbsp. fresh thyme, minced
- ½ cup grated Parmesan cheese
- Sea salt
- Freshly ground black pepper

Directions:

1. In a large slow cooker, place all ingredients except cheese and mix well.
2. Set the slow cooker on low. Cover and cook for about 3 hours.
3. Uncover and sprinkle with cheese evenly. Cover and cook for about 1½ hours.
4. Serve hot.

Nutrition: calories 90, fat 8, carbs 5, protein 6

Parmesan Tomato Eggplant

Preparation Time: 15 minutes
Cooking time: 7 hours
Servings: 6

- 2 tablespoons coconut oil
- 2 cups tomato sauce
- 8 ounces mascarpone cheese
- 8 ounces eggplant, peeled and thinly sliced
- 3 cups shredded fontina cheese
- 1 cup grated Parmesan cheese
- 1 cup coarsely ground almond meal

Directions:

1. Coat the inside of the slow cooker insert with the coconut oil.
2. In a medium bowl, stir together the tomato sauce and mascarpone. Coat the bottom of the insert with ½ cup of sauce.
3. Arrange several eggplant slices in a single layer, or slightly overlapping, over the sauce.
4. Top with a bit of fontina cheese, a bit of Parmesan cheese, a sprinkling of almond meal, and more sauce. Continue layering until you've used all the ingredients, ending with a layer of sauce, then cheese, and then almond meal. Cover and cook for 7 hours on low or 4 hours on high. Serve hot.

Nutrition: calories 542, fat 12, carbs 13, protein 22

Delicious Chili Tofu Cauliflower

Preparation Time: 6 hours
Cooking time: 6 hours on low
Servings: 4
Ingredients:

- 2 tablespoons coconut oil
- 2 cups cauliflower florets
- 8 ounces firm tofu, cut into 1-inch cubes
- ½ onion, diced
- 2 cups crumbled blue cheese, divided

- 1 cup diced tomatoes, with juice
- ¼ cup all-natural spicy hot sauce (such as Frank's RedHot)
- 1 tablespoon erythritol
- 1½ teaspoons chili powder
- 1 teaspoon ground cumin
- ¼ teaspoon kosher salt
- 2 celery stalks, finely diced

Directions:

1. In the slow cooker, combine the coconut oil, cauliflower, tofu, onion, 1 cup of blue cheese, tomatoes and their juice, hot sauce, erythritol, chili powder, cumin, and salt. Stir to mix. Cover and cook for 6 hours on low.
2. Serve the chili hot, topped with the celery and remaining 1 cup of blue cheese.

Nutrition: calories 321, fat 12, carbs 4, protein 30

Spinach Mayo Artichoke Dip

Preparation Time: 17 minutes
Cooking time: 4 hours 10 minutes
Servings: 20
Ingredients:

- 3 garlic cloves
- ½ medium onion
- 2 cans (14 ounces) artichoke hearts
- 10 ounces chopped spinach
- 10 ounces chopped kale
- 1 cup Parmesan cheese
- 1 cup shredded mozzarella cheese
- 1 cup Greek yogurt
- ¾ sour cream
- ¼ cup mayo
- Salt
- Pepper

Directions:

1. Place the artichokes, garlic, and onion in a food processor and chop finely.

2. Transfer into a slow cooker with the rest of the ingredients.
3. Cook for 4 hours on high. Stir the mix well, forming a paste. Serve with veggie sticks.

Nutrition: calories 83, fat 8, carbs 3, protein 18

Oregano Mascarpone Zucchini Lasagna

Preparation Time: 15 minutes
Cooking time: 3 hours 30 minutes
Servings: 6
Ingredients:

- Coconut oil for coating the slow cooker insert
- 1 pound mascarpone cheese
- 1 cup grated Parmesan cheese, divided
- 1 cup chopped spinach
- 1 large egg, beaten
- 1 teaspoon dried oregano
- ¾ teaspoon kosher salt
- ½ teaspoon freshly ground black pepper
- 1½ cups tomato sauce, divided
- 1 cup heavy (whipping) cream
- 2 medium zucchini, cut into ⅓-inch slices
- 4 cups shredded fontina cheese
- 2 tablespoons chopped fresh flat-leaf parsley

Directions:

1. Coat the inside of the slow cooker insert with coconut oil.
2. In a medium bowl, stir together the mascarpone cheese, ½ cup of Parmesan cheese, spinach, egg, oregano, salt, and pepper.
3. In a separate bowl, stir together the tomato sauce and heavy cream. Spoon 1 cup of the sauce into the slow cooker and spread it out to coat the bottom of the insert.

4. Arrange one-third of the zucchini slices in a single layer, or slightly overlapping, over the sauce.

5. Spread one-third of the mascarpone mixture over the zucchini slices, then top with one-third of the remaining tomato sauce, followed by one-third of the fontina cheese. Repeat the layers two more times.

6. Sprinkle the remaining ½ cup of Parmesan cheese over the top. Cover and cook for 7 hours on low or 3½ hours on high. Serve hot, garnished with the parsley.

Nutrition: calories 696, fat 31, carbs 8, protein 31

Coconut Pumpkin Curry

Preparation Time: 15 minutes

Cooking time: 6 hours

Servings: 4

Ingredients:

- 2 tablespoons coconut oil, melted
- 1½ pounds extra-firm tofu, cut into 1-inch cubes
- 12 ounces cremini or button mushrooms, halved or quartered
- ½ cup diced onion
- 2 garlic cloves, minced
- 1 tablespoon grated fresh ginger
- 3 tablespoons curry powder
- 1 teaspoon ground cumin
- 1 teaspoon kosher salt
- ½ teaspoon cayenne pepper
- 1 (14-ounce) can coconut milk
- ¼ cup chopped macadamia nuts
- ¼ cup chopped fresh cilantro

Directions:

1. Coat the inside of the slow cooker insert with the coconut oil. Add the tofu, mushrooms, onion, garlic, ginger, curry powder, cumin, salt, cayenne, and coconut milk. Cover and cook for 6 hours on low.

2. Serve hot, garnished with the macadamia nuts and cilantro.

Nutrition: calories 350, fat 29, carbs 11, protein 15

Balsamic-Glazed Pine Nuts Brussels Sprouts

Preparation Time: 15 minutes

Cooking time: 6 hours

Servings: 6

- 1 pound Brussels sprouts, halved
- 2 tablespoons coconut oil
- Kosher salt
- Freshly ground black pepper
- 2 tablespoons unsalted butter, cubed
- 2 tablespoons balsamic vinegar
- 2 tablespoons erythritol
- 2 cups grated Parmesan cheese
- ¼ cup toasted pine nuts

Directions:

1. In the slow cooker, combine the Brussels sprouts and coconut oil. Season with salt and pepper and stir to mix.

2. Top with the butter. Cover and cook for 6 hours on low or 3 hours on high.

3. To serve, drizzle the balsamic glaze over the Brussels sprouts and serve hot, garnished with the Parmesan cheese and pine nuts.

Nutrition: calories 231, fat 9, carbs 6, protein 14

Delicious Tofu & Vegetables Tofu Curry

Preparation Time: 17 minutes

Cooking time: 6 hours

Servings: 4

Ingredients:

- 2 tablespoons coconut oil
- ½ onion, diced
- 1 tablespoon minced fresh ginger

- 2 garlic cloves, minced
- 1 pound firm tofu, diced
- ½ green bell pepper, seeded and sliced
- 1 (14-ounce) can coconut milk
- ¼ cup Thai green curry paste
- 1 tablespoon erythritol
- 1 teaspoon kosher salt
- ½ teaspoon turmeric
- ¼ cup chopped fresh cilantro, for garnish

Directions:
1. In a medium skillet, heat the coconut oil over medium-high heat.
2. Add the onion and sauté until softened, about 5 minutes.
3. Stir in the ginger and garlic, and then transfer the mixture to the slow cooker.
4. Mix in the tofu, green bell pepper, coconut milk, curry paste, erythritol, salt, and turmeric. Cover and cook for 6 hours on low. Serve hot, garnished with the cilantro.

Nutrition: calories 245, fat 9, carbs 3, protein 22

Tasty Tagine Five a Day
Preparation Time: 8 minutes
Cooking time: 8 hours
Servings: 6
Ingredients:

- 4 tablespoons of olive oil
- 1 sliced red onion
- 2 cloves of crushed garlic
- 500 grams of aubergine in 1 cm-thick slices, cut lengthways
- 300 grams of quartered ripe tomatoes
- 1 small sliced fennel bulb
- 50 grams of sundried tomatoes
- 1 teaspoon of coriander seeds

Ingredients for the dressing

- 100 grams of feta cheese, and extra for topping

- 50 grams of toasted almond flakes

Directions
1. Pour 2 tablespoons of olive oil into the slow cooker and add the crushed garlic and the onions.
2. Brush the aubergines with the remaining olive oil and place them on top of the onions and garlic.
3. Arrange the sundried tomatoes, fennel slices, and tomatoes around the aubergines. Season with salt and pepper and pour the coriander seeds over the top. Cook for 6-8 hours on low.
4. Place the dressing ingredients into a food processor and work until smooth. Spoon the vegetables onto serving dishes, drizzle the dressing over the top and crumble the feta cheese on top.

Nutrition: calories: 289, fat: 20, carbs: 11, Protein: 8

Beautiful Baked Mushrooms with Pesto & Ricotta
Preparation Time: 10 minutes
Cooking time: 4 hours
Servings: 4
Ingredients

- 5 tablespoons of olive oil, extra virgin
- 16 large chestnut mushrooms
- A 250-gram tub of ricotta
- 2 tablespoons of pesto
- 2 finely chopped cloves of garlic
- 25 grams of freshly grated parmesan cheese
- 2 tablespoons of fresh, chopped parsley

Directions:
1. Trim the mushroom stems level with the caps. In a small bowl combine the garlic, pesto, and ricotta, and spoon into the mushroom heads.
2. Place the mushroom caps in a slow cooker and cook on low for 4-6 hours.

3. In the last half-hour, sprinkle the parmesan cheese over the top of the mushrooms.
4. Serve topped with the fresh parsley.

Nutrition: calories 400, fat 34, carbs 2, protein 19

Cheddar Vegetarian Chili

Preparation Time: 10 minutes
Cooking time: 7 hours 10 minutes
Servings: 8
Ingredients:

- ¼ cup coconut oil
- 1 pound firm tofu, diced
- 1 (14.5-ounce) can diced tomatoes, with juice
- 1 onion, diced - 3 garlic cloves, minced
- 1 or 2 jalapeño peppers, seeded and minced
- 3 tablespoons unsweetened cocoa powder
- 2 tablespoons chili powder
- 1½ teaspoons paprika
- 1½ teaspoons ground cumin
- 1 teaspoon ground cinnamon
- 1 teaspoon kosher salt
- ½ teaspoon dried oregano
- 2½ cups sour cream, divided
- 2 cups shredded Cheddar cheese
- 1 avocado, peeled, pitted, and sliced

Directions:

1. Combine all the ingredients and cook
2. Just before serving, stir in 1½ cups of sour cream. Serve hot, garnished with the remaining 1 cup of sour cream, Cheddar cheese, and avocado.

Nutrition: calories 342, fat 34, carbs 9, protein 15

Delicious Dal with Crispy Onions

Preparation Time: 17 minutes
Cooking time: 6 hours
Servings: 6

Ingredients

- 250 grams of black urid beans
- 100 grams of ghee or butter
- 2 large onions thinly sliced
- 3 cloves of crushed garlic
- 1 piece of ginger, thumb-sized and finely chopped
- 2 teaspoons of ground cumin
- 2 teaspoons of ground coriander
- 1 teaspoon of ground turmeric
- 1 teaspoon of paprika
- ¼ teaspoon of chili powder
- A small bunch fresh coriander, reserve the leaves and finely chop the stems
- 400 grams of passata
- 1 red chili, pierced with the tip of a knife
- 50 ml of double cream

Ingredients to serve alongside dal

- Baked sweet potato
- Naan bread
- Cooked rice
- Coriander
- Sliced red chili
- Lime wedges
- Yogurt, cream, or swirl
- Indian chutney or pickle
- Crispy salad onions

Directions

1. Soak the beans for 4 hours or overnight in cold water.
2. In a large saucepan, melt the ghee or butter, then add the ginger, onions, and garlic and cook for 15 minutes to caramelize the onions.
3. Add the coriander stems, spices, and 100ml of water.
4. Pour the ingredients into the slow cooker and add the chili, passata, beans, and 400ml of water. Season and cook for 5-6 hours on low.

KETO SLOW COOKER COOKBOOK

5. When cooked, the beans should be tender, and the dal should be very thick. Add the cream and serve with a side dish of your choice.

Nutrition: calories: 527, fat: 34, carbs: 35, protein: 19

Delicious Warming Bean and Veg Soup

Preparation Time: 15 minutes
Cooking time: 8 hours
Servings: 4
Ingredients

- 2 cloves of minced garlic
- 1 medium-sized potato, diced
- 2 carrots, peeled and sliced
- 2 celery stalks, diced
- A handful of frozen broad beans
- 2 tins of butter beans
- Paprika
- Worcestershire sauce
- Chili
- Salt and pepper
- Parmesan cheese
- Fresh herbs of your choice

Directions

1. Add all the ingredients except the Parmesan cheese and the fresh herbs to the slow cooker.
2. Cook on low for 8-10 hours.
3. Spoon onto dishes, top with Parmesan cheese and fresh herbs, and serve.

Nutrition: calories 210, fat 34, carbs 2, protein 14

Sumptuous Slow-Cooked Baked Beans

Preparation Time: 15 minutes
Cooking time: 8 hours
Servings: 8
Ingredients

- 1 pound of dried beans of your choice
- 1 diced medium onion
- 1/3 cup of brown sugar
- 1/3 cup of molasses
- ¼ cup of tomato sauce
- 2 tablespoons of yellow mustard
- 1 tablespoon of smoked paprika
- 1 tablespoon of Worcestershire sauce
- 1 tablespoon of cider vinegar or white balsamic vinegar
- Salt and pepper

Directions

1. Rinse the dried beans, and pour them into the slow cooker, cover them with 2 inches of water and leave them to soak overnight.
2. The following morning, drain the water from the slow cooker and add the remaining ingredients.
3. Add 2 ½ cups of water and salt and pepper to season.
4. Cook for 8 hours on low.
5. Spoon onto dishes and serve.

Nutrition: calories 133, fat 1, carbs 30, protein 4

Precious Peppers Stuffed with Black Beans & Quinoa

Preparation Time: 10 minutes
Cooking time: 3 hours 10 minutes
Servings: 6
Ingredients

- 6 bell peppers
- 1 cup of uncooked quinoa
- 1 14-ounce can of black beans, drained and rinsed
- 1 ½ cups of red enchilada sauce
- 1 teaspoon of cumin
- 1 teaspoon of chili powder
- 1 teaspoon of onion powder
- ½ a teaspoon of garlic salt
- 1 ½ cups of Pepperjack cheese, shredded, divided

85

- Cilantro
- Avocado
- Sour cream

Directions

1. Cut the tops off the peppers and scrape out the insides.
2. Combine 1 cup of cheese, spices, enchilada sauce, beans, and quinoa in a large bowl and stir together thoroughly.
3. Stuff the mixture into the peppers. Pour ½ cup of water into the slow cooker.
4. Arrange the peppers in the water.
5. Cover and cook on high-low for 6 hours.
6. Take the lid off and sprinkle the peppers with the remaining cheese, cover and cook for a few minutes to melt the cheese.
7. Serve with avocado, sour cream, and cilantro.

Nutrition: calories 150, fat 12, carbs 4, protein 7

Tasty Eggplant Parmesan

Preparation Time: 10 minutes
Cooking time: 8 hours
Servings: 6
Ingredients

- 4 pounds of eggplant
- 1 tablespoon of salt
- 3 large eggs
- ¼ cup of milk
- 1 ½ cup of breadcrumbs
- 3 ounces of parmesan cheese
- 2 teaspoons of Italian seasoning
- 4 cups of marinara sauce
- 16 ounces of mozzarella cheese

Directions

1. Peel the eggplant and cut it into 1/3 inch-rounds.
2. Layer the eggplant in a colander and sprinkle each layer with salt. Let sit for 30 minutes and then rinse and pat dry.
3. Spread ½ cup of sauce on the bottom of the slow cooker.
4. In a small bowl, whisk together the milk and eggs.
5. In another small bowl, whisk together the Italian seasoning, Parmesan cheese, and breadcrumbs.
6. Dip the eggplant into the egg mixture and then into the breadcrumb mixture.
7. Layer 1/3 of the slices in the slow cooker.
8. Pour 1 cup of sauce and the mozzarella cheese over the top.
9. Repeat twice, cover, and cook for 8 hours.
10. Divide onto plates and serve.

Nutrition: calories 258, fat 6, carbs 23, protein 16

Delicious Chili Lentils and Beans

Preparation Time: 15 minutes
Cooking time: 8 hours
Servings: 6
Ingredients

- 1 finely chopped onion
- 3 cloves of minced garlic
- 1 stalk of celery, chopped
- 2 chopped bell peppers
- 1 can of diced tomatoes
- 4 cups of vegetable broth
- 1 can of water
- 1 cup of dried lentils
- 1 can of Bush's Pinto Beans
- 2 tablespoons of chili powder
- 2 teaspoons of cumin
- 1 tablespoon of oregano

Directions

1. Put all of the ingredients into the slow cooker and cook for 8 hours on low.
2. Serve with a combination of the following: cilantro, green onion, avocado, sour cream, plain Greek Yogurt, and shredded cheese.

Nutrition: calories 208, fat 16, carbs 3, protein 18

Mouth-watering Butternut Macaroni Squash

Preparation Time: 15 minutes

Cooking time: 8 hours

Servings: 8

Ingredients

- 1 ½ cups of butternut squash, cubed
- ½ cup of chopped tomatoes
- 1 ½ cups of water
- 2 cloves of minced garlic
- A handful of fresh thyme, finely chopped
- A handful of fresh rosemary, finely chopped
- ¼ cup of nutritional yeast
- 1 cup of non-dairy milk
- 1 ½ cups of whole wheat macaroni
- Salt and pepper

Directions

1. Add the butternut squash, chopped tomatoes, water, garlic, thyme, and rosemary to the slow cooker. Cover and cook on low for 7-9 hours.
2. Transfer the ingredients from the slow cooker into a food processor and add the nutritional yeast, half a cup of non-dairy milk, and blend.
3. Pour the ingredients back into the slow cooker, add the macaroni, cover, and cook for a further 20 minutes on high.
4. Stir, cook for a further 25 minutes and add salt and pepper to taste.

5. Spoon onto dishes and serve.

Nutrition: calories 234, fat 2, carbs 6, protein 8

Delightful Veggie Pot Pie

Preparation Time: 15 minutes

Cooking time: 3 hours 30 minutes

Servings: 6

Ingredients

- 6 -7 cups of chopped veggies of your choice
- ½ cup of diced onions
- 4 cloves of minced garlic
- Fresh thyme, finely chopped
- ½ cup of flour
- 2 cups of chicken broth
- ¼ cup of cornstarch
- ¼ cup of heavy cream
- Salt and pepper
- 1 thawed frozen puff pastry sheet
- 2 tablespoons of butter

Directions

1. Add the chopped veggies to the slow cooker as well as the garlic and onions.
2. Add the flour. Add the broth and stir until everything is well blended.
3. Cover and cook for 3-4 hours on high.
4. In a small bowl, combine the cornstarch and ¼ cup of water and whisk together thoroughly. Add the cornstarch mix to the slow cooker.
5. Add the cream, cover, and continue to cook until the mixture thickens approximately 15 minutes.
6. Transfer the vegetable mixture into a baking dish.
7. Lay the puff pastry over the top. Melt the butter and brush it over the top of the pastry.
8. Bake at 350 degrees for 10 minutes until the pastry turns fluffy and golden. Divide onto dishes and serve.

Nutrition: calories 354, fat 2, carbs 6, protein 12

CHAPTER 10:

Side Dish Recipes

Creamy Hash Brown Mix

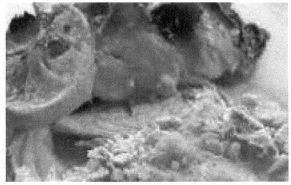

Preparation time: 10 minutes
Cooking time: 3 hours
Servings: 12
Ingredients:

- 2 pounds hash browns
- 1 and ½ cups milk
- 10 ounces cream of chicken soup
- 1 cup cheddar cheese, shredded
- ½ cup butter, melted
- Salt and black pepper to the taste
- ¾ cup cornflakes, crushed

Directions:

1. In a bowl, mix hash browns with milk, cream of chicken, cheese, butter, salt, and pepper, stir, transfer to your Slow cooker, cover and cook on Low for 3 hours.
2. Add cornflakes, divide between plates, and serve as a side dish.

Nutrition: calories 234, fat 12, carbs 22, protein 6

Broccoli Mix

Preparation time: *10 minutes*
Cooking time: *2 hours*
Servings: *10*
Ingredients:

- 6 cups broccoli florets
- 1 and ½ cups cheddar cheese, shredded
- 10 ounces canned cream of celery soup
- ½ teaspoon Worcestershire sauce
- ¼ cup yellow onion, chopped
- Salt and black pepper to the taste
- 1 cup crackers, crushed
- 2 tablespoons soft butter

Directions:

1. In a bowl, mix broccoli with cream of celery soup, cheese, salt, pepper, onion, and Worcestershire sauce, toss and transfer to your Slow cooker. Add butter, toss again, sprinkle crackers, cover, and cook on High for 2 hours.
2. Serve as a side dish.

Nutrition: calories 159, fat 11, carbs 11, protein 6

Bean Medley

Preparation time: 10 minutes
Cooking time: 5 hours
Servings: 12
Ingredients:

- 2 celery ribs, chopped
- 1 and ½ cups ketchup
- 1 green bell pepper, chopped

- 1 yellow onion, chopped
- 1 sweet red pepper, chopped
- ½ cup brown sugar
- ½ cup Italian dressing
- ½ cup water
- 1 tablespoon cider vinegar
- 2 bay leaves
- 15 ounces canned lima beans, drained
- 15 ounces canned black beans, drained

Directions:
1. In your Slow cooker, mix all the ingredients and cook

Nutrition: calories 255, fat 4, carbs 45, protein 6

Green Beans Mix

Preparation time: 10 minutes
Cooking time: 2 hours
Servings: 12
Ingredients:

- 16 ounces green beans
- ½ cup brown sugar
- ½ cup butter, melted
- ¾ teaspoon soy sauce
- Salt and black pepper to the taste

Directions:
1. In your Slow cooker, mix green beans with sugar, butter, soy sauce, salt, and pepper, stir, cover, and cook on Low for 2 hours.
2. Divide between plates and serve as a side dish.

Nutrition: calories 176, fat 4, carbs 14, protein 4

Corn and Bacon

Preparation time: 10 minutes
Cooking time: 4 hours
Servings: 20
Ingredients:

- 10 cups corn
- 24 ounces cream cheese, cubed

- ½ cup milk
- ½ cup melted butter
- ½ cup heavy cream
- ¼ cup sugar
- A pinch of salt and black pepper
- 4 bacon strips, cooked and crumbled
- 2 tablespoons green onions, chopped

Directions:
1. In your Slow cooker, mix the corn with cream cheese, milk, butter, cream, sugar, salt, pepper, bacon, and green onions, cover, and cook on Low for 4 hours.
2. Stir the corn, divide between plates and serve as a side dish.

Nutrition: calories 259, fat 20, carbs 18, protein 5

Peas and Carrots

Preparation time: 10 minutes
Cooking time: 5 hours
Servings: 12
Ingredients:

- 1 yellow onion, chopped
- 1 pound carrots, sliced
- 16 ounces peas
- ¼ cup melted butter
- ¼ cup water
- ¼ cup honey
- 4 garlic cloves, minced
- A pinch of salt and black pepper
- 1 teaspoon marjoram, dried

Directions:
1. In your Slow cooker, mix the onion with carrots, peas, butter, water, honey, garlic, salt, pepper, and marjoram, cover, and cook on Low for 5 hours.
2. Stir peas and carrots mix, divide between plates and serve as a side dish.

Nutrition: calories 105, fat 4, carbs 16, protein 4

Beans, Carrots and Spinach Salad

Preparation time: 10 minutes
Cooking time: 7 hours
Servings: *6*
Ingredients:

- 1 and ½ cups northern beans
- 1 yellow onion, chopped
- 5 carrots, chopped
- 2 garlic cloves, minced
- ½ teaspoon oregano, dried
- Salt and black pepper to the taste
- 4 and ½ cups chicken stock
- 5 ounces baby spinach
- 2 teaspoons lemon peel, grated
- 1 avocado, peeled, pitted, and chopped
- 3 tablespoons lemon juice
- ¾ cup feta cheese, crumbled
- 1/3 cup pistachios, chopped

Directions:

1. In your Slow cooker, mix beans with onion, carrots, garlic, oregano, salt, pepper, and stock, stir, cover, and cook on Low for 7 hours.
2. Drain beans and veggies, transfer them to a salad bowl, add baby spinach, lemon peel, avocado, lemon juice, pistachios, and cheese, toss, divide between plates and serve as a side dish.

Nutrition: calories 300, fat 8, fiber 14, carbs 43, protein 16

Scalloped Potatoes

Preparation time: *10 minutes*
Cooking time: *6 hours*
Servings: *6*
Ingredients:

- Cooking spray
- 2 and ½ pounds gold potatoes, sliced
- 10 ounces canned cream of potato soup
- 1 yellow onion, roughly chopped

- 8 ounces sour cream
- 1 cup Gouda cheese, shredded
- ½ cup blue cheese, crumbled
- ½ cup parmesan, grated
- ½ cup chicken stock
- Salt and black pepper to the taste
- 1 tablespoon chives, chopped

Directions:

1. Grease your Slow cooker with cooking spray and arrange potato slices on the bottom. Add cream of potato soup, onion, sour cream, Gouda cheese, blue cheese, parmesan, stock, salt and pepper, cover, and cook on Low for 6 hours.
2. Add chives, divide between plates, and serve as a side dish.

Nutrition: calories 306, fat 14, carbs 33, protein 12

Sweet Potatoes with Bacon

Preparation time: 10 minutes
Cooking time: 5 hours
Servings: 6
Ingredients:

- 4 pounds sweet potatoes, peeled and sliced
- 3 tablespoons brown sugar
- ½ cup orange juice
- ½ teaspoon sage, dried
- ½ teaspoon thyme, dried
- 4 bacon slices, cooked and crumbled
- 2 tablespoons soft butter

Directions:

1. Arrange sweet potato slices in your Slow cooker, add sugar, orange juice, sage, thyme, butter, and bacon, cover and cook on Low for 5 hours.
2. Divide between plates and serve them as a side dish.

Nutrition: calories 200, fat 4, carbs 30, protein 4

Cauliflower and Broccoli Mix

Preparation time: *10 minutes*
Cooking time: *7 hours*
Servings: *10*
Ingredients:

- 4 cups broccoli florets
- 4 cups cauliflower florets
- 7 ounces Swiss cheese, torn
- 14 ounces Alfredo sauce
- 1 yellow onion, chopped
- Salt and black pepper to the taste
- 1 teaspoon thyme, dried
- ½ cup almonds, sliced

Directions:

1. In your Slow cooker, mix broccoli with cauliflower, cheese, sauce, onion, salt, pepper, and thyme, stir, cover, and cook on Low for 7 hours.
2. Add almonds, divide between plates and serve as a side dish.

Nutrition: calories 177, fat 7, carbs 10, protein 7

Wild Rice Mix

Preparation time: *10 minutes*
Cooking time: *6 hours*
Servings: *16*
Ingredients:

- 45 ounces chicken stock
- 1 cup carrots, sliced
- 2 and ½ cups wild rice
- 4 ounces mushrooms, sliced
- 2 tablespoons butter, soft
- Salt and black pepper to the taste
- 2 teaspoons marjoram, dried
- 2/3 cup dried cherries
- 2/3 cup green onions, chopped
- ½ cup pecans, chopped

Directions:

1. In your Slow cooker, mix stock with carrots, rice, mushrooms, butter, salt, pepper, and marjoram, cover, and cook on Low for 6 hours.
2. Add cherries, green onions, and pecans, toss, divide between plates and serve as a side dish.

Nutrition: calories 169, fat 6, carbs 27, protein 5

Mashed Potatoes

Preparation time: 10 minutes
Cooking time: 4 hours
Servings: 12
Ingredients:

- 3 pounds gold potatoes, peeled and cubed
- 1 bay leaf
- 6 garlic cloves, minced
- 28 ounces chicken stock
- 1 cup milk - ¼ cup butter
- Salt and black pepper to the taste

Directions:

1. In your Slow cooker, mix potatoes with bay leaf, garlic, salt, pepper, and stock, cover, and cook on Low for 4 hours.
2. Drain potatoes, mash them, mix with butter and milk, blend really, divide between plates and serve as a side dish.

Nutrition: calories 135, fat 4, carbs 22, protein 4

Orange Glazed Carrots

Preparation time: 10 minutes
Cooking time: 8 hours
Servings: 10
Ingredients:

- 3 pounds carrots, cut into medium chunks
- 1 cup orange juice
- 2 tablespoons orange peel, grated
- ½ cup orange marmalade
- ½ cup veggie stock

- ¼ cup white wine
- 1 tablespoon tapioca, crushed
- ¼ cup parsley, chopped
- 3 tablespoons butter
- Salt and black pepper to the taste

Directions:

1. In your Slow cooker, mix carrots with orange juice, orange peel, marmalade, stock, wine, tapioca, parsley, butter, salt, and pepper, cover, and cook on Low for 8 hours. Toss carrots, divide between plates, and serve as a side dish.

Nutrition: calories 160, fat 4, carbs 31, protein 3

Creamy Risotto

Preparation time: 10 minutes
Cooking time: 1 hour
Servings: 4
Ingredients:

- 4 ounces mushrooms, sliced
- ½ quart veggie stock
- 1 teaspoon olive oil
- 2 tablespoons porcini mushrooms
- 2 cups white rice
- A small bunch of parsley, chopped

Directions:

1. In your Slow cooker, mix mushrooms with stock, oil, porcini mushrooms, and rice, stir, cover and cook on High for 1 hour. Add parsley, stir, divide between plates and serve as a side dish.

Nutrition: calories 346, fat 3, carbs 35, protein 10

Veggie and Garbanzo Mix

Preparation time: 10 minutes
Cooking time: 6 hours
Servings: 4
Ingredients:

- 15 ounces canned garbanzo beans, drained

- 3 cups cauliflower florets
- 1 cup green beans - 1 cup carrot, sliced
- 14 ounces veggie stock
- ½ cup onion, chopped
- 2 teaspoons curry powder
- ¼ cup basil, chopped
- 14 ounces coconut milk

Directions:

1. In your Slow cooker, mix beans with cauliflower, green beans, carrot, onion, stock, curry powder, basil, and milk, stir, cover, and cook on Low for 6 hours.
2. Stir veggie mix again, divide between plates and serve as a side dish.

Nutrition: calories 219, fat 5, carbs 32, protein 7

Cauliflower Pilaf

Preparation time: *10 minutes*
Cooking time: *3 hours*
Servings: *6*
Ingredients:

- 1 cup cauliflower rice
- 6 green onions, chopped
- 3 tablespoons ghee, melted
- 2 garlic cloves, minced
- ½ pound Portobello mushrooms, sliced
- 2 cups warm water
- Salt and black pepper to the taste

Directions:

1. In your Slow cooker, mix cauliflower rice with green onions, melted ghee, garlic, mushrooms, water, salt, and pepper, stir well, cover, and cook on Low for 3 hours.
2. Divide between plates and serve as a side dish.

Nutrition: calories 200, fat 5, carbs 14, protein 4

Squash Side Salad

Preparation time: 10 minutes
Cooking time: 4 hours
Servings: 8
Ingredients:

- 1 tablespoon olive oil
- 1 cup carrots, chopped
- 1 yellow onion, chopped
- 1 teaspoon sugar
- 1 and ½ teaspoons curry powder
- 1 garlic clove, minced
- 1 big butternut squash, peeled and cubed
- A pinch of sea salt and black pepper
- ¼ teaspoon ginger, grated
- ½ teaspoon cinnamon powder
- 3 cups coconut milk

Directions:

1. In your Slow cooker, mix oil with carrots, onion, sugar, curry powder, garlic, squash, salt, pepper, ginger, cinnamon, and coconut milk, stir well, cover, and cook on Low for 4 hours.
2. Stir, divide between plates, and serve as a side dish.

Nutrition: calories 200, fat 4, carbs 17, protein 4

Mushrooms and Sausage Mix

Preparation time: 10 minutes
Cooking time: 2 hours and 30 minutes
Servings: 12
Ingredients:

- ½ cup butter, melted
- 1 pound pork sausage, ground
- ½ pound mushrooms, sliced
- 6 celery ribs, chopped
- 2 yellow onions, chopped
- 2 garlic cloves, minced
- 1 tablespoon sage, chopped
- 1 cup cranberries, dried
- ½ cup cauliflower florets, chopped
- ½ cup veggie stock

Directions:

1. Heat up a pan with the butter over medium-high heat, add sausage, stir, cook for a couple of minutes and transfer to your Slow cooker.
2. Add mushrooms, celery, onion, garlic, sage, cranberries, cauliflower, and stock, stir, cover and cook on High for 2 hours and 30 minutes.
3. Divide between plates and serve as a side dish.

Nutrition: calories 200, fat 3, carbs 9, protein 4

Glazed Baby Carrots

Preparation time: 10 minutes
Cooking time: 6 hours
Servings: 6
Ingredients:

- ½ cup peach preserves
- ½ cup butter, melted
- 2 pounds baby carrots
- 2 tablespoon sugar
- 1 teaspoon vanilla extract
- A pinch of salt and black pepper
- A pinch of nutmeg, ground
- ½ teaspoon cinnamon powder
- 2 tablespoons water

Directions:

1. Put all the ingredients in a slow cooker, cover, and cook on Low for 6 hours.
2. Divide between plates and serve as a side dish.

Nutrition: calories 283, fat 14, carbs 28, protein 3

Spinach and Squash Side Salad

Preparation time: 10 minutes
Cooking time: 4 hours
Servings: 12
Ingredients:

- 3 pounds butternut squash, peeled and cubed - 1 yellow onion, chopped
- 2 teaspoons thyme, chopped
- 3 garlic cloves, minced
- A pinch of salt and black pepper
- 10 ounces veggie stock
- 6 ounces baby spinach

Directions:

1. In your Slow cooker, mix squash cubes with onion, thyme, salt, pepper, and stock, stir, cover, and cook on Low for 4 hours.
2. Transfer squash mixture to a bowl, add spinach, toss, divide between plates and serve as a side dish.

Nutrition: calories 100, fat 1, carbs 18, protein 4

Buttery Mushrooms

Preparation time: 10 minutes
Cooking time: 4 hours
Servings: 6
Ingredients:

- 1 yellow onion, chopped
- 1 pounds mushrooms, halved
- ½ cup butter, melted
- 1 teaspoon Italian seasoning
- Salt and black pepper to the taste
- 1 teaspoon sweet paprika

Directions:

1. In your Slow cooker, mix mushrooms with onion, butter, Italian seasoning, salt, pepper, and paprika, toss, cover, and cook on Low for 4 hours.
2. Divide between plates and serve as a side dish.

Nutrition: calories 120, fat 6, carbs 8, protein 4

Cauliflower Rice and Spinach

Preparation time: 10 minutes
Cooking time: 3 hours
Servings: 8
Ingredients:

- 2 garlic cloves, minced
- 2 tablespoons butter, melted
- 1 yellow onion, chopped
- ¼ teaspoon thyme, dried
- 3 cups veggie stock
- 20 ounces spinach, chopped
- 6 ounces coconut cream
- Salt and black pepper to the taste
- 2 cups cauliflower rice

Directions:

1. Heat up a pan with the butter over medium heat, add onion, stir and cook for 4 minutes.
2. Add garlic, thyme, and stock, stir, cook for 1 minute more, and transfer to your Slow cooker.
3. Add spinach, coconut cream, cauliflower rice, salt, and pepper, stir a bit, cover and cook on High for 3 hours.
4. Divide between plates and serve as a side dish.

Nutrition: calories 200, fat 4, carbs 8, protein 2

Maple Sweet Potatoes

Preparation time: *10 minutes*
Cooking time: *5 hours*
Servings: *10*
Ingredients:

- 8 sweet potatoes, halved and sliced
- 1 cup walnuts, chopped
- ½ cup cherries, dried and chopped
- ½ cup maple syrup
- ¼ cup apple juice
- A pinch of salt

Directions:

1. Arrange sweet potatoes in your slow cooker, add walnuts, dried cherries, maple syrup, apple juice, and a pinch of salt, toss a bit, cover, and cook on Low for 5 hours.

2. Divide between plates and serve as a side dish.

Nutrition: calories 271, fat 6, carbs 26, protein 6

CHAPTER 11:

Snack Recipes

Squash Salsa

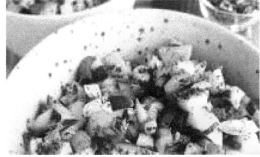

Preparation time: 10 minutes
Cooking time: 3 hours
Servings: 2
Ingredients:

- 1 cup butternut squash, peeled and cubed
- 1 cup cherry tomatoes, cubed
- 1 cup avocado, peeled, pitted, and cubed
- ½ tablespoon balsamic vinegar
- ½ tablespoon lemon juice
- 1 tablespoon lemon zest, grated
- ¼ cup veggie stock
- 1 tablespoon chives, chopped
- A pinch of rosemary, dried
- A pinch of sage, dried
- A pinch of salt and black pepper

Directions:

1. In your slow cooker, mix the squash with the tomatoes, avocado, and the other ingredients, toss, put the lid on and cook on Low for 3 hours.
2. Divide into bowls and serve as a snack.

Nutrition: calories 182, fat 5, carbs 12, protein 5

Taco Dip

Preparation time: 10 minutes
Cooking time: 2 hours and 30 minutes
Servings: 7
Ingredients:

- 1 rotisserie chicken, shredded
- 2 cups pepper jack, cheese, grated
- 15 ounces canned enchilada sauce
- 1 jalapeno, sliced
- 8 ounces cream cheese, soft
- 1 tablespoon taco seasoning

Directions:

1. In your slow cooker, mix chicken with pepper jack, enchilada sauce, jalapeno, cream, and taco seasoning, stir, cover, and cook on High for 1 hour.
2. Stir the dip, cover, and cook on Low for 1 hour and 30 minutes more.
3. Divide into bowls and serve as a snack.

Nutrition: calories 251, fat 5, carbs 17, protein 5

Beans Spread

Preparation time: 10 minutes
Cooking time: 6 hours
Servings: 2
Ingredients:

- 1 cup canned black beans, drained
- 2 tablespoons tahini paste
- ½ teaspoon balsamic vinegar
- ¼ cup veggie stock
- ½ tablespoon olive oil

Directions:

1. Transfer to your food processor, blend well, divide into bowls, and serve.

Nutrition: calories 221, fat 6, carbs 19, protein 3

Lasagna Dip

Preparation time: 10 minutes

Cooking time: 1 hour

Servings: 10

Ingredients:

- 8 ounces cream cheese
- ¾ cup parmesan, grated
- 1 and ½ cups ricotta
- ½ teaspoon red pepper flakes, crushed
- 2 garlic cloves, minced
- 3 cups marinara sauce
- 1 and ½ cups mozzarella, shredded
- 1 and ½ teaspoon oregano, chopped

Directions:

1. In your slow cooker, mix cream cheese with parmesan, ricotta, pepper flakes, garlic, marinara, mozzarella, and oregano, stir, cover, and cook on High for 1 hour.
2. Stir, divide into bowls, and serve as a dip.

Nutrition: calories 231, fat 4, carbs 21, protein 5

Rice Snack Bowls

Preparation time: 10 minutes

Cooking time: 6 hours

Servings: 2

Ingredients:

- ½ cup wild rice
- 1 red onion, sliced
- ½ cup brown rice
- 2 cups veggie stock
- ½ cup baby spinach
- ½ cup cherry tomatoes, halved
- 2 tablespoons pine nuts, toasted
- 1 tablespoon raisins

- 1 tablespoon chives, chopped
- 1 tablespoon dill, chopped
- ½ tablespoon olive oil
- A pinch of salt and black pepper

Directions:

1. In your slow cooker, mix the rice with the onion, stock, and the other ingredients, toss, put the lid on and cook on Low for 6 hours.
2. Divide into bowls and serve as a snack.

Nutrition: calories 301, fat 6, carbs 12, protein 3

Beer and Cheese Dip

Preparation time: 10 minutes

Cooking time: 1 hour

Servings: 10

Ingredients:

- 12 ounces cream cheese
- 6 ounces beer
- 4 cups cheddar cheese, shredded
- 1 tablespoon chives, chopped

Directions:

1. In your slow cooker, mix cream cheese with beer and cheddar, stir, cover, and cook on Low for 1 hour.
2. Stir your dip, add chives, divide into bowls and serve.

Nutrition: calories 212, fat 4, carbs 16, protein 5

Cauliflower Spread

Preparation time: 10 minutes

Cooking time: 7 hours

Servings: 2

Ingredients:

- 1 cup cauliflower florets
- 1 tablespoon mayonnaise
- ½ cup heavy cream
- 1 tablespoon lemon juice
- ½ teaspoon garlic powder
- ¼ teaspoon smoked paprika

- ¼ teaspoon mustard powder
- A pinch of salt and black pepper

Directions:

1. In your slow cooker, combine the cauliflower with the cream, mayonnaise, and the other ingredients, toss, put the lid on and cook on Low for 7 hours.
2. Transfer to a blender, pulse well into bowls and serve as a spread.

Nutrition: calories 152, fat 13.8, carbs 6.2, protein 2

Queso Dip

Preparation time: 10 minutes
Cooking time: 1 hour
Servings: 10
Ingredients:

- 16 ounces Velveeta
- 1 cup whole milk
- ½ cup coria
- 2 jalapenos, chopped
- 2 teaspoons sweet paprika
- 2 garlic cloves, minced
- A pinch of cayenne pepper
- 1 tablespoon cilantro, chopped

Directions:

1. In your Slow cooker, mix Velveeta with milk, cotija, jalapenos, paprika, garlic, and cayenne, stir, cover, and cook on High for 1 hour.
2. Stir the dip, add cilantro, divide into bowls and serve as a dip.

Nutrition: Calories 233, fat 4, carbs 10, Protein 10

Party Snack Mix

Preparation time: 15 minutes
Cooking time: 2 hours
Servings: 8
Ingredients:

- 4 cups rice Chex cereal

- 1 cup corn Chex cereal
- 2 cups small pretzels
- 1 cup shelled peanuts
- 2 tablespoons unsalted butter, melted, or extra-virgin olive oil
- 1 teaspoon smoked paprika
- 1 teaspoon garlic powder
- 1 teaspoon onion powder
- 1 teaspoon minced fresh rosemary (optional)
- 1 tablespoon vegetarian Worcestershire sauce

Directions

1. Place the rice cereal, corn cereal, pretzels, and peanuts in a 3-quart slow cooker. Stir to combine.
2. In a small measuring cup, whisk together the butter, paprika, garlic powder, onion powder, rosemary (if using), and Worcestershire sauce. Pour this mixture into the slow cooker on top of the cereal mixture and stir gently to thoroughly coat.
3. Cook on low, uncovered, for 2 hours. Stir several times to ensure that the mixture cooks evenly and does not stick to the slow cooker. The mix is done when the cereal is glazed.
4. Remove the mix from the slow cooker, spread it onto a parchment paper-lined baking sheet, and let cool for 2 hours before serving or storing.

Nutrition: Calories: 121; Fat: 2g; Carbohydrates: 14g; Protein: 3g;

Marinated Mushrooms

Preparation time: *15 minutes*
Cooking time: *3 hours*
Servings: *8*
Ingredients:

- 2 ounces dried mushrooms
- 2 (8-ounce) packages button mushrooms

- 2 tablespoons unsalted butter, plus more as needed
- 2 shallots, minced
- ¼ cup dry sherry (not cooking sherry)
- 1 tablespoon herbs de Provence
- ¼ teaspoon sea salt
- ¼ teaspoon freshly ground black pepper

Directions

1. Place the dried mushrooms in a small bowl and cover with hot water. Let stand for 10 minutes to rehydrate. Drain; then remove the tough ends of the stems and discard. Coarsely chop the mushrooms and set aside.
2. Slice the larger fresh mushrooms in half, leaving the smaller ones whole.
3. Place a large skillet over high heat and melt the butter. Add half the button mushrooms and cook until browned; then push the first batch to the sides and add the remaining button mushrooms, adding more butter as needed to brown them. Transfer the browned mushrooms to a 3-quart slow cooker along with the chopped rehydrated dried mushrooms.
4. In the same skillet, cook the shallots for about 3 minutes, or until slightly softened. Transfer the shallots to the slow cooker and add the sherry, herbes de Provence, salt, and pepper.
5. Cover and cook on low for 2 to 3 hours, or until the button mushrooms are tender and brown.

Nutrition: Calories: 64; Fat: 3g; Carbohydrates: 6g; Protein: 2g; Sodium: 78mg

Jalapeño Poppers

Preparation time: *30 minutes*
Cooking time: *4 hours*
Servings: *24*
Ingredients:

- 24 slices bacon

- 1 (8-ounce) package cream cheese, at room temperature
- ¼ cup sour cream
- ¼ cup grated Cheddar cheese
- 12 jalapeños, seeded and halved lengthwise
- ⅓ Cup Chicken Stock (or store-bought) or water

Directions

1. Place the bacon in a large skillet over medium heat and cook, turning frequently, until partially cooked but still bendable. Drain the bacon on paper towels and let cool. In a medium bowl, mix together the cream cheese, sour cream, and Cheddar cheese until well blended. Divide the cheese mixture evenly among the jalapeño halves. Wrap each stuffed jalapeño half with a slice of bacon; secure the bacon with a toothpick.
2. Pour the chicken stock into a 3-to 4-quart slow cooker and add the stuffed jalapeños.
3. Cover and cook on low for 4 hours or on high for 2 hours. Using a slotted spoon, remove the stuffed jalapeños from the slow cooker. Serve hot or at room temperature.

Nutrition: Calories: 89; Fat: 7g; Carbohydrates: 1g; Protein: 5g;

Spicy Cocktail Meatballs

Preparation time: *15 minutes*
Cooking time: *6 hours*
Servings: *10*
Ingredients:

- 1 large egg
- ¼ cup 2% milk
- 1 cup crisp rice cereal, finely crushed
- 2 tablespoons honey mustard
- 1 teaspoon sea salt
- ¼ teaspoon cayenne pepper
- 1 teaspoon dried thyme

- 2 pounds lean ground beef
- 2 tablespoons extra-virgin olive oil
- 1 (18-ounce) jar apple jelly
- ⅓ Cup Dijon mustard
- ⅓ Cup grainy mustard

Directions

1. In a large bowl, mix the egg, milk, cereal, honey mustard, salt, cayenne pepper, and thyme. Let stand for 5 minutes, so the cereal softens. Add the ground beef and mix gently but thoroughly with your hands. Form into 32 (1-inch) meatballs. (The meatballs can be prepared up to this point and stored in a covered container in the refrigerator for up to 2 days.)
2. Place a large skillet over medium-high heat and add the olive oil. Once hot, add the meatballs in two or three batches, and brown them for 3 to 4 minutes per batch. Once browned, place the meatballs in a 4-quart slow cooker. In the same skillet over medium-high heat, add the apple jelly, Dijon mustard, and grainy mustard, stirring occasionally to scrape up any browned bits from the bottom of the pan, until the jelly melts and the mixture is smooth.
3. .Pour the jelly mixture over the meatballs.
4. Cover and cook on low for 6 hours, stirring gently once if you are home, or until the meatballs read at least 160°F on a food thermometer. Serve with toothpicks.

Nutrition: Calories: 404; Fat: 13g; Carbohydrates: 50g; Protein: 19g;

Artichoke and Spinach Dip

Preparation time: *10 minutes*

Cooking time: 2 hours

Servings: *16*

Ingredients:

- 1 (14-ounce) can artichoke hearts, drained and chopped

- 2 cups frozen chopped spinach, thawed and squeezed dry
- 1 tablespoon minced garlic
- ½ cup 2% milk
- 1 (8-ounce) package cream cheese, at room temperature
- 1 cup grated Parmesan cheese
- ¼ teaspoon sea salt
- ⅛ teaspoon freshly ground black pepper

Directions

1. Place the artichoke hearts, spinach, garlic, milk, cream cheese, Parmesan, salt, and pepper in a 2-quart slow cooker. Stir well to combine.
2. Cover and cook on low for 2 hours, or until the cheese is melted and the dip is hot.
3. Serve the dip in the slow cooker with the heat on low or "keep warm."

Nutrition: Calories: 96; Fat: 7g; Carbohydrates: 4g; Fiber: 1g; Protein: 5g;

Mushroom Dip

Preparation time: 10 minutes

Cooking time: 5 hours

Servings: 2

Ingredients:

- 4 ounces white mushrooms, chopped
- 1 eggplant, cubed
- ½ cup heavy cream
- ½ tablespoon tahini paste
- 2 garlic cloves, minced
- A pinch of salt and black pepper
- 1 tablespoon balsamic vinegar
- ½ tablespoon basil, chopped
- ½ tablespoon oregano, chopped

Directions:

1. In your slow cooker, mix the mushrooms with the eggplant, cream, and the other

ingredients, toss, put the lid on and cook on High for 5 hours.

2. Divide the mushroom mix into bowls and serve as a dip.

Nutrition: calories 261, fat 7, carbs 10, protein 6

Raspberry Chia Pudding
Preparation time: 2 Hours
Cooking time: 2 Hours
Servings: 2
Ingredients: 4 tablespoons chia seeds
- 1 cup of coconut milk
- 2 teaspoons raspberries

Directions:
1. Put chia seeds and coconut milk in the Slow Cooker and cook it for 2 hours on Low. Then transfer the cooked chia pudding to the glasses and top with raspberries.

Nutrition: 423 calories, 7 protein, 19 carbohydrates, 37 fat

Ham Omelet
Preparation time: 3 Hours
Cooking time: 3 Hours
Servings: 2
Ingredients:
- Cooking spray
- 4 eggs, whisked
- 1 tablespoon sour cream
- 2 spring onions, chopped
- 1 small yellow onion, chopped
- ½ cup ham, chopped
- ½ cup cheddar cheese, shredded
- 1 tablespoon chives, chopped
- A pinch of salt and black pepper

Directions:
1. Grease your Slow Cooker with the cooking spray and mix the eggs with the sour cream, spring onions, and the other ingredients inside. Toss the mix, spread into the pot, put the lid on, and cook on High for 3 hours. Divide the mix between plates and serve for breakfast right away.

Nutrition: calories 192, fat 6, carbs 6, protein 12

Crab Dip
Preparation time: 10 minutes
Cooking time: 2 hours
Servings: 6
Ingredients:
- 12 ounces cream cheese
- ½ cup parmesan, grated
- ½ cup mayonnaise
- ½ cup green onions, chopped
- 2 garlic cloves, minced
- Juice of 1 lemon
- 1 and ½ tablespoon Worcestershire sauce
- 1 and ½ teaspoons old bay seasoning
- 12 ounces crabmeat

Directions:
1. In your slow cooker, mix cream cheese with parmesan, mayo, green onions, garlic, lemon juice, Worcestershire sauce, old bay seasoning, and crabmeat, stir, cover, and cook on Low for 2 hours.
2. Divide into bowls and serve as a dip.

Nutrition: calories 200, fat 4, carbs 12, protein 3

Chickpeas Spread
Preparation time: 10 minutes
Cooking time: 8 hours
Servings: 2
Ingredients:
- ½ cup chickpeas, dried
- 1 tablespoon olive oil

- 1 tablespoon lemon juice
- 1 cup veggie stock
- 1 tablespoon tahini
- A pinch of salt and black pepper
- 1 garlic clove, minced
- ½ tablespoon chives, chopped

Directions:

1. In your slow cooker, combine the chickpeas with the stock, salt, pepper, and garlic, stir, put the lid on and cook on Low for 8 hours.
2. Drain chickpeas, transfer them to a blender, add the rest of the ingredients, pulse well, divide into bowls and serve as a party spread.

Nutrition: calories 211, fat 6, carbs 8, protein 4

Corn Dip

Preparation time: 10 minutes
Cooking time: 3 hours
Servings: 12
Ingredients:

- 9 cups corn, rice, and wheat cereal
- 1 cup cheerios
- 2 cups pretzels
- 1 cup peanuts
- 6 tablespoons hot, melted butter
- 1 tablespoon salt
- ¼ cup Worcestershire sauce
- 1 teaspoon garlic powder

Directions:

1. In your slow cooker, mix cereal with cheerios, pretzels, peanuts, butter, salt, Worcestershire sauce, and garlic powder, toss well, cover, and cook on Low for 3 hours.
2. Divide into bowls and serve as a snack.

Nutrition: Calories 182, fat 4, carbs 8, protein 8

Spinach Dip

Preparation time: 10 minutes
Cooking time: 1 hour
Servings: 2
Ingredients:

- 2 tablespoons heavy cream
- ½ cup Greek yogurt
- ½ pound baby spinach
- 2 garlic cloves, minced
- Salt and black pepper to the taste

Directions:

1. In your slow cooker, mix the spinach with the cream and the other ingredients, toss, put the lid on and cook on High for 1 hour.
2. Blend using an immersion blender, divide into bowls and serve as a party dip.

Nutrition: calories 221, fat 5, carbs 12, protein 5

Candied Pecans

Preparation time: 10 minutes
Cooking time: 3 hours
Servings: 4
Ingredients:

- 1 cup white sugar
- 1 and ½ tablespoons cinnamon powder
- ½ cup brown sugar
- 1 egg white, whisked
- 4 cups pecans
- 2 teaspoons vanilla extract
- ¼ cup water

Directions:

1. In a bowl, mix white sugar with cinnamon, brown sugar, and vanilla and stir.
2. Dip pecans in egg white, then in the sugar mix and put them in your slow cooker, also add the water, cover and cook on Low for 3 hours.

3. Divide into bowls and serve as a snack.

Nutrition: Calories 152, Fat 4, Fiber 7, Carbs 16, Protein 6

Dill Potato Salad

Preparation time: 10 minutes
Cooking time: 8 hours
Servings: 2
Ingredients:

- 1 red onion, sliced
- 1 pound gold potatoes, peeled and roughly cubed
- 2 tablespoons balsamic vinegar
- ½ cup heavy cream
- 1 tablespoons mustard
- A pinch of salt and black pepper
- 1 tablespoon dill, chopped
- ½ cup celery, chopped

Directions:

1. In your slow cooker, mix the potatoes with the cream, mustard, and the other ingredients, toss, put the lid on and cook on Low for 8 hours.
2. Divide salad into bowls and serve as an appetizer.

Nutrition: Calories 251, fat 6, carbs 8, protein 7

Chicken Bites

Preparation time: 10 minutes
Cooking time: 7 hours
Servings: 4
Ingredients:

- 1 pound chicken thighs, boneless and skinless
- 1 tablespoon ginger, grated
- 1 yellow onion, sliced
- 1 tablespoon garlic, minced
- 2 teaspoons cumin, ground
- 1 teaspoon cinnamon powder
- 2 tablespoons sweet paprika

- 1 and ½ cups chicken stock
- 2 tablespoons lemon juice
- ½ cup green olives, pitted and roughly chopped
- Salt to the taste
- 3 tablespoons olive oil
- 5 pita breads, cut in quarters and heated in the oven

Directions:

1. Heat up a pan with the olive oil over medium-high heat, add onions, garlic, ginger, salt, and pepper, stir and cook for 2 minutes. Add cumin and cinnamon, stir well and take off the heat.
2. Put chicken pieces in your slow cooker, add onions mix, lemon juice, olives, and stock, stir, cover, and cook on Low for 7 hours. Shred meat, stir the whole mixture again, divide it on pita chips, and serve as a snack.

Nutrition: Calories 265, Fat 7, Carbs 14, Protein 6

Peanut Snack

Preparation time: 10 minutes
Cooking time: 1 hour and 30 minutes
Servings: 4
Ingredients:

- 1 cup peanuts
- 1 cup chocolate peanut butter
- 12 ounces dark chocolate chips
- 12 ounces white chocolate chips

Directions:

1. In your slow cooker, mix peanuts with peanut butter, dark and white chocolate chips, cover, and cook on Low for 1 hour and 30 minutes.

2. Divide this mix into small muffin cups, leave aside to cool down, and serve as a snack.

Nutrition*: Calories 200, Fat 4, Carbs 10, Protein 5

Apple Dip

Preparation time: 10 minutes

Cooking time: 1 hour and 30 minutes

Servings: 8

Ingredients:

- 5 apples, peeled and chopped
- ½ teaspoon cinnamon powder
- 12 ounces jarred caramel sauce
- A pinch of nutmeg, ground

Directions:

1. In your slow cooker, mix apples with cinnamon, caramel sauce, and nutmeg, stir, cover and cook on High for 1 hour and 30 minutes.
2. Divide into bowls and serve.

Nutrition: Calories 200, Fat 3, Fiber 6, Carbs 10, Protein 5

Tomato and Mushroom Salsa

Preparation time: 10 minutes

Cooking time: 4 hours

Servings: 2

Ingredients:

- 1 cup cherry tomatoes, halved
- 1 cup mushrooms, sliced
- 1 small yellow onion, chopped
- 1 garlic clove, minced
- 12 ounces tomato sauce
- ¼ cup cream cheese, cubed
- 1 tablespoon chives, chopped
- Salt and black pepper to the taste

Directions:

1. In your slow cooker, mix the tomatoes with the mushrooms and the other ingredients, toss, put the lid on and cook on Low for 4 hours.
2. Divide into bowls and serve as a party salsa

Nutrition: Calories 285, Fat 4, Fiber 7, Carbs 12, Protein 4

CHAPTER 12:

Desserts

Delicious Apple Crisp

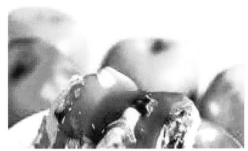

Preparation Time: 10 minutes
Cooking Time: 3 hours
Servings: 8
Ingredients:

- 2 lbs apples, peeled & sliced
- 1/2 cup butter
- 1/4 tsp ground nutmeg
- 1/2 tsp ground cinnamon
- 2/3 cup brown sugar
- 2/3 cup flour
- 2/3 cup old-fashioned oats

Directions:

1. Add sliced apples into the cooking pot.
2. In a mixing bowl, mix together flour, nutmeg, cinnamon, sugar, and oats.
3. Add butter into the flour mixture and mix until the mixture is crumbly.
4. Sprinkle flour mixture over sliced apples.
5. Cover instant pot aura with lid.
6. Select slow cook mode and cook on HIGH for 2-3 hours.
7. Top with vanilla ice-cream and serve.

Nutrition: calories 251 fat 12, carbs 33, protein 2.1 g

Easy Peach Cobbler Cake
Preparation Time: 10 minutes
Cooking Time: 45 minutes
Serve: 8
Ingredients:

- 3/4 cup butter, cut into pieces
- 1 oz yellow cake mix
- 20 oz can pineapples, crushed
- 21 oz can peach pie filling

Directions:

1. Pour crushed pineapples and peach pie filling into the cooking pot and spread evenly.
2. Sprinkle cake mix on top of pineapple mixture, then places butter pieces on top of the cake mix.
3. Cover instant pot aura with lid.
4. Select Bake mode and set the temperature to 350 F and time for 45 minutes.
5. Serve with vanilla ice cream.

Nutrition: calories 175, fat 2, carbs, 3, protein 1

Strawberry Dump Cake
Preparation Time: 10 minutes
Cooking Time: 40 minutes
Serve: 12
Ingredients:

- 16 oz box cake mix
- 20 oz can pineapple, crushed
- 2 1/2 cups strawberries, frozen, thawed, & sliced

Directions:

1. Add strawberries into the cooking pot and spread evenly.
2. Mix together cake mix and crushed pineapple and pour over sliced strawberries and spread evenly.
3. Cover instant pot aura with lid.
4. Select Bake mode and set the temperature to 350 F and time for 40 minutes.
5. Serve and enjoy.

Nutrition: calories 175, fat 2.3 g

Baked Apples

Preparation Time: 10 minutes
Cooking Time: 30 minutes
Serve: 6
Ingredients:

- 4 apples, sliced
- 1/2 tsp cinnamon
- 1 tbsp butter, melted

Directions:

1. Toss sliced apples with butter and cinnamon and place them into the cooking pot.
2. Cover instant pot aura with lid.
3. Select Bake mode and set the temperature to 375 F and time for 30 minutes.
4. Serve and enjoy.

Nutrition: calories 95, fat 2, carbs 20, protein 1

Baked Peaches

Preparation Time: 10 minutes
Cooking Time: 10 minutes
Serve: 6
Ingredients:

- 3 ripe peaches, slice in half & remove the pit
- 1/4 tsp cinnamon
- 2 tbsp brown sugar
- 1 tbsp butter

Directions:

1. Mix together butter, brown sugar, and cinnamon and place in the middle of each peach piece.
2. Place peaches in the cooking pot.
3. Cover instant pot aura with lid.
4. Select Bake mode and set the temperature to 375 F and time for 10 minutes.
5. Serve and enjoy.

Nutrition: calories 158, fat 12, carbs 6, protein 11

Delicious Peach Crisp

Preparation Time: 10 minutes
Cooking Time: 45 minutes
Serve: 8
Ingredients:

- 8 cups can peach, sliced
- 1/2 cup butter, cubed
- 1/2 cup brown sugar
- 1/2 cup all-purpose flour
- 1 1/2 cups rolled oats
- 2 tbsp cornstarch
- 1/2 cup sugar

Directions:

1. Add peaches, cornstarch, and sugar into the cooking pot and stir well.
2. Mix together butter, brown sugar, flour, and oats and sprinkle over peaches.
3. Cover instant pot aura with lid.
4. Select Bake mode and set the temperature to 350 F and time for 30-45 minutes.
5. Serve with ice cream

Nutrition: calories 478, fat 12, carbs 37, protein 3

Gingerbread Pudding Cake

Preparation Time: 10 minutes
Cooking Time: 2 hours 30 minutes
Serve: 6
Ingredients:

- 1 egg

- 1 1/4 cups whole wheat flour
- 1/8 tsp ground nutmeg
- 1/2 tsp ground ginger
- 1/2 tsp ground cinnamon
- 3/4 tsp baking soda
- 1 cup of water
- 1/2 cup molasses
- 1 tsp vanilla
- 1/4 cup sugar
- 1/4 cup butter, softened
- 1/4 tsp salt

Directions:

1. In a bowl, beat sugar and butter until combined. Add egg and beat until combined.
2. Add water, molasses, and vanilla and beat until well combined.
3. Add flour, nutmeg, ginger, cinnamon, baking soda, and salt and stir until combined. Pour batter into the cooking pot.
4. Cover instant pot aura with lid.
5. Select slow cook mode and cook on HIGH for 2 1/2 hours.
6. Serve with vanilla ice-cream.

Nutrition: calories 278, fat 8, carbs 49, protein 3

Healthy Blueberry Cobbler

Preparation Time: 10 minutes
Cooking Time: 2 hours 30 minutes
Serve: 6
Ingredients:

- 2 1/4 cups all-purpose flour
- 4 cups blueberries
- 8 tbsp butter, melted
- 1 tsp cinnamon
- 1 tbsp cornstarch
- 3 1/2 tsp baking powder
- 1 1/4 cups sugar
- 1 tsp salt

Directions:

1. Add blueberries into the cooking pot.
2. Mix together flour, cinnamon, cornstarch, baking powder, sugar, and salt and sprinkle over blueberries evenly.
3. Pour melted butter over flour mixture evenly.
4. Cover instant pot aura with lid.
5. Select slow cook mode and cook on LOW for 2 1/2 hours.
6. Serve with vanilla ice-cream.

Nutrition: calories 570, fat 16, carbs 13, protein 5

Easy Peach Cobbler

Preparation Time: 10 minutes
Cooking Time: 3 hours
Serve: 6
Ingredients:

- 1/2 cup butter, cut into pieces
- 1 box cake mix
- 30 oz can sliced peaches in syrup

Directions:

1. Add sliced peaches with syrup into the cooking pot.
2. Sprinkle cake mix on top of sliced peaches.
3. Spread butter pieces on top of the cake mix.
4. Cover instant pot aura with lid.
5. Select slow cook mode and cook on HIGH for 3 hours.
6. Serve with vanilla ice-cream.

Nutrition: calories 602, fat 12, carbs 6, protein 11

Peach Compote

Preparation Time: 10 minutes
Cooking Time: 2 hours
Serve: 8
Ingredients:

- 8 ripe peaches, peeled & sliced
- 1 tsp vanilla

- 1 tsp cinnamon
- 1/4 cup butter, cut into pieces
- 1/2 cup brown sugar
- 1/2 cup sugar

Directions:

1. Add peaches, vanilla, cinnamon, brown sugar, and sugar into the cooking pot and stir well.
2. Spread butter pieces on top of the peach mixture.
3. Cover instant pot aura with lid.
4. Select slow cook mode and cook on LOW for 2 hours.
5. Serve with vanilla ice-cream.

Nutrition: calories 193, fat 6, carbs 34, protein 3

Cinnamon Apples

Preparation Time: 10 minutes
Cooking Time: 2 hours
Servings: 5
Ingredients:

- 5 apples, peeled and sliced
- 1 1/4 tsp ground cinnamon
- 1 tbsp cornstarch
- 2 tbsp maple syrup
- 2/3 cup apple cider

Directions:

1. In a bowl, mix together apple cider, cinnamon, cornstarch, maple syrup, and 1/4 cup water.
2. Add apples into the cooking pot the pour apple cider mixture over apples.
3. Cover instant pot aura with lid.
4. Select slow cook mode and cook on LOW for 2 hours. Stir after 1 hour.
5. Stir well and serve.

Nutrition: calories 100, fat 12, carbs 4, protein 2

Choco Rice Pudding

Preparation Time: 10 minutes
Cooking Time: 2 hours 30 minutes
Servings: 8
Ingredients:

- 2 cups sticky rice, rinsed & drained
- 1/2 cup chocolate chips
- 1/2 cup brown sugar
- 14 oz coconut milk
- 12 oz can evaporate milk
- 3 cups of water
- 1/2 cup cocoa powder

Directions:

1. Add rice, water, and cocoa powder into the cooking pot and stir well.
2. Cover instant pot aura with lid.
3. Select slow cook mode and cook on HIGH for 2 hours.
4. Add remaining ingredients and stir everything well, cover, and cook for 30 minutes more.
5. Serve and enjoy.

Nutrition: calories 178, fat 12, carbs 6, protein 11

Chocolate Fudge

Preparation Time: 10 minutes
Cooking Time: 1 hour
Serve: 30
Ingredients:

- 3 cups chocolate chips
- 1 tbsp butter
- 1 tsp vanilla

Directions:

1. Add all ingredients into the cooking pot and stir well.
2. Select slow cook mode and cook on LOW for 1 hour. Stir after every 15 minutes.
3. Once done, pour into the greased tin. Place in the fridge for 2 hours or until set.
4. Cut into pieces and serve

Nutrition: calories 278, fat 6, carbs 34, protein 9

Chocolate Brownies

Preparation Time: 10 minutes
Cooking Time: 2 hours 30 minutes
Serve: 8
Ingredients:

- 3 eggs
- 1 cup butter, melted
- 1 cup peanut butter chips
- 1 tsp vanilla
- 1/3 cup all-purpose flour
- 2/3 cup unsweetened cocoa powder
- 1/3 cup brown sugar
- 1 1/4 cup sugar
- 1/2 tsp salt

Directions:

1. Line instant pot aura cooking pot with parchment paper.
2. In a mixing bowl, beat butter, sugar, brown sugar, cocoa powder, flour, eggs, vanilla, and salt until smooth.
3. Add peanut butter chips to the batter and fold well.
4. Pour batter into the cooking pot.
5. Cover instant pot aura with lid.
6. Select slow cook mode and cook on LOW for 2 1/2 hours.
7. Slice and serve.

Nutrition: calories 178, fat 12, carbs 6, protein 11

Tasty Cherry Cobbler

Preparation Time: 10 minutes
Cooking Time: 2 hours
Serve: 6
Ingredients:

- 1/2 cup butter, cut into pieces
- 1 box cake mix
- 30 oz can cherry pie filling

Directions:

1. Add cherry pie filling into the cooking pot, then sprinkle cake mix over cherry pie filling evenly.
2. Spread butter pieces on top of the cake mix. Cover instant pot aura with lid.
3. Select slow cook mode and cook on HIGH for 2 hours.
4. Serve and enjoy.

Nutrition: calories 178, fat 12, carbs 6, protein 11

Pineapple Cherry Dump Cake

Preparation Time: 10 minutes
Cooking Time: 3 hours
Serve: 6
Ingredients:

- 15 oz can pineapple, crushed
- 3/4 cup pecans, chopped
- 1 1/2 stick butter, cubed
- 1 box cake mix
- 15 oz can cherry pie filling

Directions:

1. Add cherry pie filling and crushed pineapple into the cooking pot and stir well.
2. Sprinkle cake mix over cherry pie filling mixture evenly.
3. Spread butter pieces and pecans on top of cake mix. Cover instant pot aura with lid.
4. Select slow cook mode and cook on HIGH for 3 hours.
5. Serve and enjoy.

Nutrition (Amount per Serving): Calories 79, Fat 42.7, Carbohydrates 12, Protein 6.2

White Chocolate Fudge

Preparation Time: 10 minutes
Cooking Time: 1 hour
Serve: 12
Ingredients:

- 2 cups white chocolate, chopped

- 1/2 cup white chocolate chips
- 1/4 cup heavy whipping cream
- 1/3 cup honey
- 1 tsp vanilla

Directions:

1. Add honey, heavy whipping cream, and white chocolate into the cooking pot and stir well.
2. Cover instant pot aura with lid.
3. Select slow cook mode and cook on HIGH for 1 hour.
4. Cut into squares and serve.

Nutrition: calories 220, fat 8, carbs 6, protein 10

Applesauce

Preparation Time: 10 minutes

Cooking Time: 8 hours

Serve: 6

Ingredients:

- 10 medium apples, peeled, cored, and sliced - 1/4 cup sugar
- 1/4 cup water
- 1 tsp ground cinnamon

Directions:

1. Add all ingredients into the cooking pot and stir well.
2. Cover instant pot aura with lid.
3. Select slow cook mode and cook on LOW for 8 hours.
4. Transfer apple mixture into the blender and blend until smooth.
5. Serve and enjoy.

Nutrition (Amount per Serving): Calories 226, Fat 0.7, Protein 1

Delicious Bread Pudding

Preparation Time: 10 minutes

Cooking Time: 4 hours

Serve: 8

Ingredients:

- 5 eggs

- 8 cups of bread cubes
- 1 tbsp vanilla
- 4 cups of milk
- 3/4 cup maple syrup
- 1 tbsp cinnamon

Directions:

1. In a large bowl, whisk together eggs, sugar, cinnamon, vanilla, and milk.
2. Add bread cubes into the cooking pot.
3. Pour egg mixture on top of bread cubes and let sit for 15 minutes.
4. Cover instant pot aura with lid.
5. Select slow cook mode and cook on LOW for 4 hours.
6. Serve and enjoy.

Nutrition: calories 340, fat 12, carbs 6, protein 11

Rice Pudding

Preparation Time: 10 minutes

Cooking Time: 4 hours

Serve: 6

Ingredients:

- 3/4 cup long-grain rice
- 3/4 cup sugar
- 3 cups of milk
- 1/2 tsp cinnamon
- 1 tsp vanilla
- 2 tbsp butter
- 1/4 tsp salt

Directions:

1. Add all ingredients into the cooking pot and stir well.
2. Cover instant pot aura with lid.
3. Select slow cook mode and cook on LOW for 4 hours.
4. Stir well and serve.

Nutrition: calories 178, fat 12, carbs 6, protein 11

Maple Pears

Preparation Time: 10 minutes
Cooking Time: 4 hours
Serve: 4
Ingredients:

- 4 ripe pears, peel, core, and cut the bottom
- 1/4 cup maple syrup
- 2 cups orange juice
- 1 tbsp ginger, sliced
- 1 cinnamon stick
- 5 cardamom pods

Directions:

1. Place pears into the cooking pot.
2. Mix together the remaining ingredients and pour over pears into the cooking pot.
3. Cover instant pot aura with lid.
4. Select slow cook mode and cook on LOW for 4 hours. Serve warm and enjoy.

Nutrition (Amount per Serving): Calories 242, Fat 0.8, Carbohydrates 18, Protein 2

Cinnamon Coconut Rice Pudding

Preparation Time: 10 minutes
Cooking Time: 6 hours
Serve: 8
Ingredients:

- 1 cup rice, rinsed and uncooked
- 4 cups of coconut milk
- 2 cups coconut cream
- 1 tsp ground cinnamon
- 1 tsp vanilla

Directions:

1. Add all ingredients into the cooking pot and stir well.
2. Cover instant pot aura with lid.
3. Select slow cook mode and cook on LOW for 6 hours.
4. Stir well and serve.

Nutrition: calories 432, fat 12, carbs 9, protein 19

Fruit Compote

Preparation Time: 10 minutes
Cooking Time: 6 hours
Servings: 8
Ingredients:

- 10 Cherries
- 4 tbsp raisins
- 10 oz plums, dried
- 10 oz apricots, dried
- 30 oz can peach, un-drained and sliced
- 10 oz can oranges, un-drained

Directions:

1. Add all ingredients into the cooking pot and stir well.
2. Cover instant pot aura with lid.
3. Select slow cook mode and cook on LOW for 6 hours.
4. Stir well and serve.

Nutrition: calories 345, fat 10, carbs 5, protein 18

Pumpkin Pie Pudding

Preparation Time: 10 minutes
Cooking Time: 6 hours
Servings: 8
Ingredients:

- 2 eggs, beaten
- 2 tbsp butter, melted
- 1/2 cup biscuit mix
- 3/4 cup sugar - 12 oz milk
- 15 oz can pumpkin
- 1 1/2 tsp vanilla extract
- 2 tsp pumpkin pie spice

Directions:

1. Add all ingredients into the cooking pot and mix well.
2. Cover instant pot aura with lid.
3. Select slow cook mode and cook on LOW for 6 hours.
4. Serve with ice-cream and enjoy it.

Nutrition: calories 185, fat 8, carbs 23, protein 11

Chocolate Almond Fudge

Preparation Time: 10 minutes
Cooking Time: 6 hours
Servings: 30
Ingredients:

- 8 oz chocolate chips
- 1/2 cup milk
- 2 tbsp almonds, sliced
- 2 tbsp swerve
- 1 tbsp butter, melted

Directions:

1. Add chocolate chips, milk, butter, and swerve into the cooking pot and stir well.
2. Cover instant pot aura with lid.
3. Select slow cook mode and cook on LOW for 2 hours.
4. Add almonds and stir fudge until smooth.
5. Pour fudge mixture into the greased baking dish and spread evenly.
6. Place baking dish in the refrigerator until the fudge set.
7. Cut into squares and serve.

Nutrition: calories 325, fat 7, carbs 29, protein 45

Delicious Chocolate Cake

Preparation Time: 10 minutes
Cooking Time: 2 hours 30 minutes
Serve: 10
Ingredients:

- 3 large eggs
- 1 ½ tsp baking powder
- 3 tbsp whey protein powder
- 1/2 cup cocoa powder
- 1/2 tsp vanilla
- 2/3 cup almond milk
- 6 tbsp butter, melted
- 1/2 cup Swerve
- 1 cup almond flour
- Pinch of salt

Directions:

1. Line instant pot aura cooking pot with parchment paper.
2. In a mixing bowl, whisk together almond flour, baking powder, protein powder, cocoa powder, swerve, and salt.
3. Stir in eggs, vanilla, almond milk, and butter until well combined.
4. Cover instant pot aura with lid.
5. Select slow cook mode and cook on LOW for 2 1/2 hours.
6. Serve and enjoy.

Nutrition: calories 210, fat 12, carbs 32, protein 19

Shredded Coconut-Raspberry Cake

Preparation Time: 10 minutes
Cooking time: 3 hours
Servings: 10
Ingredients:

- ½ cup melted coconut oil, plus more for coating the slow cooker insert
- 2 cups almond flour
- 1 cup unsweetened shredded coconut
- 1 cup erythritol or 1 teaspoon stevia powder
- ¼ cup unsweetened, unflavored protein powder
- 2 teaspoons baking soda
- ¼ teaspoon fine sea salt
- 4 large eggs, lightly beaten
- ¾ cup canned coconut milk
- 1 teaspoon coconut extract
- 1 cup raspberries, fresh or frozen

Directions:

1. Generously coat the inside of the slow cooker insert with coconut oil.
2. In a large bowl, stir together the almond flour, coconut, erythritol, protein powder, baking soda, and sea salt.

3. Whisk in the eggs, coconut milk, ½ cup of coconut oil, and coconut extract.

4. Gently fold in the raspberries.

5. Transfer the batter to the prepared slow cooker, cover, and cook for 3 hours on low. Turn off the slow cooker and let the cake cool for several hours to room temperature. Serve at room temperature.

Nutrition: calories 406, fat 8, carbs 13, protein 19

Vanilla Chocolate Walnut Fudge

Preparation Time: 10 minutes

Cooking time: 2 hours

Servings: 12

Ingredients:

- Coconut oil for coating the slow cooker insert and a baking dish
- 1 cup canned coconut milk
- 4 ounces unsweetened chocolate, chopped
- 1 cup erythritol
- 2 teaspoons stevia powder
- ¼ teaspoon fine sea salt
- 2 teaspoons pure vanilla extract
- 1 cup chopped toasted walnuts

Directions

1. Generously coat the inside of the slow cooker insert with coconut oil.

2. In a large bowl, whisk the coconut milk into a uniform consistency. Add the chocolate, erythritol, stevia powder, and sea salt. Stir to mix well. Pour into the slow cooker. Cover and cook for 2 hours on low.

3. When finished, stir in the vanilla.

4. Let the fudge sit in the slow cooker, with the lid off, until it cools to room temperature, about 3 hours.

5. Coat a large baking dish with coconut oil and set aside.

6. Stir the fudge until it becomes glossy, about 10 minutes.

7. Stir in the walnuts. Transfer the mixture to the prepared baking dish and smooth it into an even layer with a rubber spatula. Refrigerate overnight. Serve chilled, cut into small pieces.

Nutrition: calories 126, fat 6, carbs 3, protein 7

Delicious Chocolate Peanut Butter Fudge

Preparation Time: 17 minutes

Cooking time: 2 hours

Servings: 12

Ingredients:

- Coconut oil for coating the slow cooker insert
- 1½ cups heavy (whipping) cream
- 1 cup all-natural peanut butter
- 1 tablespoon unsalted butter, melted
- 1 teaspoon pure vanilla extract
- 4 ounces unsweetened chocolate, chopped
- ½ cup erythritol
- 1 teaspoon stevia powder

Directions:

1. Generously coat the inside of the slow cooker insert with coconut oil.

2. In the slow cooker, stir together the heavy cream, peanut butter, butter, vanilla, chocolate, erythritol, and stevia. Cover and cook for 2 hours on low, stirring occasionally.

3. Line a small, rimmed baking sheet with parchment or wax paper.

4. Transfer the cooked fudge to the prepared sheet and refrigerate for at least 4 hours.

5. Cut into squares and serve chilled.

Nutrition: calories 246, fat 23, carbs 7, protein 9

White Chocolate Fudge

Preparation Time: 10 minutes

Cooking Time: 1 hour

Servings: 12

Ingredients:

- 2 cups white chocolate, chopped
- 1/2 cup white chocolate chips
- 1/4 cup heavy whipping cream
- 1/3 cup honey
- 1 tsp vanilla

Directions:

1. Add honey, heavy whipping cream, and white chocolate into the cooking pot and stir well.
2. Cover instant pot aura with lid.
3. Select slow cook mode and cook on HIGH for 1 hour.
4. Pour melted chocolate into the parchment-lined baking dish and place it in the fridge until set.
5. Cut into squares and serve.

Nutrition: calories 229, fat 12, carbs 13, protein 1

Delicious Bread Pudding

Preparation Time: 10 minutes

Cooking Time: 4 hours

Servings: 8

Ingredients:

- 5 eggs
- 8 cups of bread cubes
- 1 tbsp vanilla
- 4 cups of milk
- 3/4 cup maple syrup
- 1 tbsp cinnamon

Directions:

1. In a large bowl, whisk together eggs, sugar, cinnamon, vanilla, and milk.
2. Add bread cubes into the cooking pot.
3. Pour egg mixture on top of bread cubes and let sit for 15 minutes.
4. Cover instant pot aura with lid.
5. Select slow cook mode and cook on LOW for 4 hours.
6. Serve and enjoy.

Nutrition: Calories: 212 Protein: 17.3g Carbs: 14.6g Fat: 11.8g

Vanilla Pudding

Preparation Time: 10 minutes

Cooking Time: 4 hours

Servings: 6

Ingredients:

- 3/4 cup Vanilla
- 3/4 cup sugar
- 3 cups of milk
- 1/2 tsp cinnamon
- 1 tsp vanilla
- 2 tbsp butter
- 1/4 tsp salt

Directions:

1. Add all ingredients into the cooking pot and stir well.
2. Cover instant pot aura with lid.
3. Select slow cook mode and cook on LOW for 4 hours.
4. Stir well and serve.

Nutrition: calories 276, fat 6, carbs 13, protein 14

Conclusion

A Slow cooker might be exactly what you need in your life right now! This diet is easy to follow, and it brings you so many health benefits! On the other hand, slow cookers are some of the most popular kitchen appliances available on the market these days. These wonderful tools help you cook delicious and healthy meals for all your loved ones. Now, we ask you: what do you get from combining one of the healthiest diets with the best cooking tool?

Well, the answer is pretty simple: you get the cooking experience of a lifetime! So, don't hesitate! Get your hands on this amazing cooking journal and start your new and improved life!

CPSIA information can be obtained
at www.ICGtesting.com
Printed in the USA
BVHW020301090221
599628BV00020B/2302

Tower

2-Basket Air Fryer
Cookbook for Beginners and Pros

600
Affordable, Quick & Easy Recipes for Beginners and Pros. Tips and Tricks for Perfect Frying

Eloise Marshall

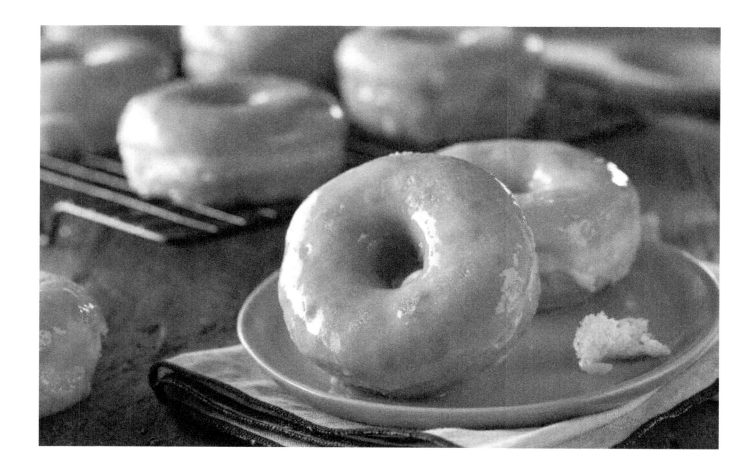

Table of Contents

Vegetarians Recipes 46

Desserts And Sweets 126

RECIPE INDEX 143

Introduction

Life is too busy today, and there is no time to cook for a long day. If you want to eat delicious and healthy meals, the Tower Dual Zone Air Fryer solves your problem. The Tower Dual Zone Air Fryer is a new arrival amongst diversified air fryers. Now, you can cook a large amount of food because it has two baskets. You can cook two different food items with two same or different settings. It is different from a single basket air fryer. This appliance targets people who want to enjoy delicious and healthy but less fatty meals with a crispy texture. The Tower Dual Zone Air Fryer is an excellent appliance to fulfill all the cooking needs. You can create excellent restaurant-style meals in your kitchen with the Tower Dual Zone Air Fryer.

No doubt, the Tower Dual Zone Air Fryer plays a vital role in making healthy and delicious foods. You don't need to stand

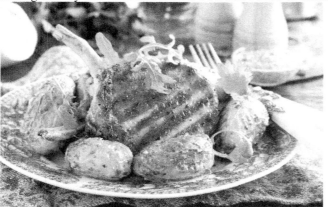

in your kitchen cooking food for a long time. The benefits of this appliance are that it is easily washable and requires less oil to cook food. The Tower Dual Zone Air Fryer works on dual zone technology. It allows you to prepare double dishes at the same time with two different cooking baskets and temperatures. If you have a big family, then you can cook food for them at the same time. The cooking zones have a separate temperature controller and cyclonic fan that spread heat evenly into the cooking baskets. The Tower Dual Zone Air Fryer cooks your favorite food in less oil. It gives you crispy food without changing the taste and texture.

You can create different dishes for any occasion or picnic. The Tower Dual Zone Air Fryer has useful cooking functions, such as max crisp, air fry, roast, reheat, dehydrate, and bake. All valuable functions are present in one appliance. You don't need to purchase separate appliances for baking or dehydrating food. You can roast chicken, beef, and fish using this appliance. Bake the cake, muffins, cupcakes, pancakes using bake cooking functions.

This Tower Dual Zone Air Fryer cookbook will introduce you to the features and benefits of this revolutionary appliance. Apart from that, the functions of the Tower Dual Zone Air Fryer are discussed in this cookbook, helping you unleash its full potential. And, of course, I'll introduce you to a wide variety of recipes so you can use it every day. The air fryer is pretty simple to use. Once you understand the Tower Dual Zone Air Fryer, you can prepare delicious food for your family and friends without any hesitation. Cook food with the Tower Dual Zone Air Fryer!

Getting Started with the Tower Dual Zone Air Fryer

What is the Tower Dual Zone Air Fryer

The new Tower Dual Zone Air Fryer has a DUAL-ZONE technology that includes a smart finish button that cooks two food items in two different ways at the same time. It has a MATCH button that cooks food by copying the setting across both zones.

The 8 –quart air fryer has a capacity that can cook full family meals up to 4 pounds. The two zones have their separate baskets that cook food using cyclonic fans that heat food rapidly with circulating hot air all-around. The baskets are very easy to clean and dishwasher safe. The Tower Dual Zone Air Fryer has a range of 105-450°F/40 - 230°C temperature. The Tower Dual Zone Air Fryer is easily available at an affordable price online and at local stores.

If you are always worried about the lack of time to prepare two different meals or a large number of meals in a single go, then this appliance is a must to have. It can hold plenty of food that can feed a large family.

The Features and Benefits of the Tower Dual Zone Air Fryers

The Tower Dual Zone Air Fryer is one of the innovative product designs manufactured. If you are looking for a perfect air fryer for your family, then the Tower Dual Zone Air Fryer is one of the best options available for you. Some of the important features and benefits of the Tower Dual Zone Air Fryer are mentioned as follows.

1. **8-Quart Capacity XL**
The enormous 8-quart capacity, which can be divided into two sections, provides ample area for cooking both large and small amounts of food. This oven can cook 2 pounds of fries and 2 pounds of wings and drumettes.
2. **Multifunctional Air Fryer**
The Tower Dual Zone Air Fryer comes with 6 preset functions. These easily customizable functions include max crisp, air fry, roast, bake, reheat and dehydrate. You never need to buy separate appliances for a single cooking function.
3. **Safer Than Deep Fryer**
Traditional deep frying method involves a large container full of sizzling oil. This can increase the safety risk of splashing hot oil over the skin. While the Tower Dual Zone Air Fryer is

close from all the sides when getting hot, there is no risk of splashing, spilling or accidental burn during the cooking process.

4.   Smart Finish

This culinary marvel can intelligently sync the cook timings of both cooking zones, allowing you to prepare multiple items at the same time while maintaining the same finish time.

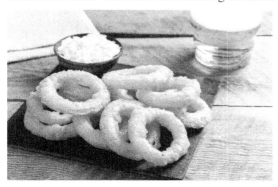

So, here's how it's done! When you put various foods in the baskets, each one takes a different amount of time to cook. When you use the smart cooking feature and start the operation, the basket with the longer cooking time will run first, while the other basket will remain on hold until the other chamber reaches the same cooking duration. Both sides finish cooking at the same time in this manner.

5.   Match Cook

This air fryer's total 8 quartz capacity is divided into two 4-quart air fryer baskets, allowing you to cook various foods and the same dish in both baskets at the same time. You can utilize the same cooking mode for both baskets and utilize the XL capacity with the match cook technology.

6.   Reduce the Risk of Acrylamide Formation

Deep frying is one of the high heat cooking methods in which harmful acrylamide is formed. It is one of the causes of developing some cancer like ovarian, endometrial, oesophageal and breast cancer. On the other side, this air fryer cooks your food into very little oil and fat by circulating hot air around the food. This process lowers the risk of acrylamide formation.

7.   Use Less Oil and Fats

The cooking basket of the oven comes with ceramic non-stick coatings and allows you to prepare your favorite food using up to 75 to 80 % less fat and oils than the traditional deep frying method.

8.   Wide Temperature Range

The Tower Dual Zone Air Fryer offers a range of 105 °F to 400 °F temperature. The lower temperature range is suitable for dehydrating your favorite fruits, vegetable, and meat slices, and the higher temperature range allows you to cook thick cuts of meat.

9.   Easy to Clean

The interior of this air fryer is made up of a non-stick coating so that you can clean it easily. The cooking tray comes in metallic and dishwasher safe, but you can easily clean it by hand if you want to.

Main Functions of the Tower Dual Zone Air Fryers

The Tower Dual Zone Air Fryer has six cooking functions: max crisp, air fry, roast, reheat, dehydrate and bake. This appliance has a large capacity. You can prepare food for your big family. If you want to bake a cake with the Tower Dual Zone Air Fryer, you can select "bake" cooking mode.

1.   Max Crisp

This cooking function is perfect for frozen foods such as chicken nuggets and French fries etc. Using this function,

you will get crispy and tender food. With less time, you will get crispy and tender food.

2.   Air Fry

This cooking function will allow you to cook food with less oil and fat than other cooking methods. Using this function, you will get crunchy and crispy food from the outside and juicy and tender food from the inside. You can prepare chicken, beef, lamb, pork, and seafood using this cooking option.

3.   Roast

Now, you didn't need an oven to roast food. The Tower Dual Zone Air Fryer has useful cooking function, "roast". With this function, you can roast chicken, lamb, seafood, and vegetable dishes. It is one of the dry cooking methods that give you a nice brown texture to the food and increase the flavor of your foods.

4.   Reheat

The reheat function can quickly warm your food without changing its texture and flavor if you have leftover food. Now, you didn't need to place food onto the stovetop for reheating.

5.   Dehydrate

This cooking function is used to dehydrate fruits, meat, and vegetables. Using this cooking method, you can preserve food for a long time. It takes hours to dehydrate the food but gives you a delicious and crispy texture.

6.   Bake

This cooking method allows you to bake cakes, muffins, cupcakes, and any other dessert on any occasion or regular day. You didn't need an oven to bake the food. The Tower Dual Zone Air Fryer has a baking option for baking your food with delicious texture.

Maintaining and Cleaning the Appliance

1.   Maintaining

● It is very important to check that the voltage indication is corresponding to the main voltage from the switch.

● Do not immerse the appliance in water.

● Keep the cord away from the hot area.

● Do not touch the outer surface of the air fryer hen using for cooking purposes.

● Put the appliance on a horizontal and flat surface.

● Unplug the appliance after use.

2. Cleaning

● First, unplug the power cord of the air fryer.

● Make sure the appliance is cooled before cleaning.

● The air fryer should be cleaning after every use.

● To clean the outer surface, use a damp towel.

● Clean the inside of the air fryer with a nonabrasive sponge.

● The accessories of the air fryer are dishwasher safe, but to extend the life of the drawers, it's recommended to wash them manually.

Tips for Cooking Success

Remember these nifty tips whenever you are cooking with your new air fryer.

1.   Pressing the Start/Pause button while using the Smart Finish will pause the cooking process on both zones. Press the same button to resume cooking.

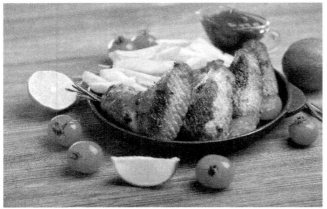

2. If at any time you need to pause the cooking process in one of the baskets, first select the zone, then the Start/Pause button.

3. To stop or end the cooking process, select the zone, then set the time to zero using the arrow down button. The display should show End after a few seconds, and the cooking process in this zone will stop.

4. You can adjust the temperature and time in each zone at any time during the cooking process. Select the zone, then adjust the setting using the arrow buttons.

5. Place a single layer of food and avoid stacking whenever possible.

6. To get the best results, toss or shake the food at least twice within the cooking cycle, especially for foods that overlap, like French fries. This will produce a more even cooking throughout.

7. When cooking fresh vegetables, add at least one tablespoon of cooking oil. More oil can be added to create a crispier texture.

8. Use the crisper plates when you want your food to become crunchy. Note that the crisper plates will slightly elevate your food to allow hot air to permeate the bottom and result in a crispier texture.

9. Follow the correct breading technique for wet battered food. Coat the food with flour first, then with egg, and finally with bread crumbs. Press the crumbs into the food to avoid it from flying around when air frying.

10. It is best to regularly check the progress to avoid overcooking.

11. A food-safe temperature must be reached to avoid any foodborne illness. Use a thermometer to check for doneness, especially when cooking raw meat. Instant-read thermometers are your best choice for this. Once cooking time is up or when the desired browning is achieved, promptly remove the food from the unit.

12. Do not use metal cutleries or tools that can damage the non-stick coating. Dump the food directly on a plate or use silicon-tipped tongs.

13. Small bits of food may be blown away while cooking. You can avoid this by securing pieces of food with toothpicks.

14. To cook recipes intended for traditional ovens, simply reduce the temperature by 25 °F and regularly check for doneness.

15. Do not let food touch the heating elements.

16. Never overload the baskets. Not only will this result in uneven cooking, but it may also cause the appliance to malfunction as well.

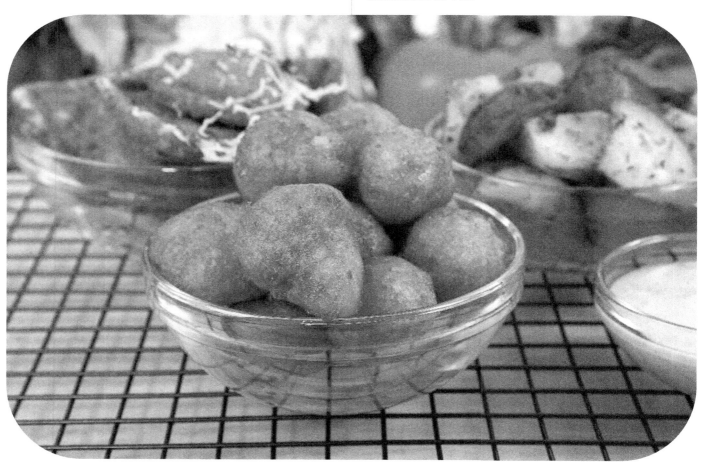

Measurement Conversions

BASIC KITCHEN CONVERSIONS & EQUIVALENTS

DRY MEASUREMENTS CONVERSION CHART
3 TEASPOONS = 1 TABLESPOON = 1/16 CUP
6 TEASPOONS = 2 TABLESPOONS = 1/8 CUP
12 TEASPOONS = 4 TABLESPOONS = 1/4 CUP
24 TEASPOONS = 8 TABLESPOONS = 1/2 CUP
36 TEASPOONS = 12 TABLESPOONS = 3/4 CUP
48 TEASPOONS = 16 TABLESPOONS = 1 CUP

METRIC TO US COOKING CONVER SIONS
OVEN TEMPERATURES
120 °C = 250 °F
160 °C = 320 °F
180° C = 360 °F
205 °C = 400 °F
220 °C = 425 °F

LIQUID MEASUREMENTS CONVERSION CHART
8 FLUID OUNCES = 1 CUP = 1/2 PINT = 1/4 QUART
16 FLUID OUNCES = 2 CUPS = 1 PINT = 1/2 QUART
32 FLUID OUNCES = 4 CUPS = 2 PINTS = 1 QUART = 1/4 GALLON
128 FLUID OUNCES = 16 CUPS = 8 PINTS = 4 QUARTS = 1 GALLON

BAKING IN GRAMS
1 CUP FLOUR = 140 GRAMS
1 CUP SUGAR = 150 GRAMS
1 CUP POWDERED SUGAR = 160 GRAMS
1 CUP HEAVY CREAM = 235 GRAMS

VOLUME
1 MILLILITER = 1/5 TEASPOON
5 ML = 1 TEASPOON
15 ML = 1 TABLESPOON
240 ML = 1 CUP OR 8 FLUID OUNCES
1 LITER = 34 FL. OUNCES
WEIGHT
1 GRAM = .035 OUNCES

100 GRAMS = 3.5 OUNCES
500 GRAMS = 1.1 POUNDS
1 KILOGRAM = 35 OUNCES

US TO METRIC COOKING CONVERSIONS
1/5 TSP = 1 ML
1 TSP = 5 ML
1 TBSP = 15 ML
1 FL OUNCE = 30 ML
1 CUP = 237 ML
1 PINT (2 CUPS) = 473 ML
1 QUART (4 CUPS) = .95 LITER
1 GALLON (16 CUPS) = 3.8 LITERS
1 OZ = 28 GRAMS
1 POUND = 454 GRAMS

BUTTER
1 CUP BUTTER = 2 STICKS = 8 OUNCES = 230 GRAMS = 8 TABLESPOONS

WHAT DOES 1 CUP EQUAL
1 CUP = 8 FLUID OUNCES
1 CUP = 16 TABLESPOONS
1 CUP = 48 TEASPOONS
1 CUP = 1/2 PINT
1 CUP = 1/4 QUART
1 CUP = 1/16 GALLON
1 CUP = 240 ML

BAKING PAN CONVERSIONS
1 CUP ALL-PURPOSE FLOUR = 4.5 OZ
1 CUP ROLLED OATS = 3 OZ 1 LARGE EGG = 1.7 OZ
1 CUP BUTTER = 8 OZ 1 CUP MILK = 8 OZ
1 CUP HEAVY CREAM = 8.4 OZ
1 CUP GRANULATED SUGAR = 7.1 OZ
1 CUP PACKED BROWN SUGAR = 7.75 OZ
1 CUP VEGETABLE OIL = 7.7 OZ
1 CUP UNSIFTED POWDERED SUGAR = 4.4 OZ

BAKING PAN CONVERSIONS
9-INCH ROUND CAKE PAN = 12 CUPS
10-INCH TUBE PAN =16 CUPS
11-INCH BUNDT PAN = 12 CUPS
9-INCH SPRINGFORM PAN = 10 CUPS
9 X 5 INCH LOAF PAN = 8 CUPS
9-INCH SQUARE PAN = 8 CUPS

Appetizers And Snacks

Buffalo Bites

Servings: 16
Cooking Time: 12 Minutes
Ingredients:
- 1 pound ground chicken
- 8 tablespoons buffalo wing sauce
- 2 ounces Gruyère cheese, cut into 16 cubes
- 1 tablespoon maple syrup

Directions:
1. Mix 4 tablespoons buffalo wing sauce into all the ground chicken.
2. Shape chicken into a log and divide into 16 equal portions.
3. With slightly damp hands, mold each chicken portion around a cube of cheese and shape into a firm ball. When you have shaped 8 meatballs, place them in air fryer basket.
4. Cook at 390°F/200°C for approximately 5minutes. Shake basket, reduce temperature to 360°F/180°C, and cook for 5 minutes longer.
5. While the first batch is cooking, shape remaining chicken and cheese into 8 more meatballs.
6. Repeat step 4 to cook second batch of meatballs.
7. In a medium bowl, mix the remaining 4 tablespoons of buffalo wing sauce with the maple syrup. Add all the cooked meatballs and toss to coat.
8. Place meatballs back into air fryer basket and cook at 390°F/200°C for 2 minutes to set the glaze. Skewer each with a toothpick and serve.

Mozzarella Sticks

Servings: 4
Cooking Time: 5 Minutes
Ingredients:
- 1 egg
- 1 tablespoon water
- 8 eggroll wraps
- 8 mozzarella string cheese "sticks"
- sauce for dipping

Directions:
1. Beat together egg and water in a small bowl.
2. Lay out egg roll wraps and moisten edges with egg wash.
3. Place one piece of string cheese on each wrap near one end.
4. Fold in sides of egg roll wrap over ends of cheese, and then roll up.
5. Brush outside of wrap with egg wash and press gently to seal well.
6. Place in air fryer basket in single layer and cook 390°F/200°C for 5 minutes. Cook an additional 1 or 2minutes, if necessary, until they are golden brown and crispy.
7. Serve with your favorite dipping sauce.

Fried Bananas

Servings: 4
Cooking Time: 8 Minutes
Ingredients:
- ½ cup panko breadcrumbs
- ½ cup sweetened coconut flakes
- ¼ cup sliced almonds
- ½ cup cornstarch
- 2 egg whites
- 1 tablespoon water
- 2 firm bananas
- oil for misting or cooking spray

Directions:
1. In food processor, combine panko, coconut, and almonds. Process to make small crumbs.
2. Place cornstarch in a shallow dish. In another shallow dish, beat together the egg whites and water until slightly foamy.
3. Preheat air fryer to 390°F/200°C.
4. Cut bananas in half crosswise. Cut each half in quarters lengthwise so you have 16 "sticks."
5. Dip banana sticks in cornstarch and tap to shake off excess. Then dip bananas in egg wash and roll in crumb mixture. Spray with oil.
6. Place bananas in air fryer basket in single layer and cook for 4minutes. If any spots have not browned, spritz with oil. Cook for 4 more minutes, until golden brown and crispy.
7. Repeat step 6 to cook remaining bananas.

Stuffed Prunes In Bacon

Servings: 6
Cooking Time: 20 Minutes
Ingredients:
- 12 bacon slices, halved
- 24 pitted prunes
- 3 tbsp crumbled blue cheese
- 1 tbsp cream cheese

Directions:
1. Cut prunes in half lengthwise, but do not cut all the way through. Add ½ tsp of blue cheese and cream cheese to the center of each prune. Wrap each prune with a slice of bacon and seal with a toothpick.
2. Preheat air fryer to 400°F/205°C. Place the prunes on the bottom of the greased frying basket in a single layer. Bake for 6-8 minutes, flipping the prunes once until the bacon is cooked and crispy. Allow to cool and serve warm.

Middle Eastern Phyllo Rolls

Servings: 6
Cooking Time: 5 Minutes
Ingredients:
- 6 ounces Lean ground beef or ground lamb
- 3 tablespoons Sliced almonds
- 1 tablespoon Chutney (any variety), finely chopped
- ¼ teaspoon Ground cinnamon
- ¼ teaspoon Ground coriander
- ¼ teaspoon Ground cumin
- ¼ teaspoon Ground dried turmeric
- ¼ teaspoon Table salt
- ¼ teaspoon Ground black pepper
- 6 18 × 14-inch phyllo sheets (thawed, if necessary)
- Olive oil spray

Directions:
1. Set a medium skillet over medium heat for a minute or two, then crumble in the ground meat. Cook for 3 minutes, stirring often, or until well browned. Stir in the almonds,

chutney, cinnamon, coriander, cumin, turmeric, salt, and pepper until well combined. Remove from the heat, scrape the cooked ground meat mixture into a bowl, and cool for 15 minutes.

2. Preheat the air fryer to 400°F/205°C.

3. Place one sheet of phyllo dough on a clean, dry work surface. (Keep the others covered.) Lightly coat it with olive oil spray, then fold it in half by bringing the short ends together. Place about 3 tablespoons of the ground meat mixture along one of the longer edges, then fold both of the shorter sides of the dough up and over the meat to partially enclose it (and become a border along the sheet of dough). Roll the dough closed, coat it with olive oil spray on all sides, and set it aside seam side down. Repeat this filling and spraying process with the remaining phyllo sheets.

4. Set the rolls seam side down in the basket in one layer with some air space between them. Air-fry undisturbed for 5 minutes, or until very crisp and golden brown.

5. Use kitchen tongs to transfer the rolls to a wire rack. Cool for only 2 or 3 minutes before serving hot.

Savory Sausage Balls

Servings: 10
Cooking Time: 8 Minutes
Ingredients:
- 2 cups all-purpose flour
- 1 tablespoon baking powder
- ½ teaspoon garlic powder
- ¼ teaspoon onion powder
- ½ teaspoon salt
- 3 tablespoons milk
- 2½ cups grated pepper jack cheese
- 1 pound fresh sausage, casing removed

Directions:
1. Preheat the air fryer to 370°F/185°C.

2. In a large bowl, whisk together the flour, baking powder, garlic powder, onion powder, and salt. Add in the milk, grated cheese, and sausage.

3. Using a tablespoon, scoop out the sausage and roll it between your hands to form a rounded ball. You should end up with approximately 32 balls. Place them in the air fryer basket in a single layer and working in batches as necessary.

4. Cook for 8 minutes, or until the outer coating turns light brown.

5. Carefully remove, repeating with the remaining sausage balls.

Hawaiian Ahi Tuna Bowls

Servings: 4
Cooking Time: 20 Minutes
Ingredients:
- 8 oz sushi-grade tuna steaks, cubed
- ½ peeled cucumber, diced
- 12 wonton wrappers
- ¾ cup dried beans
- 2 tbsp soy sauce
- 1 tsp toasted sesame oil
- ½ tsp Sriracha sauce
- 1 chili, minced
- 2 oz avocado, cubed
- ¼ cup sliced scallions
- 1 tbsp toasted sesame seeds

Directions:
1. Make wonton bowls by placing each wonton wrapper in a foil-lined baking cup. Press gently in the middle and against

the sides. Use a light coating of cooking spray. Spoon a heaping tbsp of dried beans into the wonton cup.

2. Preheat air fryer to 280°F/195°C. Place the cups in a single layer on the frying basket. Bake until brown and crispy, 9-11 minutes. Using tongs, carefully remove the cups and allow them to cool slightly. Remove the beans and place the cups to the side. In a bowl, whisk together the chili, soy sauce, sesame oil, and sriracha. Toss in tuna, cucumber, avocado, and scallions. Place 2 heaping tbsp of the tuna mixture into each wonton cup. Top with sesame seeds and serve immediately.

Goat Cheese & Zucchini Roulades

Servings: 6
Cooking Time: 20 Minutes
Ingredients:
- ½ cup goat cheese
- 1 garlic clove, minced
- 2 tbsp basil, minced
- 1 tbsp capers, minced
- 1 tbsp dill pickles, chopped
- ⅛ tsp salt
- ⅛ tsp red pepper flakes
- 1 tbsp lemon juice
- 2 zucchini, cut into strips

Directions:
1. Preheat air fryer to 360°F/180°C. Place the goat cheese, garlic, basil, capers, dill pickles, salt, red pepper flakes, and lemon juice in a bowl and stir to combine. Divide the filling between zucchini slices, then roll up and secure with a toothpick through the middle. Arrange the zucchini roulades on the greased frying basket. Bake for 10 minutes. When ready, gently remove the toothpicks and serve.

Crunchy Tortellini Bites

Servings: 5
Cooking Time: 10 Minutes
Ingredients:
- 10 ounces (about 2½ cups) Cheese tortellini
- ⅓ cup Yellow cornmeal
- ⅓ cup Seasoned Italian-style dried bread crumbs
- ⅓ cup (about 1 ounce) Finely grated Parmesan cheese
- 1 Large egg
- Olive oil spray

Directions:
1. Bring a large pot of water to a boil over high heat. Add the tortellini and cook for 3 minutes. Drain in a colander set in the sink, then spread out the tortellini on a large baking sheet and cool for 15 minutes.

2. Preheat the air fryer to 400°F/205°C.

3. Mix the cornmeal, bread crumbs, and cheese in a large zip-closed plastic bag.

4. Whisk the egg in a medium bowl until uniform. Add the tortellini and toss well to coat, even along the inside curve of the pasta. Use a slotted spoon or kitchen tongs to transfer 5 or 6 tortellini to the plastic bag, seal, and shake gently to coat thoroughly and evenly. Set the coated tortellini aside on a cutting board and continue coating the rest in the same way.

5. Generously coat the tortellini on all sides with the olive oil spray, then set them in one layer in the basket. Air-fry undisturbed for 10 minutes, gently tossing the basket and rearranging the tortellini at the 4- and 7-minute marks, until brown and crisp.

6. Pour the contents of the basket onto a wire rack. Cool for 5 minutes before serving.

Avocado Fries

Servings: 8
Cooking Time: 8 Minutes
Ingredients:
- 2 medium avocados, firm but ripe
- 1 large egg
- ½ teaspoon garlic powder
- ¼ teaspoon cayenne pepper
- ¼ teaspoon salt
- ¾ cup almond flour
- ½ cup finely grated Parmesan cheese
- ½ cup gluten-free breadcrumbs

Directions:
1. Preheat the air fryer to 370°F185°C.
2. Rinse the outside of the avocado with water. Slice the avocado in half, slice it in half again, and then slice it in half once more to get 8 slices. Remove the outer skin. Repeat for the other avocado. Set the avocado slices aside.
3. In a small bowl, whisk the egg, garlic powder, cayenne pepper, and salt in a small bowl. Set aside.
4. In a separate bowl, pour the almond flour.
5. In a third bowl, mix the Parmesan cheese and breadcrumbs.
6. Carefully roll the avocado slices in the almond flour, then dip them in the egg wash, and coat them in the cheese and breadcrumb topping. Repeat until all 16 fries are coated.
7. Liberally spray the air fryer basket with olive oil spray and place the avocado fries into the basket, leaving a little space around the sides between fries. Depending on the size of your air fryer, you may need to cook these in batches.
8. Cook fries for 8 minutes, or until the outer coating turns light brown.
9. Carefully remove, repeat with remaining slices, and then serve warm.

Thai-style Crabwontons

Servings: 4
Cooking Time: 20 Minutes
Ingredients:
- 4 oz cottage cheese, softened
- 2 ½ oz lump crabmeat
- 2 scallions, chopped
- 2 garlic cloves, minced
- 2 tsp tamari sauce
- 12 wonton wrappers
- 1 egg white, beaten
- 5 tbsp Thai sweet chili sauce

Directions:
1. Using a fork, mix together cottage cheese, crabmeat, scallions, garlic, and tamari sauce in a bowl. Set it near your workspace along with a small bowl of water. Place one wonton wrapper on a clean surface. The points should be facing so that it looks like a diamond. Put 1 level tbsp of the crab and cheese mix onto the center of the wonton wrapper. Dip your finger into the water and run the moist finger along the edges of the wrapper.
2. Fold one corner of the wrapper to the opposite side and make a triangle. From the center out, press out any air and seal the edges. Continue this process until all of the wontons have been filled and sealed. Brush both sides of the wontons with beaten egg white.
3. Preheat air fryer to 340°F/170°C. Place the wontons on the bottom of the greased frying basket in a single layer. Bake for 8 minutes, flipping the wontons once until golden brown and crispy. Serve hot and enjoy!

Indian Cauliflower Tikka Bites

Servings: 6
Cooking Time: 20 Minutes
Ingredients:
- 1 cup plain Greek yogurt
- 1 teaspoon fresh ginger
- 1 teaspoon minced garlic
- 1 teaspoon vindaloo
- ½ teaspoon cardamom
- ½ teaspoon paprika
- ½ teaspoon turmeric powder
- ½ teaspoon cumin powder
- 1 large head of cauliflower, washed and cut into medium-size florets
- ½ cup panko breadcrumbs
- 1 lemon, quartered

Directions:
1. Preheat the air fryer to 350°F/175°C.
2. In a large bowl, mix the yogurt, ginger, garlic, vindaloo, cardamom, paprika, turmeric, and cumin. Add the cauliflower florets to the bowl, and coat them with the yogurt.
3. Remove the cauliflower florets from the bowl and place them on a baking sheet. Sprinkle the panko breadcrumbs over the top. Place the cauliflower bites into the air fryer basket, leaving space between the florets. Depending on the size of your air fryer, you may need to make more than one batch.
4. Cook the cauliflower for 10 minutes, shake the basket, and continue cooking another 10 minutes (or until the florets are lightly browned).
5. Remove from the air fryer and keep warm. Continue to cook until all the florets are done.
6. Before serving, lightly squeeze lemon over the top. Serve warm.

Cajun-spiced Pickle Chips

Servings: 4
Cooking Time: 20 Minutes
Ingredients:
- 16 oz canned pickle slices
- ½ cup flour
- 2 tbsp cornmeal
- 3 tsp Cajun seasoning
- 1 tbsp dried parsley
- 1 egg, beaten
- ¼ tsp hot sauce
- ½ cup buttermilk
- 3 tbsp light mayonnaise
- 3 tbsp chopped chives
- ⅛ tsp garlic powder
- ⅛ tsp onion powder
- Salt and pepper to taste

Directions:
1. Preheat air fryer to 350°F/175°C. Mix flour, cornmeal, Cajun seasoning, and parsley in a bowl. Put the beaten egg in a small bowl nearby. One at a time, dip a pickle slice in the egg, then roll in the crumb mixture. Gently press the crumbs, so they stick to the pickle. Place the chips in the greased frying basket and Air Fry for 7-9 minutes, flipping once until golden and crispy. In a bowl, whisk hot sauce, buttermilk, mayonnaise, chives, garlic and onion powder, salt, and pepper. Serve with pickles.

Fried String Beans With Greek Sauce

Servings: 4
Cooking Time: 10 Minutes
Ingredients:
- 1 egg
- 1 tbsp flour
- ¼ tsp paprika
- ½ tsp garlic powder
- Salt to taste
- ¼ cup bread crumbs
- ¼ lemon zest
- ½ lb whole string beans
- ½ cup Greek yogurt
- 1 tbsp lemon juice
- ⅛ tsp cayenne pepper

Directions:
1. Preheat air fryer to 380°F195°C. Whisk the egg and 2 tbsp of water in a bowl until frothy. Sift the flour, paprika, garlic powder, and salt in another bowl, then stir in the bread crumbs. Dip each string bean into the egg mixture, then roll into the bread crumb mixture. Put the string beans in a single layer in the greased frying basket. Air Fry them for 5 minutes until the breading is golden brown. Stir the yogurt, lemon juice and zest, salt, and cayenne in a small bowl. Serve the bean fries with lemon-yogurt sauce.

Green Olive And Mushroom Tapenade

Servings: 1
Cooking Time: 10 Minutes
Ingredients:
- ¾ pound Brown or Baby Bella mushrooms, sliced
- 1½ cups (about ½ pound) Pitted green olives
- 3 tablespoons Olive oil
- 1½ tablespoons Fresh oregano leaves, loosely packed
- ¼ teaspoon Ground black pepper

Directions:
1. Preheat the air fryer to 400°F/205°C.
2. When the machine is at temperature, arrange the mushroom slices in as close to an even layer as possible in the basket. They will overlap and even stack on top of each other.
3. Air-fry for 10 minutes, tossing the basket and rearranging the mushrooms every 2 minutes, until shriveled but with still-noticeable moisture.
4. Pour the mushrooms into a food processor. Add the olives, olive oil, oregano leaves, and pepper. Cover and process until grainy, not too much, just not fully smooth for better texture, stopping the machine at least once to scrape down the inside of the canister. Scrape the tapenade into a bowl and serve warm, or cover and refrigerate for up to 4 days. (The tapenade will taste better if it comes back to room temperature before serving.)

Chinese-style Potstickers

Servings: 6
Cooking Time: 30 Minutes
Ingredients:
- 1 cup shredded Chinese cabbage
- ¼ cup chopped shiitake mushrooms
- ¼ cup grated carrots
- 2 tbsp minced chives
- 2 garlic cloves, minced
- 2 tsp grated fresh ginger
- 12 dumpling wrappers
- 2 tsp sesame oil

Directions:
1. Preheat air fryer to 370°F/185°C. Toss the Chinese cabbage, shiitake mushrooms, carrots, chives, garlic, and ginger in a baking pan and stir. Place the pan in the fryer and Bake for 3-6 minutes. Put a dumpling wrapper on a clean workspace, then top with a tablespoon of the veggie mix.
2. Fold the wrapper in half to form a half-circle and use water to seal the edges. Repeat with remaining wrappers and filling. Brush the potstickers with sesame oil and arrange them on the frying basket. Air Fry for 5 minutes until the bottoms should are golden brown. Take the pan out, add 1 tbsp of water, and put it back in the fryer to Air Fry for 4-6 minutes longer. Serve hot.

Oregano Cheese Rolls

Servings: 4
Cooking Time: 25 Minutes
Ingredients:
- ¼ cup grated cheddar cheese
- ¼ cup blue cheese, crumbled
- 8 flaky pastry dough sheets
- 1 tbsp vegetable oil
- 1 tsp dry oregano

Directions:
1. Preheat air fryer to 350°F/175°C. Mix the cheddar cheese, blue cheese, and oregano in a bowl. Divide the cheese mixture between pastry sheets and seal the seams with a touch of water. Brush the pastry rolls with vegetable oil. Arrange them on the greased frying basket and Bake for 15 minutes or until the pastry crust is golden brown and the cheese is melted. Serve hot.

Wrapped Shrimp Bites

Servings: 4
Cooking Time: 15 Minutes
Ingredients:
- 2 jumbo shrimp, peeled
- 2 bacon strips, sliced
- 2 tbsp lemon juice
- ½ tsp chipotle powder
- ½ tsp garlic salt

Directions:
1. Preheat air fryer to 350°F/175°C. Wrap the bacon around the shrimp and place the shrimp in the foil-lined frying basket, seam side down. Drizzle with lemon juice, chipotle powder and garlic salt. Air Fry for 10 minutes, turning the shrimp once until cooked through and bacon is crispy. Serve hot.

Piri Piri Chicken Wings

Servings: 4
Cooking Time: 45 Minutes
Ingredients:
- 1 cup crushed cracker crumbs
- 1 tbsp sweet paprika
- 1 tbsp smoked paprika
- 1 tbsp Piri Piri seasoning
- 1 tsp sea salt
- 2 tsp onion powder
- 1 tsp garlic powder
- 2 lb chicken drumettes
- 2 tbsp olive oil

Directions:
1. Preheat the air fryer to 380°F/195°C. Combine the cracker crumbs, paprikas, Piri Piri seasoning, sea salt, onion and garlic powders in a bowl and mix well. Pour into a screw-top glass jar and set aside. Put the drumettes in a large bowl, drizzle with the olive oil, and toss to coat. Sprinkle 1/3 cup of the breading mix over the meat and press the mix into the drumettes. Put half the drumettes in the frying basket and Air Fry for 20-25 minutes, shaking the basket once until golden and crisp. Serve hot.

Asian Five-spice Wings

Servings: 4
Cooking Time: 15 Minutes
Ingredients:
- 2 pounds chicken wings
- ½ cup Asian-style salad dressing
- 2 tablespoons Chinese five-spice powder

Directions:
1. Cut off wing tips and discard or freeze for stock. Cut remaining wing pieces in two at the joint.
2. Place wing pieces in a large sealable plastic bag. Pour in the Asian dressing, seal bag, and massage the marinade into the wings until well coated. Refrigerate for at least an hour.
3. Remove wings from bag, drain off excess marinade, and place wings in air fryer basket.
4. Cook at 360°F/180°C for 15minutes or until juices run clear. About halfway through cooking time, shake the basket or stir wings for more even cooking.
5. Transfer cooked wings to plate in a single layer. Sprinkle half of the Chinese five-spice powder on the wings, turn, and sprinkle other side with remaining seasoning.

Cheeseburger Slider Pockets

Servings: 4
Cooking Time: 13 Minutes
Ingredients:
- 1 pound extra lean ground beef
- 2 teaspoons steak seasoning
- 2 tablespoons Worcestershire sauce
- 8 ounces Cheddar cheese
- ⅓ cup ketchup
- ¼ cup light mayonnaise
- 1 tablespoon pickle relish
- 1 pound frozen bread dough, defrosted
- 1 egg, beaten
- sesame seeds
- vegetable or olive oil, in a spray bottle

Directions:
1. Combine the ground beef, steak seasoning and Worcestershire sauce in a large bowl. Divide the meat mixture into 12 equal portions. Cut the Cheddar cheese into twelve 2-inch squares, about ¼-inch thick. Stuff a square of cheese into the center of each portion of meat and shape into a 3-inch patty.
2. Make the slider sauce by combining the ketchup, mayonnaise, and relish in a small bowl. Set aside.
3. Cut the bread dough into twelve pieces. Shape each piece of dough into a ball and use a rolling pin to roll them out into 4-inch circles. Dollop ½ teaspoon of the slider sauce into the center of each dough circle. Place a beef patty on top of the sauce and wrap the dough around the patty, pinching the dough together to seal the pocket shut. Try not to stretch the dough too much when bringing the edges together. Brush both sides of the slider pocket with the beaten egg. Sprinkle sesame seeds on top of each pocket.
4. Preheat the air fryer to 350°F/175°C.
5. Spray or brush the bottom of the air fryer basket with oil. Air-fry the slider pockets four at a time. Transfer the slider pockets to the air fryer basket, seam side down and air-fry at 350°F/175°C for 10 minutes, until the dough is golden brown. Flip the slider pockets over and air-fry for another 3 minutes. When all the batches are done, pop all the sliders into the air fryer for a few minutes to re-heat and serve them hot out of the fryer.

Prosciutto Mozzarella Bites

Servings: 8
Cooking Time: 6 Minutes
Ingredients:
- 8 pieces full-fat mozzarella string cheese
- 8 thin slices prosciutto
- 16 basil leaves

Directions:
1. Preheat the air fryer to 360°F/180°C.
2. Cut the string cheese in half across the center, not lengthwise. Do the same with the prosciutto.
3. Place a piece of prosciutto onto a clean workspace. Top the prosciutto with a basil leaf and then a piece of string cheese. Roll up the string cheese inside the prosciutto and secure with a wooden toothpick. Repeat with the remaining cheese sticks.
4. Place the prosciutto mozzarella bites into the air fryer basket and cook for 6 minutes, checking for doneness at 4 minutes.

Grilled Ham & Muenster Cheese On Raisin Bread

Servings: 1
Cooking Time: 10 Minutes
Ingredients:
- 2 slices raisin bread
- 2 tablespoons butter, softened
- 2 teaspoons honey mustard
- 3 slices thinly sliced honey ham (about 3 ounces)
- 4 slices Muenster cheese (about 3 ounces)
- 2 toothpicks

Directions:
1. Preheat the air fryer to 370°F/185°C.
2. Spread the softened butter on one side of both slices of raisin bread and place the bread, buttered side down on the counter. Spread the honey mustard on the other side of each slice of bread. Layer 2 slices of cheese, the ham and the remaining 2 slices of cheese on one slice of bread and top with the other slice of bread. Remember to leave the buttered side of the bread on the outside.
3. Transfer the sandwich to the air fryer basket and secure the sandwich with toothpicks.
4. Air-fry at 370°F/185°C for 5 minutes. Flip the sandwich over, remove the toothpicks and air-fry for another 5 minutes. Cut the sandwich in half and enjoy!!

Cholula Avocado Fries

Servings: 2
Cooking Time: 20 Minutes
Ingredients:
- 1 egg, beaten
- ¼ cup flour
- 2 tbsp ground flaxseed
- ¼ tsp Cholula sauce
- Salt to taste
- 1 avocado, cut into fries

Directions:
1. Preheat air fryer to 375°F/190°C. Mix the egg and Cholula sauce in a bowl. In another bowl, combine the remaining ingredients, except for the avocado. Submerge avocado slices in the egg mixture and dredge them into the flour to coat. Place the fries in the lightly greased frying basket and Air Fry for 5 minutes. Serve immediately.

Crispy Curried Sweet Potato Fries

Servings: 4
Cooking Time: 20 Minutes
Ingredients:
- ½ cup sour cream
- ½ cup peach chutney
- 3 tsp curry powder
- 2 sweet potatoes, julienned
- 1 tbsp olive oil
- Salt and pepper to taste

Directions:
1. Preheat air fryer to 390°F/200°C. Mix together sour cream, peach chutney, and 1 ½ tsp curry powder in a small bowl. Set aside. In a medium bowl, add sweet potatoes, olive oil, the rest of the curry powder, salt, and pepper. Toss to coat. Place the potatoes in the frying basket. Bake for about 6 minutes, then shake the basket once. Cook for an additional 4 -6 minutes or until the potatoes are golden and crispy. Serve the fries hot in a basket along with the chutney sauce for dipping.

Tomato & Halloumi Bruschetta

Servings: 4
Cooking Time: 20 Minutes
Ingredients:
- 2 tbsp softened butter
- 8 French bread slices
- 1 cup grated halloumi cheese
- ½ cup basil pesto
- 12 chopped cherry tomatoes
- 2 green onions, thinly sliced

Directions:
1. Preheat air fryer to 350°F/175°C. Spread butter on one side of the bread. Place butter-side up in the frying basket. Bake until the bread is slightly brown, 3-5 minutes. Remove the bread and top it with halloumi cheese. Melt the cheese on the bread in the air fryer for another 1-3 minutes.
2. Meanwhile, mix pesto, cherry tomatoes, and green onions in a small bowl. When the cheese has melted, take the bread out of the fryer and arrange on a plate. Top with pesto mix and serve.

Marmalade-almond Topped Brie

Servings:6
Cooking Time: 35 Minutes
Ingredients:
- 1 cup almonds
- 1 egg white, beaten
- ⅛ tsp ground cumin
- ⅛ tsp cayenne pepper
- 1 tsp ground cinnamon
- ¼ tsp powdered sugar
- 1 round Brie cheese
- 2 tbsp orange marmalade

Directions:
1. Preheat air fryer to 325ºF/160°C. In a bowl, mix the beaten egg white and almonds. In another bowl, mix the spices and sugar. Stir in almonds, drained of excess egg white. Transfer the almonds to the frying basket and Bake for 12 minutes, tossing once. Let cool for 5 minutes. When cooled, chop into smaller bits. Adjust the air fryer temperature to 400°F/205°C. Place the Brie on a parchment-lined pizza pan and Bake for 10 minutes. Transfer the Brie to a serving plate, spread orange marmalade on top, and garnish with spiced walnuts. Serve and enjoy!

Corn Tortilla Chips

Servings: 4
Cooking Time: 12 Minutes
Ingredients:
- Eight 6-inch corn tortillas
- ½ teaspoon sea salt
- ¼ teaspoon ground cumin
- ¼ teaspoon chili powder
- ¼ teaspoon garlic powder
- ⅛ teaspoon onion powder
- 1 tablespoon avocado oil

Directions:
1. Cut each corn tortilla into quarters, creating 32 chips in total.
2. Preheat the air fryer to 350°F/175°C.
3. In a small bowl, mix together the sea salt, cumin, chili powder, garlic powder, and onion powder.
4. Spray or brush one side of the tortillas with avocado oil. Sprinkle the seasoning mixture evenly over the oiled side of the chips.
5. Working in batches, place half the chips in the air fryer basket. Cook for 8 minutes, shake the basket, and cook another 2 to 4 minutes, checking for crispness. When the chips are golden brown, spread them out onto paper towels and allow them to cool for 3 minutes before serving. Repeat with the remaining chips.

Cinnamon Sweet Potato Fries

Servings: 5
Cooking Time: 30 Minutes
Ingredients:
- 3 sweet potatoes
- 2 tsp butter, melted
- 1 tsp cinnamon
- Salt and pepper to taste

Directions:
1. Preheat air fryer to 400°F/205°C. Peel the potatoes and slice them thinly crosswise. Transfer the slices to a large bowl. Toss with butter, cinnamon, salt, and pepper until fully coated. Place half of the slices into the air fryer. Stacking is ok. Air Fry for 10 minutes. Shake the basket, and cook for another 10 -12 minutes until crispy. Serve hot.

Onion Puffs

Servings: 14
Cooking Time: 8 Minutes
Ingredients:
- Vegetable oil spray
- ¾ cup Chopped yellow or white onion
- ½ cup Seasoned Italian-style panko bread crumbs
- 4½ tablespoons All-purpose flour
- 4½ tablespoons Whole, low-fat, or fat-free milk
- 1½ tablespoons Yellow cornmeal
- 1¼ teaspoons Granulated white sugar
- ½ teaspoon Baking powder
- ¼ teaspoon Table salt

Directions:
1. Cut or tear a piece of aluminum foil so that it lines the air fryer's basket with a ½-inch space on each of its four sides. Lightly coat the foil with vegetable oil spray, then set the foil sprayed side up inside the basket.
2. Preheat the air fryer to 400°F/205°C.
3. Stir the onion, bread crumbs, flour, milk, cornmeal, sugar, baking powder, and salt in a bowl to form a thick batter.

4. Remove the basket from the machine. Drop the onion batter by 2-tablespoon measures onto the foil, spacing the mounds evenly across its surface. Return the basket to the machine and air-fry undisturbed for 4 minutes.

5. Remove the basket from the machine. Lightly coat the puffs with vegetable oil spray. Use kitchen tongs to pick up a corner of the foil, then gently pull it out of the basket, letting the puffs slip onto the basket directly. Return the basket to the machine and continue air-frying undisturbed for 8 minutes, or until brown and crunchy.

6. Use kitchen tongs to transfer the puffs to a wire rack or a serving platter. Cool for 5 minutes before serving.

Crispy Ravioli Bites

Servings: 5
Cooking Time: 7 Minutes
Ingredients:
- ⅓ cup All-purpose flour
- 1 Large egg(s), well beaten
- ⅔ cup Seasoned Italian-style dried bread crumbs
- 10 ounces (about 20) Frozen mini ravioli, meat or cheese, thawed
- Olive oil spray

Directions:
1. Preheat the air fryer to 400°F/205°C.
2. Pour the flour into a medium bowl. Set up and fill two shallow soup plates or small pie plates on your counter: one with the beaten egg(s) and one with the bread crumbs.
3. Pour all the ravioli into the flour and toss well to coat. Pick up 1 ravioli, gently shake off any excess flour, and dip the ravioli in the egg(s), coating both sides. Let any excess egg slip back into the rest, then set the ravioli in the bread crumbs, turning it several times until lightly and evenly coated on all sides. Set aside on a cutting board and continue on with the remaining ravioli.
4. Lightly coat the ravioli on both sides with olive oil spray, then set them in the basket in as close to a single layer as you can. Some can lean up against the side of the basket. Air-fry for 7 minutes, tossing the basket at the 4-minute mark to rearrange the pieces, until brown and crisp.
5. Pour the contents of the basket onto a wire rack. Cool for 5 minutes before serving.

Cinnamon Pita Chips

Servings: 4
Cooking Time: 6 Minutes
Ingredients:
- 2 tablespoons sugar
- 2 teaspoons cinnamon
- 2 whole 6-inch pitas, whole grain or white
- oil for misting or cooking spray

Directions:
1. Mix sugar and cinnamon together.
2. Cut each pita in half and each half into 4 wedges. Break apart each wedge at the fold.
3. Mist one side of pita wedges with oil or cooking spray. Sprinkle them all with half of the cinnamon sugar.
4. Turn the wedges over, mist the other side with oil or cooking spray, and sprinkle with the remaining cinnamon sugar.
5. Place pita wedges in air fryer basket and cook at 330°F/165°C for 2minutes.
6. Shake basket and cook 2 more minutes. Shake again, and if needed cook 2 more minutes, until crisp. Watch carefully because at this point they will cook very quickly.

Artichoke Samosas

Servings: 6
Cooking Time: 25 Minutes

Ingredients:
- ½ cup minced artichoke hearts
- ¼ cup ricotta cheese
- 1 egg white
- 3 tbsp grated mozzarella
- ½ tsp dried thyme
- 6 phyllo dough sheets
- 2 tbsp melted butter
- 1 cup mango chutney

Directions:
1. Preheat air fryer to 400°F/205°C. Mix together ricotta cheese, egg white, artichoke hearts, mozzarella cheese, and thyme in a small bowl until well blended. When you bring out the phyllo dough, cover it with a damp kitchen towel so that it doesn't dry out while you are working with it. Take one sheet of phyllo and place it on the work surface.
2. Cut it into thirds lengthwise. At the base of each strip, place about 1 ½ tsp of filling. Fold the bottom right-hand tip of the strip over to the left-hand side to make a triangle. Continue flipping and folding triangles along the strip. Brush the triangle with butter to seal the edges. Place triangles in the greased frying basket and Bake until golden and crisp, 4 minutes. Serve with mango chutney.

Hot Shrimp

Servings: 4
Cooking Time: 15 Minutes
Ingredients:
- 1 lb shrimp, cleaned and deveined
- 4 tbsp olive oil
- ½ lime, juiced
- 3 garlic cloves, minced
- ½ tsp salt
- ¼ tsp chili powder

Directions:
1. Preheat air fryer to 380°F/195°C. Toss the shrimp with 2 tbsp of olive oil, lime juice, 1/3 of garlic, salt, and red chili powder in a bowl. Mix the remaining olive oil and garlic in a small ramekin. Pour the shrimp into the center of a piece of aluminum foil, then fold the sides up and crimp the edges so that it forms an aluminum foil bowl that is open on top. Put the resulting packet into the frying basket.

Cheesy Spinach Dip(1)

Servings: 6
Cooking Time: 35 Minutes
Ingredients:
- ½ can refrigerated breadstick dough
- 8 oz feta cheese, cubed
- ¼ cup sour cream
- ½ cup baby spinach
- ½ cup grated Swiss cheese
- 2 green onions, chopped
- 2 tbsp melted butter
- 4 tsp grated Parmesan cheese

Directions:
1. Preheat air fryer to 320°F/160°C. Blend together feta, sour cream, spinach, Swiss cheese, and green onions in a bowl. Spread into the pan and Bake until hot, about 8 minutes. Unroll six of the breadsticks and cut in half crosswise to make 12 pieces. Carefully stretch each piece and tie into a loose knot. Tuck in the ends to prevent burning.
2. When the dip is ready, remove the pan from the air fryer and place each bread knot on top of the dip until the dip is covered. Brush melted butter on each knot and sprinkle with Parmesan. Bake until the knots are golden, 8-13 minutes. Serve warm.

Cocktail Beef Bites

Servings: 4
Cooking Time: 30 Minutes
Ingredients:
- 1 lb sirloin tip, cubed
- 1 cup cheese pasta sauce
- 1 ½ cups soft bread crumbs
- 2 tbsp olive oil
- ½ tsp garlic powder
- ½ tsp dried thyme

Directions:
1. Preheat air fryer to 360°F/180°C. Toss the beef and the pasta sauce in a medium bowl. Set aside. In a shallow bowl, mix bread crumbs, oil, garlic, and thyme until well combined. Drop the cubes in the crumb mixture to coat. Place them in the greased frying basket and Bake for 6-8 minutes, shaking once until the beef is crisp and browned. Serve warm with cocktail forks or toothpicks.

Crab Toasts

Servings: 15
Cooking Time: 5 Minutes
Ingredients:
- 1 6-ounce can flaked crabmeat, well drained
- 3 tablespoons light mayonnaise
- ½ teaspoon lemon juice
- 1 teaspoon Worcestershire sauce
- ¼ cup shredded sharp Cheddar cheese
- ¼ cup shredded Parmesan cheese
- 1 loaf artisan bread, French bread, or baguette, cut into slices ⅜-inch thick

Directions:
1. Mix together all ingredients except the bread slices.
2. Spread each slice of bread with a thin layer of crabmeat mixture. (For a bread slice measuring 2 x 1½ inches you will need about ½ tablespoon of crab mixture.)
3. Place in air fryer basket in single layer and cook at 360°F/180°C for 5minutes or until tops brown and toast is crispy.
4. Repeat step 3 to cook remaining crab toasts.

Olive & Pepper Tapenade

Servings: 4
Cooking Time: 10 Minutes
Ingredients:
- 1 red bell pepper
- 3 tbsp olive oil
- ½ cup black olives, chopped
- 1 garlic clove, minced
- ½ tsp dried oregano
- 1 tbsp white wine juice

Directions:
1. Preheat air fryer to 380°F/195°C. Lightly brush the outside of the bell pepper with some olive oil and put it in the frying basket. Roast for 5 minutes. Combine the remaining olive oil with olives, garlic, oregano, and white wine in a bowl. Remove the red pepper from the air fryer, then gently slice off the stem and discard the seeds. Chop into small pieces. Add the chopped pepper to the olive mixture and stir all together until combined. Serve and enjoy!

Asian-style Shrimp Toast

Servings: 4
Cooking Time: 25 Minutes
Ingredients:
- 8 large raw shrimp, chopped
- 1 egg white
- 2 garlic cloves, minced
- 1 red chili, minced
- 1 celery stalk, minced
- 2 tbsp cornstarch
- ¼ tsp Chinese five-spice
- 3 firm bread slices

Directions:
1. Preheat air fryer to 350°F/175°C. Add the shrimp, egg white, garlic, red chili, celery, corn starch, and five-spice powder in a bowl and combine. Place 1/3 of the shrimp mix on a slice of bread, smearing it to the edges, then slice the bread into 4 strips. Lay the strips in the frying basket in a single layer and Air Fry for 3-6 minutes until golden and crispy. Repeat until all strips are cooked. Serve hot.

Sausage And Cheese Rolls

Servings: 3
Cooking Time: 18 Minutes
Ingredients:
- 3 3- to 3½-ounce sweet or hot Italian sausage links
- 2 1-ounce string cheese stick(s), unwrapped and cut in half lengthwise
- Three quarters from one thawed sheet (cut the sheet into four quarters; wrap and refreeze one of them) A 17.25-ounce box frozen puff pastry

Directions:
1. Preheat the air fryer to 400°F/205°C.
2. When the machine is at temperature, set the sausage links in the basket and air-fry undisturbed for 12 minutes, or until cooked through.
3. Use kitchen tongs to transfer the links to a wire rack. Cool for 15 minutes. (If necessary, pour out any rendered fat that has collected below the basket in the machine.)
4. Cut the sausage links in half lengthwise. Sandwich half a string cheese stick between two sausage halves, trimming the ends so the cheese doesn't stick out beyond the meat.
5. Roll each piece of puff pastry into a 6 x 6-inch square on a clean, dry work surface. Set the sausage-cheese sandwich at one edge and roll it up in the dough. The ends will be open like a pig-in-a-blanket. Repeat with the remaining puff pastry, sausage, and cheese.
6. Set the rolls seam side down in the basket. Air-fry undisturbed for 6 minutes, or until puffed and golden brown.
7. Use a nonstick-safe spatula, and perhaps a flatware fork for balance, to transfer the rolls to a wire rack. Cool for at least 5 minutes before serving.

Cheesy Green Wonton Triangles

Servings: 20 Wontons
Cooking Time: 55 Minutes
Ingredients:
- 6 oz marinated artichoke hearts
- 6 oz cream cheese
- ¼ cup sour cream
- ¼ cup grated Parmesan
- ¼ cup grated cheddar
- 5 oz chopped kale
- 2 garlic cloves, chopped
- Salt and pepper to taste
- 20 wonton wrappers

Directions:
1. Microwave cream cheese in a bowl for 20 seconds. Combine with sour cream, Parmesan, cheddar, kale, artichoke hearts, garlic, salt, and pepper. Lay out the wrappers on a cutting board. Scoop 1 ½ tsp of cream cheese mixture on top of the wrapper. Fold up diagonally to form a triangle. Bring together the two bottom corners. Squeeze out any air and press together to seal the edges.
2. Preheat air fryer to 375°F/190°C. Place a batch of wonton in the greased frying basket and Bake for 10 minutes. Flip them and cook for 5-8 minutes until crisp and golden. Serve.

Barbecue Chicken Nachos

Servings: 3
Cooking Time: 5 Minutes
Ingredients:
- 3 heaping cups (a little more than 3 ounces) Corn tortilla chips (gluten-free, if a concern)
- ¾ cup Shredded deboned and skinned rotisserie chicken meat (gluten-free, if a concern)
- 3 tablespoons Canned black beans, drained and rinsed
- 9 rings Pickled jalapeño slices
- 4 Small pickled cocktail onions, halved
- 3 tablespoons Barbecue sauce (any sort)
- ¾ cup (about 3 ounces) Shredded Cheddar cheese

Directions:
1. Preheat the air fryer to 400°F/205°C.
2. Cut a circle of parchment paper to line a 6-inch round cake pan for a small air fryer, a 7-inch round cake pan for a medium air fryer, or an 8-inch round cake pan for a large machine.
3. Fill the pan with an even layer of about two-thirds of the chips. Sprinkle the chicken evenly over the chips. Set the pan in the basket and air-fry undisturbed for 2 minutes.
4. Remove the basket from the machine. Scatter the beans, jalapeño rings, and pickled onion halves over the chicken. Drizzle the barbecue sauce over everything, then sprinkle the cheese on top.
5. Return the basket to the machine and air-fry undisturbed for 3 minutes, or until the cheese has melted and is bubbly. Remove the pan from the machine and cool for a couple of minutes before serving.

Chili Black Bean Empanadas

Servings: 4
Cooking Time: 20 Minutes
Ingredients:
- ½ cup cooked black beans
- ¼ cup white onions, diced
- 1 tsp red chili powder
- ½ tsp paprika
- ½ tsp garlic salt
- ½ tsp ground cumin
- ½ tsp ground cinnamon
- 4 empanada dough shells

Directions:
1. Preheat air fryer to 350°F/175°C. Stir-fry black beans and onions in a pan over medium heat for 5 minutes. Add chili, paprika, garlic salt, cumin, and cinnamon. Set aside covered when onions are soft and the beans are hot.
2. On a clean workspace, lay the empanada shells. Spoon bean mixture onto shells without spilling. Fold the shells over to cover fully. Seal the edges with water and press with a fork. Transfer the empanadas to the foil-lined frying basket and Bake for 15 minutes, flipping once halfway through cooking. Cook until golden. Serve.

Spicy Pearl Onion Dip

Servings: 4
Cooking Time: 20 Minutes+chilling Time
Ingredients:
- 2 cups peeled pearl onions
- 3 garlic cloves
- 3 tbsp olive oil
- Salt and pepper to taste
- 1 cup Greek yogurt
- ¼ tsp Worcestershire sauce
- 1 tbsp lemon juice
- ⅛ tsp red pepper flakes
- 1 tbsp chives, chopped

Directions:
1. Preheat air fryer to 360°F/180°C. Place the onions, garlic, and 2 tbsp of olive oil in a bowl and combine until the onions are well coated. Pour the mixture into the frying basket and Roast for 11-13 minutes. Transfer the garlic and onions to your food processor. Pulse the vegetables several times until the onions are minced but still have some chunks.
2. Combine the garlic and onions and the remaining olive oil, along with the salt, yogurt, Worcestershire sauce, lemon juice, black pepper, chives and red pepper flakes in a bowl. Cover and chill for at least 1 hour. Serve with toasted bread if desired.

Shrimp Egg Rolls

Servings: 8
Cooking Time: 10 Minutes
Ingredients:
- 1 tablespoon vegetable oil
- ½ head green or savoy cabbage, finely shredded
- 1 cup shredded carrots
- 1 cup canned bean sprouts, drained
- 1 tablespoon soy sauce
- ½ teaspoon sugar
- 1 teaspoon sesame oil
- ¼ cup hoisin sauce
- freshly ground black pepper
- 1 pound cooked shrimp, diced
- ¼ cup scallions
- 8 egg roll wrappers
- vegetable oil
- duck sauce

Directions:
1. Preheat a large sauté pan over medium-high heat. Add the oil and cook the cabbage, carrots and bean sprouts until they start to wilt – about 3 minutes. Add the soy sauce, sugar, sesame oil, hoisin sauce and black pepper. Sauté for a few more minutes. Stir in the shrimp and scallions and cook until the vegetables are just tender. Transfer the mixture to a colander in a bowl to cool. Press or squeeze out any excess water from the filling so that you don't end up with soggy egg rolls.
2. To make the egg rolls, place the egg roll wrappers on a flat surface with one of the points facing towards you so they look like diamonds. Dividing the filling evenly between the eight wrappers, spoon the mixture onto the center of the egg roll wrappers. Spread the filling across the center of the wrappers from the left corner to the right corner, but leave 2 inches from each corner empty. Brush the empty sides of the wrapper with a little water. Fold the bottom corner of the wrapper tightly up over the filling, trying to avoid making any air pockets. Fold the left corner in toward the center and then the right corner toward the center. It should now look like an envelope. Tightly roll the egg roll from the bottom to the top open corner. Press to seal the egg roll together, brushing with a little extra water if need be. Repeat this technique with all 8 egg rolls.
3. Preheat the air fryer to 370°F/185°C.
4. Spray or brush all sides of the egg rolls with vegetable oil. Air-fry four egg rolls at a time for 10 minutes, turning them over halfway through the cooking time.
5. Serve hot with duck sauce or your favorite dipping sauce.

Blooming Onion

Servings: 4
Cooking Time: 25 Minutes
Ingredients:
- 1 large Vidalia onion, peeled
- 2 eggs
- ½ cup milk
- 1 cup flour
- 1 teaspoon salt
- ½ teaspoon freshly ground black pepper
- ¼ teaspoon ground cayenne pepper
- ½ teaspoon paprika
- ½ teaspoon garlic powder
- Dipping Sauce:
- ½ cup mayonnaise
- ½ cup ketchup
- 1 teaspoon Worcestershire sauce
- ½ teaspoon ground cayenne pepper
- ½ teaspoon paprika
- ½ teaspoon onion powder

Directions:
1. Cut off the top inch of the onion, leaving the root end of the onion intact. Place the now flat, stem end of the onion down on a cutting board with the root end facing up. Make 16 slices around the onion, starting with your knife tip ½-inch away from the root so that you never slice through the root. Begin by making slices at 12, 3, 6 and 9 o'clock around the onion. Then make three slices down the onion in between each of the original four slices. Turn the onion over, gently separate the onion petals, and remove the loose pieces of onion in the center.
2. Combine the eggs and milk in a bowl. In a second bowl, combine the flour, salt, black pepper, cayenne pepper, paprika, and garlic powder.
3. Preheat the air fryer to 350°F/175°C.
4. Place the onion cut side up into a third empty bowl. Sprinkle the flour mixture all over the onion to cover it and get in between the onion petals. Turn the onion over to carefully shake off the excess flour and then transfer the onion to the empty flour bowl, again cut side up.
5. Pour the egg mixture all over the onion to cover all the flour. Let it soak for a minute in the mixture. Carefully remove the onion, tipping it upside down to drain off any excess egg, and transfer it to the empty egg bowl, again cut side up.
6. Finally, sprinkle the flour mixture over the onion a second time, making sure the onion is well coated and all the petals have the seasoned flour mixture on them. Carefully turn the onion over, shake off any excess flour and transfer it to a plate or baking sheet. Spray the onion generously with vegetable oil.
7. Transfer the onion, cut side up to the air fryer basket and air-fry for 25 minutes. The onion petals will open more fully as it cooks, so spray with more vegetable oil at least twice during the cooking time.
8. While the onion is cooking, make the dipping sauce by combining all the dip ingredients and mixing well. Serve the Blooming Onion as soon as it comes out of the air fryer with dipping sauce on the side.

Chicken Shawarma Bites

Servings: 6
Cooking Time: 22 Minutes
Ingredients:
- 1½ pounds Boneless skinless chicken thighs, trimmed of any fat and cut into 1-inch pieces
- 1½ tablespoons Olive oil
- Up to 1½ tablespoons Minced garlic
- ½ teaspoon Table salt
- ¼ teaspoon Ground cardamom
- ¼ teaspoon Ground cinnamon
- ¼ teaspoon Ground cumin
- ¼ teaspoon Mild paprika
- Up to a ¼ teaspoon Grated nutmeg
- ¼ teaspoon Ground black pepper

Directions:
1. Preheat the air fryer to 400°F/205°C.
2. Mix all the ingredients in a large bowl until the chicken is thoroughly and evenly coated in the oil and spices.
3. When the machine is at temperature, scrape the coated chicken pieces into the basket and spread them out into one layer as much as you can. Air-fry for 22 minutes, shaking the basket at least three times during cooking to rearrange the pieces, until well browned and crisp.
4. Pour the chicken pieces onto a wire rack. Cool for 5 minutes before serving.

Fiery Cheese Sticks

Servings: 4
Cooking Time: 20 Minutes + Freezing Time
Ingredients:
- 1 egg, beaten
- ½ cup dried bread crumbs
- ¼ cup ground peanuts
- 1 tbsp chili powder
- ¼ tsp ground coriander
- ¼ tsp red pepper flakes
- ⅛ tsp cayenne pepper
- 8 mozzarella cheese sticks

Directions:
1. Preheat the air fryer to 375°F/190°C. Beat the egg in a bowl, and on a plate, combine the breadcrumbs, peanuts, coriander, chili powder, pepper flakes, and cayenne. Dip each piece of string cheese in the egg, then in the breadcrumb mix. After lining a baking sheet with parchment paper, put the sticks on it and freeze them for 30 minutes. Get the sticks out of the freezer and set in the frying basket in a single layer. Spritz them with cooking oil. Air Fry for 7-9 minutes until the exterior is golden and the interior is hot and melted. Serve hot with marinara or ranch sauce.

Prosciutto Polenta Rounds

Servings: 6
Cooking Time: 40 Minutes + 10 Minutes To Cool
Ingredients:
- 1 tube precooked polenta
- 1 tbsp garlic oil
- 4 oz cream cheese, softened
- 3 tbsp mayonnaise
- 2 scallions, sliced
- 1 tbsp minced fresh chives
- 6 prosciutto slices, chopped

Directions:
1. Preheat the air fryer to 400°F/205°C. Slice the polenta crosswise into 12 rounds. Brush both sides of each round with garlic oil and put 6 of them in the frying basket. Put a rack in the basket over the polenta and add the other 6 rounds. Bake for 15 minutes, flip, and cook for 10-15 more minutes or until the polenta is crispy and golden. While the polenta is cooking, beat the cream cheese and mayo and stir in the scallions, chives, and prosciutto. When the polenta is cooked, lay out on a wire rack to cool for 15 minutes. Top with the cream cheese mix and serve.

Home-style Buffalo Chicken Wings

Servings: 4
Cooking Time: 35 Minutes
Ingredients:
- 2 lb chicken wing portions
- 6 tbsp chili sauce
- 1 tsp dried oregano
- 1 tsp smoked paprika
- 1tsp garlic powder
- ½ tsp salt
- ¼ cup crumbled blue cheese
- 1/3 cup low-fat yogurt
- ½ tbsp lemon juice
- ½ tbsp white wine vinegar
- 2 celery stalks, cut into sticks
- 2 carrots, cut into sticks

Directions:
1. Add chicken with 1 tbsp of chili sauce, oregano, garlic, paprika, and salt to a large bowl. Toss to coat well, then set aside. In a small bowl, mash blue cheese and yogurt with a fork. Stir lemon juice and vinegar until smooth and blended. Refrigerate covered until it is time to serve.
2. Preheat air fryer to 300°F/150°C. Place the chicken in the greased frying basket and Air Fry for 22 minutes, flipping the chicken once until crispy and browned. Set aside in a clean bowl. Coat with the remaining tbsp of chili sauce. Serve with celery, carrot sticks and the blue cheese dip.

Mini Frank Rolls

Servings: 4
Cooking Time: 30 Minutes
Ingredients:
- ½ can crescent rolls
- 8 mini smoked hot dogs
- ½ tsp dried rosemary

Directions:
1. Preheat air fryer to 350°F/175°C. Roll out the crescent roll dough and separate into 8 triangles. Cut each triangle in half. Place 1 hot dog at the base of the triangle and roll it up in the dough; gently press the tip in. Repeat for the rest of the rolls. Place the rolls in the greased frying basket and sprinkle with rosemary. Bake for 8-10 minutes. Serve warm. Enjoy!

Italian-style Fried Olives

Servings: 4
Cooking Time: 25 Minutes
Ingredients:
- 1 jar pitted green olives
- ½ cup all-purpose flour
- Salt and pepper to taste
- 1 tsp Italian seasoning
- ½ cup bread crumbs
- 1 egg

Directions:
1. Preheat air fryer to 400°F/205°C. Set out three small bowls. In the first, mix flour, Italian seasoning, salt and pepper. In the bowl, beat the egg. In the third bowl, add bread crumbs. Dip the olives in the flour, then the egg, then in the crumbs. When all of the olives are breaded, place them in the greased frying basket and Air Fry for 6 minutes. Turn them and cook for another 2 minutes or until brown and crispy. Serve chilled.

Shrimp Pirogues

Servings: 8
Cooking Time: 5 Minutes

Ingredients:
- 12 ounces small, peeled, and deveined raw shrimp
- 3 ounces cream cheese, room temperature
- 2 tablespoons plain yogurt
- 1 teaspoon lemon juice
- 1 teaspoon dried dill weed, crushed
- salt
- 4 small hothouse cucumbers, each approximately 6 inches long

Directions:
1. Pour 4 tablespoons water in bottom of air fryer drawer.
2. Place shrimp in air fryer basket in single layer and cook at 390°F/200°C for 5 minutes, just until done. Watch carefully because shrimp cooks quickly, and overcooking makes it tough.
3. Chop shrimp into small pieces, no larger than ½ inch. Refrigerate while mixing the remaining ingredients.
4. With a fork, mash and whip the cream cheese until smooth.
5. Stir in the yogurt and beat until smooth. Stir in lemon juice, dill weed, and chopped shrimp.
6. Taste for seasoning. If needed, add ¼ to ½ teaspoon salt to suit your taste.
7. Store in refrigerator until serving time.
8. When ready to serve, wash and dry cucumbers and split them lengthwise. Scoop out the seeds and turn cucumbers upside down on paper towels to drain for 10minutes.
9. Just before filling, wipe centers of cucumbers dry. Spoon the shrimp mixture into the pirogues and cut in half crosswise. Serve immediately.

Individual Pizzas

Servings: 2
Cooking Time: 7 Minutes
Ingredients:
- 6 ounces Purchased fresh pizza dough (not a prebaked crust)
- Olive oil spray
- 4½ tablespoons Purchased pizza sauce or purchased pesto
- ½ cup (about 2 ounces) Shredded semi-firm mozzarella

Directions:
1. Preheat the air fryer to 400°F/205°C.
2. Press the pizza dough into a 5-inch circle for a small air fryer, a 6-inch circle for a medium air fryer, or a 7-inch circle for a large machine. Generously coat the top of the dough with olive oil spray.
3. Remove the basket from the machine and set the dough oil side down in the basket. Smear the sauce or pesto over the dough, then sprinkle with the cheese.
4. Return the basket to the machine and air-fry undisturbed for 7 minutes, or until the dough is puffed and browned and the cheese has melted. (Extra toppings will not increase the cooking time, provided you add no extra cheese.)
5. Remove the basket from the machine and cool the pizza in it for 5 minutes. Use a large nonstick-safe spatula to transfer the pizza from the basket to a wire rack. Cool for 5 minutes more before serving.

Avocado Toast With Lemony Shrimp

Servings: 4
Cooking Time: 6 Minutes
Ingredients:
- 6 ounces Raw medium shrimp (30 to 35 per pound), peeled and deveined
- 1½ teaspoons Finely grated lemon zest
- 2 teaspoons Lemon juice

- 1½ teaspoons Minced garlic
- 1½ teaspoons Ground black pepper
- 4 Rye or whole-wheat bread slices (gluten-free, if a concern)
- 2 Ripe Hass avocado(s), halved, pitted, peeled and roughly chopped
- For garnishing Coarse sea salt or kosher salt

Directions:
1. Preheat the air fryer to 400°F/205°C.
2. Toss the shrimp, lemon zest, lemon juice, garlic, and pepper in a bowl until the shrimp are evenly coated.
3. When the machine is at temperature, use kitchen tongs to place the shrimp in a single layer in the basket. Air-fry undisturbed for 4 minutes, or until the shrimp are pink and barely firm. Use kitchen tongs to transfer the shrimp to a cutting board.
4. Working in batches, set as many slices of bread as will fit in the basket in one layer. Air-fry undisturbed for 2 minutes, just until warmed through and crisp. The bread will not brown much.
5. Arrange the bread slices on a clean, dry work surface. Divide the avocado bits among them and gently smash the avocado into a coarse paste with the tines of a flatware fork. Top the toasts with the shrimp and sprinkle with salt as a garnish.

Roasted Red Pepper Dip

Servings: 2
Cooking Time: 15 Minutes
Ingredients:
- 2 Medium-size red bell pepper(s)
- 1¾ cups (one 15-ounce can) Canned white beans, drained and rinsed
- 1 tablespoon Fresh oregano leaves, packed
- 3 tablespoons Olive oil
- 1 tablespoon Lemon juice
- ½ teaspoon Table salt
- ½ teaspoon Ground black pepper

Directions:
1. Preheat the air fryer to 400°F/205°C.
2. Set the pepper(s) in the basket and air-fry undisturbed for 15 minutes, until blistered and even blackened.
3. Use kitchen tongs to transfer the pepper(s) to a zip-closed plastic bag or small bowl. Seal the bag or cover the bowl with plastic wrap. Set aside for 20 minutes.
4. Peel each pepper, then stem it, cut it in half, and remove all its seeds and their white membranes.
5. Set the pieces of the pepper in a food processor. Add the beans, oregano, olive oil, lemon juice, salt, and pepper. Cover and process until smooth, stopping the machine at least once to scrape down the inside of the canister. Scrape the dip into a bowl and serve warm, or cover and refrigerate for up to 3 days (although the dip tastes best if it's allowed to come back to room temperature).

Yellow Onion Rings

Servings: 3
Cooking Time: 30 Minutes
Ingredients:
- ½ sweet yellow onion
- ½ cup buttermilk
- ¾ cup flour
- 1 tbsp cornstarch
- Salt and pepper to taste
- ¾ tsp garlic powder
- ½ tsp dried oregano

- 1 cup bread crumbs

Directions:
1. Preheat air fryer to 390°F/200°C. Cut the onion into ½-inch slices. Separate the onion slices into rings. Place the buttermilk in a bowl and set aside. In another bowl, combine the flour, cornstarch, salt, pepper, and garlic. Stir well and set aside. In a separate bowl, combine the breadcrumbs with oregano and salt.
2. Dip the rings into the buttermilk, dredge in flour, dip into the buttermilk again, and then coat into the crumb mixture. Put in the greased frying basket without overlapping. Spritz them with cooking oil and Air Fry for 13-16 minutes, shaking once or twice until the rings are crunchy and browned. Serve hot.

Classic Chicken Wings

Servings: 8
Cooking Time: 20 Minutes
Ingredients:
- 16 chicken wings
- ¼ cup all-purpose flour
- ¼ teaspoon garlic powder
- ¼ teaspoon paprika
- ½ teaspoon salt
- ½ teaspoon black pepper
- ¼ cup butter
- ½ cup hot sauce
- ½ teaspoon Worcestershire sauce
- 2 ounces crumbled blue cheese, for garnish

Directions:
1. Preheat the air fryer to 380°F/195°C.
2. Pat the chicken wings dry with paper towels.
3. In a medium bowl, mix together the flour, garlic powder, paprika, salt, and pepper. Toss the chicken wings with the flour mixture, dusting off any excess.
4. Place the chicken wings in the air fryer basket, making sure that the chicken wings aren't touching. Cook the chicken wings for 10 minutes, turn over, and cook another 5 minutes. Raise the temperature to 400°F/205°C and continue crisping the chicken wings for an additional 3 to 5 minutes.
5. Meanwhile, in a microwave-safe bowl, melt the butter and hot sauce for 1 to 2 minutes in the microwave. Remove from the microwave and stir in the Worcestershire sauce.
6. When the chicken wings have cooked, immediately transfer the chicken wings into the hot sauce mixture. Serve the coated chicken wings on a plate, and top with crumbled blue cheese.

Avocado Balls

Servings: 6
Cooking Time: 25 Minutes + Freezing Time
Ingredients:
- 2 avocados, peeled
- 1 tbsp minced cilantro
- 1 tbsp lime juice
- ½ tsp salt
- 1 egg, beaten
- 1 tbsp milk
- ¼ cup almond flour
- ½ cup ground almonds

Directions:
1. Preheat the air fryer to 400°F/205°C. Mash the avocados in a bowl with cilantro, lime juice, and salt. Line a baking sheet with parchment paper and form the mix into 12 balls. Use an ice cream scoop or ⅛-cup measure. Put them on the baking sheet and freeze for 2 hours. Beat the egg with milk in

a shallow bowl, then combine the almond flour and almonds on a plate. Dip the frozen guac balls in the egg mix, then roll them in the almond mix, coating evenly. Put half the bombs in the freezer while you cook the first group. The other 6 go in the frying basket. Mist with olive oil and Air Fry for 4-5 minutes or until they are golden. Repeat with the second batch and serve. Enjoy!

Fried Cheese Ravioli With Marinara Sauce

Servings: 4
Cooking Time: 7 Minutes
Ingredients:
- 1 pound cheese ravioli, fresh or frozen
- 2 eggs, lightly beaten
- 1 cup plain breadcrumbs
- ½ teaspoon paprika
- ½ teaspoon dried oregano
- ½ teaspoon salt
- grated Parmesan cheese
- chopped fresh parsley
- 1 to 2 cups marinara sauce (jarred or homemade)

Directions:
1. Bring a stockpot of salted water to a boil. Boil the ravioli according to the package directions and then drain. Let the cooked ravioli cool to a temperature where you can comfortably handle them.
2. While the pasta is cooking, set up a dredging station with two shallow dishes. Place the eggs into one dish. Combine the breadcrumbs, paprika, dried oregano and salt in the other dish.
3. Preheat the air fryer to 380°F/195°C.
4. Working with one at a time, dip the cooked ravioli into the egg, coating all sides. Then press the ravioli into the breadcrumbs, making sure that all sides are covered. Transfer the ravioli to the air fryer basket, cooking in batches, one layer at a time. Air-fry at 380°F/195°C for 7 minutes.
5. While the ravioli is air-frying, bring the marinara sauce to a simmer on the stovetop. Transfer to a small bowl.
6. Sprinkle a little Parmesan cheese and chopped parsley on top of the fried ravioli and serve warm with the marinara sauce on the side for dipping.

Mediterranean Potato Skins

Servings: 4
Cooking Time: 50 Minutes
Ingredients:
- 2 russet potatoes
- 3 tbsp olive oil
- Salt and pepper to taste
- 2 tbsp rosemary, chopped
- 10 Kalamata olives, diced
- ¼ cup crumbled feta
- 2 tbsp chopped dill

Directions:
1. Preheat air fryer to 380°F/195°C. Poke 2-3 holes in the potatoes with a fork. Drizzle them with some olive oil and sprinkle with salt. Put the potatoes into the frying basket and Bake for 30 minutes. When the potatoes are ready, remove them from the fryer and slice in half. Scoop out the flesh of the potatoes with a spoon, leaving a ½-inch layer of potato inside the skins, and set the skins aside.
2. Combine the scooped potato middles with the remaining olive oil, salt, black pepper, and rosemary in a medium bowl. Mix until well combined. Spoon the potato filling into the potato skins, spreading it evenly over them. Top with olives,

dill and feta. Put the loaded potato skins back into the air fryer and Bake for 15 minutes. Enjoy!

Curried Veggie Samosas

Servings: 4
Cooking Time: 30 Minutes
Ingredients:
- 4 cooked potatoes, mashed
- ¼ cup peas
- 2 tsp coconut oil
- 3 garlic cloves, minced
- 1 ½ tbsp lemon juice
- 1 ½ tsp cumin powder
- 1 tsp onion powder
- 1 tsp ground coriander
- Salt to taste
- ½ tsp curry powder
- ¼ tsp cayenne powder
- 10 rice paper wrappers
- 1 cup cilantro chutney

Directions:
1. Preheat air fryer to 390°F/200°C. In a bowl, place the mashed potatoes, peas, oil, garlic, lemon juice, cumin, onion powder, coriander, salt, curry powder, and cayenne. Stir.
2. Fill a bowl with water. Soak a rice paper wrapper in the water for a few seconds. Lay it on a flat surface. Place ¼ cup of the potato filling in the center of the wrapper and roll like a burrito or spring roll. Repeat the process until you run out of ingredients. Place the "samosas" inside in the greased frying basket, separating them. Air Fry for 8-10 minutes or until hot and crispy around the edges. Let cool for a few minutes. Enjoy with the cilantro chutney.

Jalapeño & Mozzarella Stuffed Mushrooms

Servings: 4
Cooking Time: 30 Minutes
Ingredients:
- 16 button mushrooms
- 1/3 cup salsa
- 3 garlic cloves, minced
- 1 onion, finely chopped
- 1 jalapeño pepper, minced
- ⅛ tsp cayenne pepper
- 3 tbsp shredded mozzarella
- 2 tsp olive oil

Directions:
1. Preheat air fryer to 350°F/175°C. Cut the stem off the mushrooms, then slice them finely. Set the caps aside. Combine the salsa, garlic, onion, jalapeño, cayenne, and mozzarella cheese in a bowl, then add the stems. Fill the mushroom caps with the mixture, making sure to overfill so the mix is coming out of the top. Drizzle with olive oil. Place the caps in the air fryer and Bake for 8-12 minutes. The filling should be hot and the mushrooms soft. Serve warm.

Fiery Sweet Chicken Wings

Servings: 4
Cooking Time: 30 Minutes
Ingredients:
- 8 chicken wings
- 1 tbsp olive oil
- 3 tbsp brown sugar
- 2 tbsp maple syrup
- ½ cup apple cider vinegar

- ½ tsp Aleppo pepper flakes
- Salt to taste

Directions:
1. Preheat air fryer to 390°F/200°C. Toss the wings with olive oil in a bowl. Bake in the air fryer for 20 minutes, shaking the basket twice. While the chicken is cooking, whisk together sugar, maple syrup, vinegar, Aleppo pepper flakes, and salt in a small bowl. Transfer the wings to a baking pan, then pour the sauce over the wings. Toss well to coat. Cook in the air fryer until the wings are glazed, or for another 5 minutes. Serve hot.

Fried Wontons

Servings: 24
Cooking Time: 6 Minutes
Ingredients:
- 6 ounces Lean ground beef, pork, or turkey
- 1 tablespoon Regular or reduced-sodium soy sauce or tamari sauce
- 1½ teaspoons Minced garlic
- ¾ teaspoon Ground dried ginger
- ½ teaspoon Ground white pepper
- 24 Wonton wrappers (thawed, if necessary)
- Vegetable oil spray

Directions:
1. Preheat the air fryer to 350°F/175°C .
2. Stir the ground meat, soy or tamari sauce, garlic, ginger, and white pepper in a bowl until the spices are uniformly distributed in the mixture.
3. Set a small bowl of water on a clean, dry surface or next to a clean, dry cutting board. Set one wonton wrapper on the surface. Dip your clean finger in the water, then run it along the edges of the wrapper. Set 1 teaspoon of the ground meat mixture in the center of the wrapper. Fold it over, corner to corner, to create a filled triangle. Press to seal the edges, then pull the corners on the longest side up and together over the filling to create the classic wonton shape. Press the corners together to seal. Set aside and continue filling and making more filled wontons.
4. Generously coat the filled wontons on all sides with vegetable oil spray. Arrange them in the basket in one layer and air-fry for 6 minutes, shaking the basket gently at the 2- and 4-minute marks to rearrange the wontons (but always making sure they're still in one layer), until golden brown and crisp.
5. Pour the wontons in the basket onto a wire rack or even into a serving bowl. Cool for 2 or 3 minutes (but not much longer) and serve hot.

Halloumi Fries

Servings: 3
Cooking Time: 12 Minutes
Ingredients:
- 1½ tablespoons Olive oil
- 1½ teaspoons Minced garlic
- ⅛ teaspoon Dried oregano
- ⅛ teaspoon Dried thyme
- ⅛ teaspoon Table salt
- ⅛ teaspoon Ground black pepper
- ¾ pound Halloumi

Directions:
1. Preheat the air fryer to 400°F/205°C.
2. Whisk the oil, garlic, oregano, thyme, salt, and pepper in a medium bowl.
3. Lay the piece of halloumi flat on a cutting board. Slice it widthwise into ½-inch-thick sticks. Cut each stick lengthwise into ½-inch-thick batons.

4. Put these batons into the olive oil mixture. Toss gently but well to coat.
5. Place the batons in the basket in a single layer. Air-fry undisturbed for 12 minutes, or until lightly browned, particularly at the edges.
6. Dump the fries out onto a wire rack. They may need a little coaxing with a nonstick-safe spatula to come free. Cool for a couple of minutes before serving hot.

Cheesy Pigs In A Blanket

Servings: 4
Cooking Time: 7 Minutes
Ingredients:
- 24 cocktail size smoked sausages
- 6 slices deli-sliced Cheddar cheese, each cut into 8 rectangular pieces
- 1 (8-ounce) tube refrigerated crescent roll dough
- ketchup or mustard for dipping

Directions:
1. Unroll the crescent roll dough into one large sheet. If your crescent roll dough has perforated seams, pinch or roll all the perforated seams together. Cut the large sheet of dough into 4 rectangles. Then cut each rectangle into 6 pieces by making one slice lengthwise in the middle and 2 slices horizontally. You should have 24 pieces of dough.
2. Make a deep slit lengthwise down the center of the cocktail sausage. Stuff two pieces of cheese into the slit in the sausage. Roll one piece of crescent dough around the stuffed cocktail sausage leaving the ends of the sausage exposed. Pinch the seam together. Repeat with the remaining sausages.
3. Preheat the air fryer to 350°F/175°C.
4. Air-fry in 2 batches, placing the sausages seam side down in the basket. Air-fry for 7 minutes. Serve hot with ketchup or your favorite mustard for dipping.

Pork Pot Stickers With Yum Yum Sauce

Servings: 48
Cooking Time: 8 Minutes
Ingredients:
- 1 pound ground pork
- 2 cups shredded green cabbage
- ¼ cup shredded carrot
- ½ cup finely chopped water chestnuts
- 2 teaspoons minced fresh ginger
- ¼ cup hoisin sauce
- 2 tablespoons soy sauce
- 1 tablespoon sesame oil
- freshly ground black pepper
- 3 scallions, minced
- 48 round dumpling wrappers (or wonton wrappers with the corners cut off to make them round)
- 1 tablespoon vegetable oil
- soy sauce, for serving
- Yum Yum Sauce:
- 1½ cups mayonnaise
- 2 tablespoons sugar
- 3 tablespoons rice vinegar
- 1 teaspoon soy sauce
- 2 tablespoons ketchup
- 1½ teaspoons paprika
- ¼ teaspoon ground cayenne pepper
- ¼ teaspoon garlic powder

Directions:

1. Preheat a large sauté pan over medium-high heat. Add the ground pork and brown for a few minutes. Remove the cooked pork to a bowl using a slotted spoon and discard the fat from the pan. Return the cooked pork to the sauté pan and add the cabbage, carrots and water chestnuts. Sauté for a minute and then add the fresh ginger, hoisin sauce, soy sauce, sesame oil, and freshly ground black pepper. Sauté for a few more minutes, just until cabbage and carrots are soft. Then stir in the scallions and transfer the pork filling to a bowl to cool.
2. Make the pot stickers in batches of 1 Place 12 dumpling wrappers on a flat surface. Brush a little water around the perimeter of the wrappers. Place a rounded teaspoon of the filling into the center of each wrapper. Fold the wrapper over the filling, bringing the edges together to form a half moon, sealing the edges shut. Brush a little more water on the top surface of the sealed edge of the pot sticker. Make pleats in the dough around the sealed edge by pinching the dough and folding the edge over on itself. You should have about 5 to 6 pleats in the dough. Repeat this three times until you have 48 pot stickers. Freeze the pot stickers for 2 hours (or as long as 3 weeks in an airtight container).
3. Preheat the air fryer to 400°F/205°C.
4. Air-fry the pot stickers in batches of 16. Brush or spray the pot stickers with vegetable oil just before putting them in the air fryer basket. Air-fry for 8 minutes, turning the pot stickers once or twice during the cooking process.
5. While the pot stickers are cooking, combine all the ingredients for the Yum Yum sauce in a bowl. Serve the pot stickers warm with the Yum Yum sauce and soy sauce for dipping.

Turkey Bacon Dates

Servings: 16
Cooking Time: 7 Minutes
Ingredients:
- 16 whole, pitted dates
- 16 whole almonds
- 6 to 8 strips turkey bacon

Directions:
1. Stuff each date with a whole almond.
2. Depending on the size of your stuffed dates, cut bacon strips into halves or thirds. Each strip should be long enough to wrap completely around a date.
3. Wrap each date in a strip of bacon with ends overlapping and secure with toothpicks.
4. Place in air fryer basket and cook at 390°F/200°C for 7 minutes, until bacon is as crispy as you like.
5. Drain on paper towels or wire rack. Serve hot or at room temperature.

Sweet Potato Chips

Servings: 4
Cooking Time: 10 Minutes
Ingredients:
- 2 medium sweet potatoes, washed
- 2 cups filtered water
- 1 tablespoon avocado oil
- 2 teaspoons brown sugar
- ½ teaspoon salt

Directions:
1. Using a mandolin, slice the potatoes into ⅛-inch pieces.
2. Add the water to a large bowl. Place the potatoes in the bowl, and soak for at least 30 minutes.
3. Preheat the air fryer to 350°F/175°C.
4. Drain the water and pat the chips dry with a paper towel or kitchen cloth. Toss the chips with the avocado oil, brown sugar, and salt. Liberally spray the air fryer basket with olive oil mist.
5. Set the chips inside the air fryer, separating them so they're not on top of each other. Cook for 5 minutes, shake the basket, and cook another 5 minutes, or until browned.
6. Remove and let cool a few minutes prior to serving. Repeat until all the chips are cooked.

Turkey Burger Sliders

Servings: 8
Cooking Time: 7 Minutes
Ingredients:
- 1 pound ground turkey
- ¼ teaspoon curry powder
- 1 teaspoon Hoisin sauce
- ½ teaspoon salt
- 8 slider buns
- ½ cup slivered red onions
- ½ cup slivered green or red bell pepper
- ½ cup fresh chopped pineapple (or pineapple tidbits from kids' fruit cups, drained)
- light cream cheese, softened

Directions:
1. Combine turkey, curry powder, Hoisin sauce, and salt and mix together well.
2. Shape turkey mixture into 8 small patties.
3. Place patties in air fryer basket and cook at 360°F/180°C for 7minutes, until patties are well done and juices run clear.
4. Place each patty on the bottom half of a slider bun and top with onions, peppers, and pineapple. Spread the remaining bun halves with cream cheese to taste, place on top, and serve.

Homemade French Fries

Servings: 2
Cooking Time: 25 Minutes
Ingredients:
- 2 to 3 russet potatoes, peeled and cut into ½-inch sticks
- 2 to 3 teaspoons olive or vegetable oil
- salt

Directions:
1. Bring a large saucepan of salted water to a boil on the stovetop while you peel and cut the potatoes. Blanch the potatoes in the boiling salted water for 4 minutes while you Preheat the air fryer to 400°F/205°C. Strain the potatoes and rinse them with cold water. Dry them well with a clean kitchen towel.
2. Toss the dried potato sticks gently with the oil and place them in the air fryer basket. Air-fry for 25 minutes, shaking the basket a few times while the fries cook to help them brown evenly. Season the fries with salt mid-way through cooking and serve them warm with tomato ketchup, Sriracha mayonnaise or a mix of lemon zest, Parmesan cheese and parsley.

Arancini With Sun-dried Tomatoes And Mozzarella

Servings: 6
Cooking Time: 15 Minutes
Ingredients:
- 1 tablespoon olive oil
- ½ small onion, finely chopped
- 1 cup Arborio rice
- ¼ cup white wine or dry vermouth
- 1 cup vegetable or chicken stock
- 1½ cups water

- 1 teaspoon salt
- freshly ground black pepper
- ⅓ cup grated Parmigiano-Reggiano cheese
- 2 to 3 ounces mozzarella cheese
- 2 eggs, lightly beaten
- ¼ cup chopped oil-packed sun-dried tomatoes
- 1½ cups Italian seasoned breadcrumbs, divided
- olive oil
- marinara sauce, for serving

Directions:
1. .Start by cooking the Arborio rice.
2. Stovetop Method: Preheat a medium saucepan over medium heat. Add the olive oil and sauté the onion until it starts to become tender – about 5 minutes. Add the rice and stir well to coat all the grains of rice. Add the white wine or vermouth. Let this simmer and get absorbed by the rice. Then add the stock and water, cover, reduce the heat to low and simmer for 20 minutes.
3. Pressure-Cooker Method: Preheat the pressure cooker using the BROWN setting. Add the oil and cook the onion for a few minutes. Add the rice, wine, stock, water, salt and freshly ground black pepper, give everything one good stir and lock the lid in place. Pressure cook on HIGH for 7 minutes. Reduce the pressure with the QUICK-RELEASE method and carefully remove the lid.
4. Taste the rice to make sure it is tender. Season with salt and freshly ground black pepper and stir in the grated Parmigiano-Reggiano cheese. Spread the rice out onto a baking sheet to cool.
5. While the rice is cooling, cut the mozzarella into ¾-inch cubes.
6. Once the rice has cooled, combine the rice with the eggs, sun-dried tomatoes and ½ cup of the breadcrumbs. Place the remaining breadcrumbs in a shallow dish. Shape the rice mixture into 12 balls. Press a hole in the rice ball with your finger and push one or two cubes of mozzarella cheese into the hole. Mold the rice back into a ball, enclosing the cheese. Roll the finished rice balls in the breadcrumbs and place them on a baking sheet while you make the remaining rice balls. Spray or brush the rice balls with olive oil.
7. Preheat the air fryer to 380°F/195°C.
8. Cook 6 arancini at a time. Air-fry for 10 minutes. Gently turn the arancini over, brush or spray with oil again and air-fry for another 5 minutes. Serve warm with the marinara sauce.

String Bean Fries

Servings: 4
Cooking Time: 6 Minutes
Ingredients:
- ½ pound fresh string beans
- 2 eggs
- 4 teaspoons water
- ½ cup white flour
- ½ cup breadcrumbs
- ¼ teaspoon salt
- ¼ teaspoon ground black pepper
- ¼ teaspoon dry mustard (optional)
- oil for misting or cooking spray

Directions:
1. Preheat air fryer to 360°F/180°C.
2. Trim stem ends from string beans, wash, and pat dry.
3. In a shallow dish, beat eggs and water together until well blended.
4. Place flour in a second shallow dish.
5. In a third shallow dish, stir together the breadcrumbs, salt, pepper, and dry mustard if using.

6. Dip each string bean in egg mixture, flour, egg mixture again, then breadcrumbs.
7. When you finish coating all the string beans, open air fryer and place them in basket.
8. Cook for 3minutes.
9. Stop and mist string beans with oil or cooking spray.
10. Cook for 3 moreminutes or until string beans are crispy and nicely browned.

Eggs In Avocado Halves

Servings: 3
Cooking Time: 23 Minutes
Ingredients:
- 3 Hass avocados, halved and pitted but not peeled
- 6 Medium eggs
- Vegetable oil spray
- 3 tablespoons Heavy or light cream (not fat-free cream)
- To taste Table salt
- To taste Ground black pepper

Directions:
1. Preheat the air fryer to 350°F/175°C .
2. Slice a small amount off the (skin) side of each avocado half so it can sit stable, without rocking. Lightly coat the skin of the avocado half (the side that will now sit stable) with vegetable oil spray.
3. Arrange the avocado halves open side up on a cutting board, then crack an egg into the indentation in each where the pit had been. If any white overflows the avocado half, wipe that bit of white off the cut edge of the avocado before proceeding.
4. Remove the basket (or its attachment) from the machine and set the filled avocado halves in it in one layer. Return it to the machine without pushing it in. Drizzle each avocado half with about 1½ teaspoons cream, a little salt, and a little ground black pepper.
5. Air-fry undisturbed for 10 minutes for a soft-set yolk, or air-fry for 13 minutes for more-set eggs.
6. Use a nonstick-safe spatula and a flatware fork for balance to transfer the avocado halves to serving plates. Cool a minute or two before serving.

Nicoise Deviled Eggs

Servings:4
Cooking Time: 20 Minutes
Ingredients:
- 4 eggs
- 2 tbsp mayonnaise
- 10 chopped Nicoise olives
- 2 tbsp goat cheese crumbles
- Salt and pepper to taste
- 2 tbsp chopped parsley

Directions:
1. Preheat air fryer to 260ºF/180°C. Place the eggs in silicone muffin cups to avoid bumping around and cracking during the cooking process. Add silicone cups to the frying basket and Air Fry for 15 minutes. Remove and run the eggs under cold water. When cool, remove the shells and halve them lengthwise.
2. Spoon yolks into a separate medium bowl and arrange white halves on a large plate. Mash the yolks with a fork. Stir in the remaining ingredients. Spoon mixture into white halves and scatter with mint to serve.

Turkey Spring Rolls

Servings: 4
Cooking Time: 20 Minutes
Ingredients:
- 1 lb turkey breast, grilled, cut into chunks
- 1 celery stalk, julienned
- 1 carrot, grated
- 1 tsp fresh ginger, minced
- 1 tsp sugar
- 1 tsp chicken stock powder
- 1 egg
- 1 tsp corn starch
- 6 spring roll wrappers

Directions:
1. Preheat the air fryer to 360°F/180°C. Mix the turkey, celery, carrot, ginger, sugar, and chicken stock powder in a large bowl. Combine thoroughly and set aside. In another bowl, beat the egg, and stir in the cornstarch. On a clean surface, spoon the turkey filling into each spring roll, roll up and seal the seams with the egg-cornstarch mixture. Put each roll in the greased frying basket and Air Fry for 7-8 minutes, flipping once until golden brown. Serve hot.

Mozzarella En Carrozza With Puttanesca Sauce

Servings: 6
Cooking Time: 8 Minutes
Ingredients:
- Puttanesca Sauce
- 2 teaspoons olive oil
- 1 anchovy, chopped (optional)
- 2 cloves garlic, minced
- 1 (14-ounce) can petite diced tomatoes
- ½ cup chicken stock or water
- ⅓ cup Kalamata olives, chopped
- 2 tablespoons capers
- ½ teaspoon dried oregano
- ¼ teaspoon crushed red pepper flakes
- salt and freshly ground black pepper
- 1 tablespoon fresh parsley, chopped
- 8 slices of thinly sliced white bread (Pepperidge Farm®)
- 8 ounces mozzarella cheese, cut into ¼-inch slices
- ½ cup all-purpose flour
- 3 eggs, beaten
- 1½ cups seasoned panko breadcrumbs
- ½ teaspoon garlic powder
- ½ teaspoon salt
- freshly ground black pepper
- olive oil, in a spray bottle

Directions:
1. Start by making the puttanesca sauce. Heat the olive oil in a medium saucepan on the stovetop. Add the anchovies (if using, and I really think you should!) and garlic and sauté for 3 minutes, or until the anchovies have "melted" into the oil. Add the tomatoes, chicken stock, olives, capers, oregano and crushed red pepper flakes and simmer the sauce for 20 minutes. Season with salt and freshly ground black pepper and stir in the fresh parsley.
2. Cut the crusts off the slices of bread. Place four slices of the bread on a cutting board. Divide the cheese between the four slices of bread. Top the cheese with the remaining four slices of bread to make little sandwiches and cut each sandwich into 4 triangles.
3. Set up a dredging station using three shallow dishes. Place the flour in the first shallow dish, the eggs in the second dish and in the third dish, combine the panko breadcrumbs, garlic powder, salt and black pepper. Dredge each little triangle in the flour first (you might think this is redundant, but it helps to get the coating to adhere to the edges of the sandwiches) and then dip them into the egg, making sure both the sides and the edges are coated. Let the excess egg drip off and then press the triangles into the breadcrumb mixture, pressing the crumbs on with your hands so they adhere. Place the coated triangles in the freezer for 2 hours, until the cheese is frozen.
4. Preheat the air fryer to 390°F/200°C. Spray all sides of the mozzarella triangles with oil and transfer a single layer of triangles to the air fryer basket. Air-fry in batches at 390°F/200°C for 5 minutes. Turn the triangles over and air-fry for an additional 3 minutes.
5. Serve mozzarella triangles immediately with the warm puttanesca sauce.

Maple Loaded Sweet Potatoes

Servings: 4
Cooking Time: 45 Minutes
Ingredients:
- 4 sweet potatoes
- 2 tbsp butter
- 2 tbsp maple syrup
- 1 tsp cinnamon
- 1 tsp lemon zest
- ½ tsp vanilla extract

Directions:
1. Preheat air fryer to 390°F/200°C. Poke three holes on the top of each of the sweet potatoes using a fork. Arrange in air fryer and Bake for 40 minutes. Remove and let cool for 5 minutes. While the sweet potatoes cool, melt butter and maple syrup together in the microwave for 15-20 seconds. Remove from microwave and stir in cinnamon, lemon zest, and vanilla. When the sweet potatoes are cool, cut open and drizzle the cinnamon butter mixture over each and serve immediately.

"fried" Pickles With Homemade Ranch

Servings: 8
Cooking Time: 8 Minutes
Ingredients:
- 1 cup all-purpose flour
- 2 teaspoons dried dill
- ½ teaspoon paprika
- ¾ cup buttermilk
- 1 egg
- 4 large kosher dill pickles, sliced ¼-inch thick
- 2 cups panko breadcrumbs

Directions:
1. Preheat the air fryer to 380°F/195°C.
2. In a medium bowl, whisk together the flour, dill, paprika, buttermilk, and egg.
3. Dip and coat thick slices of dill pickles into the batter. Next, dredge into the panko breadcrumbs.
4. Place a single layer of breaded pickles into the air fryer basket. Spray the pickles with cooking spray. Cook for 4 minutes, turn over, and cook another 4 minutes. Repeat until all the pickle chips have been cooked.

Bread And Breakfast

Chili Hash Browns

Servings: 4
Cooking Time: 45 Minutes
Ingredients:
- 1 tbsp ancho chili powder
- 1 tbsp chipotle powder
- 2 tsp ground cumin
- 2 tsp smoked paprika
- 1 tsp garlic powder
- 1 tsp cayenne pepper
- Salt and pepper to taste
- 2 peeled russet potatoes, grated
- 2 tbsp olive oil
- 1/3 cup chopped onion
- 3 garlic cloves, minced

Directions:
1. Preheat the air fryer to 400°F/205°C. Combine chili powder, cumin, paprika, garlic powder, chipotle, cayenne, and black pepper in a small bowl, then pour into a glass jar with a lid and store in a cool, dry place. Add the olive oil, onion, and garlic to a cake pan, put it in the air fryer, and Bake for 3 minutes. Put the grated potatoes in a bowl and sprinkle with 2 tsp of the spice mixture, toss and add them to the cake pan along with the onion mix. Bake for 20-23 minutes, stirring once or until the potatoes are crispy and golden. Season with salt and serve.

Vodka Basil Muffins With Strawberries

Servings:6
Cooking Time: 20 Minutes
Ingredients:
- ½ cup flour
- ½ cup granular sugar
- ½ tsp baking powder
- ⅛ tsp salt
- ½ cup chopped strawberries
- ¼ tsp vanilla extract
- 3 tbsp butter, melted
- 2 eggs
- ¼ tsp vodka
- 1 tbsp chopped basil

Directions:
1. Preheat air fryer to 375°F/190°C. Combine the dry ingredients in a bowl. Set aside. In another bowl, whisk the wet ingredients. Pour wet ingredients into the bowl with the dry ingredients and gently combine. Add basil and vodka to the batter. Do not overmix and spoon batter into six silicone cupcake liners lightly greased with olive oil. Place liners in the frying basket and Bake for 7 minutes. Let cool for 5 minutes onto a cooling rack before serving.

Cheesy Egg Popovers

Servings:6
Cooking Time: 30 Minutes
Ingredients:
- 5 eggs

- 1 tbsp milk
- 2 tbsp heavy cream
- Salt and pepper to taste
- ⅛ tsp ground nutmeg
- ¼ cup grated Swiss cheese

Directions:
1. Preheat air fryer to 350°F/175°C. Beat all ingredients in a bowl. Divide between greased muffin cups and place them in the frying basket. Bake for 9 minutes. Let cool slightly before serving.

Green Egg Quiche

Servings: 4
Cooking Time: 30 Minutes
Ingredients:
- 1 cup broccoli florets
- 2 cups baby spinach
- 2 garlic cloves, minced
- ¼ tsp ground nutmeg
- 1 tbsp olive oil
- Salt and pepper to taste
- 4 eggs
- 2 scallions, chopped
- 1 red onion, chopped
- 1 tbsp sour cream
- ½ cup grated fontina cheese

Directions:
1. Preheat air fryer to 375°F/190°C. Combine broccoli, spinach, onion, garlic, nutmeg, olive oil, and salt in a medium bowl, tossing to coat. Arrange the broccoli in a single layer in the parchment-lined frying basket and cook for 5 minutes. Remove and set to the side.
2. Use the same medium bowl to whisk eggs, salt, pepper, scallions, and sour cream. Add the roasted broccoli and ¼ cup fontina cheese until all ingredients are well combined. Pour the mixture into a greased baking dish and top with cheese. Bake in the air fryer for 15-18 minutes until the center is set. Serve and enjoy.

Cinnamon Rolls With Cream Cheese Glaze

Servings: 8
Cooking Time: 9 Minutes
Ingredients:
- 1 pound frozen bread dough, thawed
- ¼ cup butter, melted and cooled
- ¾ cup brown sugar
- 1½ tablespoons ground cinnamon
- Cream Cheese Glaze:
- 4 ounces cream cheese, softened
- 2 tablespoons butter, softened
- 1¼ cups powdered sugar
- ½ teaspoon vanilla

Directions:
1. Let the bread dough come to room temperature on the counter. On a lightly floured surface roll the dough into a 13-inch by 11-inch rectangle. Position the rectangle so the 13-inch side is facing you. Brush the melted butter all over the

dough, leaving a 1-inch border uncovered along the edge farthest away from you.

2. Combine the brown sugar and cinnamon in a small bowl. Sprinkle the mixture evenly over the buttered dough, keeping the 1-inch border uncovered. Roll the dough into a log starting with the edge closest to you. Roll the dough tightly, making sure to roll evenly and push out any air pockets. When you get to the uncovered edge of the dough, press the dough onto the roll to seal it together.

3. Cut the log into 8 pieces slicing slowly with a sawing motion so you don't flatten the dough. Turn the slices on their sides and cover with a clean kitchen towel. Let the rolls sit in the warmest part of your kitchen for 1½ to 2 hours to rise.

4. To make the glaze, place the cream cheese and butter in a microwave-safe bowl. Soften the mixture in the microwave for 30 seconds at a time until it is easy to stir. Gradually add the powdered sugar and stir to combine. Add the vanilla extract and whisk until smooth. Set aside.

5. When the rolls have risen, Preheat the air fryer to 350°F/175°C.

6. Transfer 4 of the rolls to the air fryer basket. Air-fry for 5 minutes. Turn the rolls over and air-fry for another 4 minutes. Repeat with the remaining 4 rolls.

7. Let the rolls cool for a couple of minutes before glazing. Spread large dollops of cream cheese glaze on top of the warm cinnamon rolls, allowing some of the glaze to drip down the side of the rolls. Serve warm and enjoy!

Fried Pb&j

Servings: 4
Cooking Time: 8 Minutes
Ingredients:
- ½ cup cornflakes, crushed
- ¼ cup shredded coconut
- 8 slices oat nut bread or any whole-grain, oversize bread
- 6 tablespoons peanut butter
- 2 medium bananas, cut into ½-inch-thick slices
- 6 tablespoons pineapple preserves
- 1 egg, beaten
- oil for misting or cooking spray

Directions:
1. Preheat air fryer to 360°F/180°C.
2. In a shallow dish, mix together the cornflake crumbs and coconut.
3. For each sandwich, spread one bread slice with 1½ tablespoons of peanut butter. Top with banana slices. Spread another bread slice with 1½ tablespoons of preserves. Combine to make a sandwich.
4. Using a pastry brush, brush top of sandwich lightly with beaten egg. Sprinkle with about 1½ tablespoons of crumb coating, pressing it in to make it stick. Spray with oil.
5. Turn sandwich over and repeat to coat and spray the other side.
6. Cooking 2 at a time, place sandwiches in air fryer basket and cook for 6 to 7minutes or until coating is golden brown and crispy. If sandwich doesn't brown enough, spray with a little more oil and cook at 390°F/200°C for another minute.
7. Cut cooked sandwiches in half and serve warm.

Egg Muffins

Servings: 4
Cooking Time: 11 Minutes
Ingredients:
- 4 eggs
- salt and pepper
- olive oil
- 4 English muffins, split

- 1 cup shredded Colby Jack cheese
- 4 slices ham or Canadian bacon

Directions:
1. Preheat air fryer to 390°F/200°C.
2. Beat together eggs and add salt and pepper to taste. Spray air fryer baking pan lightly with oil and add eggs. Cook for 2minutes, stir, and continue cooking for 4minutes, stirring every minute, until eggs are scrambled to your preference. Remove pan from air fryer.
3. Place bottom halves of English muffins in air fryer basket. Take half of the shredded cheese and divide it among the muffins. Top each with a slice of ham and one-quarter of the eggs. Sprinkle remaining cheese on top of the eggs. Use a fork to press the cheese into the egg a little so it doesn't slip off before it melts.
4. Cook at 360°F/180°C for 1 minute. Add English muffin tops and cook for 4minutes to heat through and toast the muffins.

English Breakfast

Servings: 2
Cooking Time: 30 Minutes
Ingredients:
- 6 bacon strips
- 1 cup cooked white beans
- 1 tbsp melted butter
- ½ tbsp flour
- Salt and pepper to taste
- 2 eggs

Directions:
1. Preheat air fryer to 360°F/180°C. In a second bowl, combine the beans, butter, flour, salt, and pepper. Mix well. Put the bacon in the frying basket and Air Fry for 10 minutes, flipping once. Remove the bacon and stir in the beans. Crack the eggs on top and cook for 10-12 minutes until the eggs are set. Serve with bacon.

Southwest Cornbread

Servings: 6
Cooking Time: 18 Minutes
Ingredients:
- cooking spray
- ½ cup yellow cornmeal
- ½ cup flour
- 2 teaspoons baking powder
- ½ teaspoon salt
- ½ cup frozen corn kernels, thawed and drained
- ¼ cup finely chopped onion
- 1 or 2 small jalapeño peppers, seeded and chopped
- 1 egg
- ½ cup milk
- 2 tablespoons melted butter
- 2 ounces sharp Cheddar cheese, grated

Directions:
1. Preheat air fryer to 360°F/180°C.
2. Spray air fryer baking pan with nonstick cooking spray.
3. In a medium bowl, stir together the cornmeal, flour, baking powder, and salt.
4. Stir in the corn, onion, and peppers.
5. In a small bowl, beat together the egg, milk, and butter. Stir into dry ingredients until well combined.
6. Spoon half the batter into prepared baking pan, spreading to edges. Top with grated cheese. Spoon remaining batter on top of cheese and gently spread to edges of pan so it completely covers the cheese.
7. Cook at 360°F/180°C for 18 minutes, until cornbread is done and top is crispy brown.

Oat & Nut Granola

Servings: 6
Cooking Time: 25 Minutes
Ingredients:
- 2 cups rolled oats
- ¼ cup pistachios
- ¼ cup chopped almonds
- ¼ cup chopped cashews
- ¼ cup honey
- 2 tbsp light brown sugar
- 3 tbsp butter
- ½ tsp ground cinnamon
- ½ cup dried figs

Directions:
1. Preheat the air fryer to 325°F/160°C. Combine the oats, pistachios, almonds, and cashews in a bowl and toss, then set aside. In a saucepan, cook the honey, brown sugar, butter, and cinnamon and over low heat, stirring frequently, 4 minutes. Melt the butter completely and make sure the mixture is smooth, then pour over the oat mix and stir.
2. Scoop the granola mixture in a greased baking pan. Put the pan in the frying basket and Bake for 7 minutes, then remove the pan and stir. Cook for another 6-9 minutes or until the granola is golden, then add the dried figs and stir. Remove the pan and let cool. Store in a covered container at room temperature for up to 3 days.

Cheesy Olive And Roasted Pepper Bread

Servings: 8
Cooking Time: 7 Minutes
Ingredients:
- 7-inch round bread boule
- olive oil
- ½ cup mayonnaise
- 2 tablespoons butter, melted
- 1 cup grated mozzarella or Fontina cheese
- ¼ cup grated Parmesan cheese
- ½ teaspoon dried oregano
- ½ cup black olives, sliced
- ½ cup green olives, sliced
- ½ cup coarsely chopped roasted red peppers
- 2 tablespoons minced red onion
- freshly ground black pepper

Directions:
1. Preheat the air fryer to 370°F/185°C.
2. Cut the bread boule in half horizontally. If your bread boule has a rounded top, trim the top of the boule so that the top half will lie flat with the cut side facing up. Lightly brush both sides of the boule halves with olive oil.
3. Place one half of the boule into the air fryer basket with the center cut side facing down. Air-fry at 370°F for 2 minutes to lightly toast the bread. Repeat with the other half of the bread boule.
4. Combine the mayonnaise, butter, mozzarella cheese, Parmesan cheese and dried oregano in a small bowl. Fold in the black and green olives, roasted red peppers and red onion and season with freshly ground black pepper. Spread the cheese mixture over the untoasted side of the bread, covering the entire surface.
5. Air-fry at 350°F/175°C for 5 minutes until the cheese is melted and browned. Repeat with the other half. Cut into slices and serve warm.

Smoked Salmon Croissant Sandwich

Servings: 1
Cooking Time: 30 Minutes
Ingredients:
- 1 croissant, halved
- 2 eggs
- 1 tbsp guacamole
- 1 smoked salmon slice
- Salt and pepper to taste

Directions:
1. Preheat air fryer to 360°F/180°C. Place the croissant, crusty side up, in the frying basket side by side. Whisk the eggs in a small ceramic dish until fluffy. Place in the air fryer. Bake for 10 minutes. Gently scramble the half-cooked egg in the baking dish with a fork. Flip the croissant and cook for another 10 minutes until the scrambled eggs are cooked, but still fluffy, and the croissant is toasted.
2. Place one croissant on a serving plate, then spread the guacamole on top. Scoop the scrambled eggs onto guacamole, then top with smoked salmon. Sprinkle with salt and pepper. Top with the second slice of toasted croissant, close sandwich, and serve hot.

Mascarpone Iced Cinnamon Rolls

Servings: 6
Cooking Time: 40 Minutes
Ingredients:
- ¼ cup mascarpone cheese, softened
- 9 oz puff pastry sheet
- 3 tbsp light brown sugar
- 2 tsp ground cinnamon
- 2 tsp butter, melted
- ¼ tsp vanilla extract
- ¼ tsp salt
- 2 tbsp milk
- 1 tbsp lemon zest
- ¼ cup confectioners' sugar

Directions:
1. Preheat air fryer to 320°F/160°C. Mix the brown sugar and cinnamon in a small bowl. Unroll the pastry sheet on its paper and brush it with melted butter. Then sprinkle with cinnamon sugar. Roll up the dough tightly, then cut into rolls about 1-inch wide. Put into a greased baking pan with the spiral side showing. Put the pan into the air fryer and Bake until golden brown, 18-20 minutes. Set aside to cool for 5-10 minutes.
2. Meanwhile, add the mascarpone cheese, vanilla, and salt in a small bowl, whisking until smooth and creamy. Add the confectioners' sugar and continue whisking until fully blended. Pour and mix in 1 tsp of milk at a time until the glaze is pourable but still with some thickness. Spread the glaze over the warm cinnamon rolls and scatter with lemon zest. Serve and enjoy!

Spinach-bacon Rollups

Servings: 4
Cooking Time: 9 Minutes
Ingredients:
- 4 flour tortillas (6- or 7-inch size)
- 4 slices Swiss cheese
- 1 cup baby spinach leaves
- 4 slices turkey bacon

Directions:
1. Preheat air fryer to 390°F/200°C.
2. On each tortilla, place one slice of cheese and ¼ cup of spinach.

3. Roll up tortillas and wrap each with a strip of bacon. Secure each end with a toothpick.
4. Place rollups in air fryer basket, leaving a little space in between them.
5. Cook for 4minutes. Turn and rearrange rollups (for more even cooking) and cook for 5minutes longer, until bacon is crisp.

Holiday Breakfast Casserole

Servings:2
Cooking Time: 25 Minutes
Ingredients:
- ¼ cup cooked spicy breakfast sausage
- 5 eggs
- 2 tbsp heavy cream
- ½ tsp ground cumin
- Salt and pepper to taste
- ½ cup feta cheese crumbles
- 1 tomato, diced
- 1 can green chiles, including juice
- 1 zucchini, diced

Directions:
1. Preheat air fryer to 325ºF/160°C. Mix all ingredients in a bowl and pour into a greased baking pan. Place the pan in the frying basket and Bake for 14 minutes. Let cool for 5 minutes before slicing. Serve right away.

Morning Apple Biscuits

Servings: 6
Cooking Time: 15 Minutes
Ingredients:
- 1 apple, grated
- 1 cup oat flour
- 2 tbsp honey
- ¼ cup peanut butter
- 1/3 cup raisins
- ½ tsp ground cinnamon

Directions:
1. Preheat air fryer to 350°F/175°C. Combine the apple, flour, honey, peanut butter, raisins, and cinnamon in a bowl until combined. Make balls out of the mixture. Place them onto parchment paper and flatten them. Bake for 9 minutes until slightly brown. Serve warm.

Farmers Market Quiche

Servings: 4
Cooking Time: 35 Minutes
Ingredients:
- 4 button mushrooms
- ¼ medium red bell pepper
- 1 teaspoon extra-virgin olive oil
- One 9-inch pie crust, at room temperature
- ¼ cup grated carrot
- ¼ cup chopped, fresh baby spinach leaves
- 3 eggs, whisked
- ¼ cup half-and-half
- ½ teaspoon thyme
- ½ teaspoon sea salt
- 2 ounces crumbled goat cheese or feta

Directions:
1. In a medium bowl, toss the mushrooms and bell pepper with extra-virgin olive oil; place into the air fryer basket. Set the temperature to 400°F/205°C for 8 minutes, stirring after 4 minutes. Remove from the air fryer, and roughly chop the mushrooms and bell peppers. Wipe the air fryer clean.

2. Prep a 7-inch oven-safe baking dish by spraying the bottom of the pan with cooking spray.
3. Place the pie crust into the baking dish; fold over and crimp the edges or use a fork to press to give the edges some shape.
4. In a medium bowl, mix together the mushrooms, bell peppers, carrots, spinach, and eggs. Stir in the half-and-half, thyme, and salt.
5. Pour the quiche mixture into the base of the pie shell. Top with crumbled cheese.
6. Place the quiche into the air fryer basket. Set the temperature to 325°F/160°C for 30 minutes.
7. When complete, turn the quiche halfway and cook an additional 5 minutes. Allow the quiche to rest 20 minutes prior to slicing and serving.

Honey Oatmeal

Servings: 6
Cooking Time: 35 Minutes
Ingredients:
- 2 cups rolled oats
- 2 cups oat milk
- ¼ cup honey
- ½ cup Greek yogurt
- 1 tsp vanilla extract
- ½ tsp ground cinnamon
- ¼ tsp salt
- 1 ½ cups diced mango

Directions:
1. Preheat air fryer to 380°F/195°C. Stir together the oats, milk, honey, yogurt, vanilla, cinnamon, and salt in a large bowl until well combined. Fold in ¾ cup of the mango and then pour the mixture into a greased cake pan. Sprinkle the remaining manog across the top of the oatmeal mixture. Bake in the air fryer for 30 minutes. Leave to set and cool for 5 minutes. Serve and enjoy!

Cinnamon Pear Oat Muffins

Servings: 6
Cooking Time: 30 Minutes + Cooling Time
Ingredients:
- ½ cup apple sauce
- 1 large egg
- 1/3 cup brown sugar
- 2 tbsp butter, melted
- ½ cup milk
- 11/3 cups rolled oats
- 1 tsp ground cinnamon
- ½ tsp baking powder
- Pinch of salt
- ½ cup diced peeled pears

Directions:
1. Preheat the air fryer to 350°F/175°C. Place the apple sauce, egg, brown sugar, melted butter, and milk into a bowl and mix to combine. Stir in the oats, cinnamon, baking powder, and salt and mix well, then fold in the pears.
2. Grease 6 silicone muffin cups with baking spray, then spoon the batter in equal portions into the cups. Put the muffin cups in the frying basket and Bake for 13-18 minutes or until set. Leave to cool for 15 minutes. Serve.

Chocolate Chip Banana Muffins

Servings: 12
Cooking Time: 14 Minutes
Ingredients:
- 2 medium bananas, mashed
- ¼ cup brown sugar
- 1½ teaspoons vanilla extract
- ⅔ cup milk
- 2 tablespoons butter
- 1 large egg
- 1 cup white whole-wheat flour
- ½ cup old-fashioned oats
- 1 teaspoon baking soda
- ½ teaspoon baking powder
- ⅛ teaspoon sea salt
- ¼ cup mini chocolate chips

Directions:
1. Preheat the air fryer to 330°F/165°C.
2. In a large bowl, combine the bananas, brown sugar, vanilla extract, milk, butter, and egg; set aside.
3. In a separate bowl, combine the flour, oats, baking soda, baking powder, and salt.
4. Slowly add the dry ingredients into the wet ingredients, folding in the flour mixture ⅓ cup at a time.
5. Mix in the chocolate chips and set aside.
6. Using silicone muffin liners, fill 6 muffin liners two-thirds full. Carefully place the muffin liners in the air fryer basket and bake for 20 minutes (or until the tops are browned and a toothpick inserted in the center comes out clean). Carefully remove the muffins from the basket and repeat with the remaining batter.
7. Serve warm.

Breakfast Sausage Bites

Servings: 4
Cooking Time: 30 Minutes
Ingredients:
- 1 lb ground pork sausages
- ¼ cup diced onions
- 1 tsp rubbed sage
- ¼ tsp ground nutmeg
- ½ tsp fennel
- ¼ tsp garlic powder
- 2 tbsp parsley, chopped
- Salt and pepper to taste

Directions:
1. Preheat air fryer at 350°F/175°C. Combine all ingredients, except the parsley, in a bowl. Form mixture into balls. Place them in the greased frying basket and Air Fry for 10 minutes, flipping once. Sprinkle with parsley and serve immediately.

Ham & Cheese Sandwiches

Servings: 2
Cooking Time: 15 Minutes
Ingredients:
- 1 tsp butter
- 4 bread slices
- 4 deli ham slices
- 4 Cheddar cheese slices
- 4 thick tomato slices
- 1 tsp dried oregano

Directions:
1. Preheat air fryer to 370°F/185°C. Smear ½ tsp of butter on only one side of each slice of bread and sprinkle with oregano. On one of the slices, layer 2 slices of ham, 2 slices of cheese, and 2 slices of tomato on the unbuttered side. Place the unbuttered side of another piece of bread onto the toppings. Place the sandwiches butter side down into the air fryer. Bake for 8 minutes, flipping once until crispy. Let cool slightly, cut in half and serve.

Seasoned Herbed Sourdough Croutons

Servings: 4
Cooking Time: 7 Minutes
Ingredients:
- 4 cups cubed sourdough bread, 1-inch cubes (about 8 ounces)
- 1 tablespoon olive oil
- 1 teaspoon fresh thyme leaves
- ¼ – ½ teaspoon salt
- freshly ground black pepper

Directions:
1. Combine all ingredients in a bowl and taste to make sure it is seasoned to your liking.
2. Preheat the air fryer to 400°F/205°C.
3. Toss the bread cubes into the air fryer and air-fry for 7 minutes, shaking the basket once or twice while they cook.
4. Serve warm or store in an airtight container.

Christmas Eggnog Bread

Servings: 6
Cooking Time: 18 Minutes
Ingredients:
- 1 cup flour, plus more for dusting
- ¼ cup sugar
- 1 teaspoon baking powder
- ¼ teaspoon salt
- ¼ teaspoon nutmeg
- ½ cup eggnog
- 1 egg yolk
- 1 tablespoon butter, plus 1 teaspoon, melted
- ¼ cup pecans
- ¼ cup chopped candied fruit (cherries, pineapple, or mixed fruits)
- cooking spray

Directions:
1. Preheat air fryer to 360°F/180°C.
2. In a medium bowl, stir together the flour, sugar, baking powder, salt, and nutmeg.
3. Add eggnog, egg yolk, and butter. Mix well but do not beat.
4. Stir in nuts and fruit.
5. Spray a 6 x 6-inch baking pan with cooking spray and dust with flour.
6. Spread batter into prepared pan and cook at 360°F/180°C for 18 minutes or until top is dark golden brown and bread starts to pull away from sides of pan.

Morning Potato Cakes

Servings: 6
Cooking Time: 50 Minutes
Ingredients:
- 4 Yukon Gold potatoes
- 2 cups kale, chopped
- 1 cup rice flour
- ¼ cup cornstarch
- ¾ cup milk
- 2 tbsp lemon juice
- 2 tsp dried rosemary

- 2 tsp shallot powder
- Salt and pepper to taste
- ½ tsp turmeric powder

Directions:
1. Preheat air fryer to 390°F/200°C. Scrub the potatoes and put them in the air fryer. Bake for 30 minutes or until soft. When cool, chop them into small pieces and place them in a bowl. Mash with a potato masher or fork. Add kale, rice flour, cornstarch, milk, lemon juice, rosemary, shallot powder, salt, pepper, and turmeric. Stir well.
2. Make 12 balls out of the mixture and smash them lightly with your hands to make patties. Place them in the greased frying basket, and Air Fry for 10-12 minutes, flipping once, until golden and cooked through. Serve.

Cheddar & Egg Scramble

Servings: 4
Cooking Time: 20 Minutes
Ingredients:
- 8 eggs
- ¼ cup buttermilk
- ¼ cup milk
- Salt and pepper to taste
- 3 tbsp butter, melted
- 1 cup grated cheddar
- 1 tbsp minced parsley

Directions:
1. Preheat the air fryer to 350°F/175°C. Whisk the eggs with buttermilk, milk, salt, and pepper until foamy and set aside. Put the melted butter in a cake pan and pour in the egg mixture. Return the pan into the fryer and cook for 7 minutes, stirring occasionally. Stir in the cheddar cheese and cook for 2-4 more minutes or until the eggs have set. Remove the cake pan and scoop the eggs into a serving plate. Scatter with freshly minced parsley and serve.

Coffee Cake

Servings: 8
Cooking Time: 35 Minutes
Ingredients:
- 4 tablespoons butter, melted and divided
- ⅓ cup cane sugar
- ¼ cup brown sugar
- 1 large egg
- 1 cup plus 6 teaspoons milk, divided
- 1 teaspoon vanilla extract
- 2 cups all-purpose flour
- 1½ teaspoons baking powder
- ¼ teaspoon salt
- 2 teaspoons ground cinnamon
- ⅓ cup chopped pecans
- ⅓ cup powdered sugar

Directions:
1. Preheat the air fryer to 325°F/160°C.
2. Using a hand mixer or stand mixer, in a medium bowl, cream together the butter, cane sugar, brown sugar, the egg, 1 cup of the milk, and the vanilla. Set aside.
3. In a small bowl, mix together the flour, baking powder, salt, and cinnamon. Slowly combine the dry ingredients into the wet. Fold in the pecans.
4. Liberally spray a 7-inch springform pan with cooking spray. Pour the batter into the pan and place in the air fryer basket.
5. Bake for 30 to 35 minutes. While the cake is baking, in a small bowl, add the powdered sugar and whisk together with the remaining 6 teaspoons of milk. Set aside.

6. When the cake is done baking, remove the pan from the basket and let cool on a wire rack. After 10 minutes, remove and invert the cake from pan. Drizzle with the powdered sugar glaze and serve.

Cinnamon-coconut Doughnuts

Servings: 6
Cooking Time: 35 Minutes
Ingredients:
- 1 egg, beaten
- ¼ cup milk
- 2 tbsp safflower oil
- 1 ½ tsp vanilla
- ½ tsp lemon zest
- 1 ½ cups all-purpose flour
- ¾ cup coconut sugar
- 2 ½ tsp cinnamon
- ½ tsp ground nutmeg
- ¼ tsp salt
- ¾ tsp baking powder

Directions:
1. Preheat air fryer to 350°F/175°C. Add the egg, milk, oil, vanilla, and lemon zest. Stir well and set this wet mixture aside. In a different bowl, combine the flour, ½ cup coconut sugar, ½ teaspoon cinnamon, nutmeg, salt, and baking powder. Stir well. Add this mixture to the wet mix and blend. Pull off bits of the dough and roll into balls.
2. Place in the greased frying basket, leaving room between as they get bigger. Spray the tops with oil and Air Fry for 8-10 minutes, flipping once. During the last 2 minutes of frying, place 4 tbsp of coconut sugar and 2 tsp of cinnamon in a bowl and stir to combine. After frying, coat each donut by spraying with oil and toss in the cinnamon-sugar mix. Serve and enjoy!

Smooth Walnut-banana Loaf

Servings: 4
Cooking Time: 40 Minutes
Ingredients:
- 1/3 cup peanut butter, melted
- 2 tbsp butter, melted and cooled
- ¾ cup flour
- ½ tsp salt
- ¼ tsp baking soda
- 2 ripe bananas
- 2 eggs
- 1 tsp lemon juice
- ½ cup evaporated cane sugar
- ½ cup ground walnuts
- 1 tbsp blackstrap molasses
- 1 tsp vanilla extract

Directions:
1. Preheat air fryer to 310°F/155°C. Mix flour, salt, and baking soda in a small bowl. Mash together bananas and eggs in a large bowl, then stir in sugar, peanut butter, lemon juice, butter, walnuts, molasses, and vanilla. When it is well incorporated, stir in the flour mixture until just combined. Transfer the batter to a parchment-lined baking dish and make sure it is even. Bake in the air fryer for 30 to 35 minutes until a toothpick in the middle comes out clean, and the top is golden. Serve and enjoy.

Mushroom & Cavolo Nero Egg Muffins

Servings: 6
Cooking Time: 20 Minutes
Ingredients:
- 8 oz baby Bella mushrooms, sliced
- 6 eggs, beaten
- 1 garlic clove, minced
- Salt and pepper to taste
- ½ tsp chili powder
- 1 cup cavolo nero
- 2 scallions, diced

Directions:
1. Preheat air fryer to 320°F/160°C. Place the eggs, garlic, salt, pepper, and chili powder in a bowl and beat until well combined. Fold in the mushrooms, cavolo nero, and scallions. Divide the mixture between greased muffin cups. Place into the air fryer and Bake for 12-15 minutes, or until the eggs are set. Cool for 5 minutes. Enjoy!

Buttermilk Biscuits

Servings: 4
Cooking Time: 9 Minutes
Ingredients:
- 1 cup flour
- 1½ teaspoons baking powder
- ¼ teaspoon baking soda
- ¼ teaspoon salt
- ¼ cup butter, cut into tiny cubes
- ¼ cup buttermilk, plus 2 tablespoons
- cooking spray

Directions:
1. Preheat air fryer to 330°F/165°C.
2. Combine flour, baking powder, soda, and salt in a medium bowl. Stir together.
3. Add cubed butter and cut into flour using knives or a pastry blender.
4. Add buttermilk and stir into a stiff dough.
5. Divide dough into 4 portions and shape each into a large biscuit. If dough is too sticky to handle, stir in 1 or 2 more tablespoons of flour before shaping. Biscuits should be firm enough to hold their shape. Otherwise they will stick to the air fryer basket.
6. Spray air fryer basket with nonstick cooking spray.
7. Place biscuits in basket and cook at 330°F for 9 minutes.

Pesto Egg & Ham Sandwiches

Servings: 2
Cooking Time: 20 Minutes
Ingredients:
- 4 sandwich bread slices
- 2 tbsp butter, melted
- 4 eggs, scrambled
- 4 deli ham slices
- 2 Colby cheese slices
- 4 tsp basil pesto sauce
- ¼ tsp red chili flakes
- ¼ sliced avocado

Directions:
1. Preheat air fryer at 370ºF/185°C. Brush 2 pieces of bread with half of the butter and place them, butter side down, into the frying basket. Divide eggs, chili flakes, sliced avocado, ham, and cheese on each bread slice.
2. Spread pesto on the remaining bread slices and place them, pesto side-down, onto the sandwiches. Brush the remaining butter on the tops of the sandwiches and Bake for 6 minutes, flipping once. Serve immediately.

Fruity Blueberry Muffin Cups

Servings: 2
Cooking Time: 30 Minutes
Ingredients:
- ½ cup white sugar
- 1 ½ cups all-purpose flour
- 2 tsp baking powder
- ½ tsp salt
- 1/3 cup vegetable oil
- 1 egg
- ¼ cup unsweetened yogurt
- 2 tsp vanilla extract
- 1 cup blueberries
- 1 banana, mashed
- 1 tbsp brown sugar

Directions:
1. Preheat air fryer to 350°F/175°C. In a bowl, add 1 tbsp of flour and throw in the blueberries and bananas to coat. In another bowl, combine white sugar, baking powder, remaining flour and salt. Mix well. In a third bowl, add oil, egg, yogurt and vanilla. Beat until well combined.
2. Add the wet into the dry mixture and whisk with a fork. Put in the blueberries-banana mix and stir. Spoon the batter into muffin cups, 3/4th way up. Top with brown sugar and Bake for 10-12 minutes until a toothpick inserted comes out clean.

Apple Fritters

Servings: 6
Cooking Time: 12 Minutes
Ingredients:
- 1 cup all-purpose flour
- 1½ teaspoons baking powder
- ¼ teaspoon salt
- 2 tablespoon brown sugar
- 1 teaspoon vanilla extract
- ¾ cup plain Greek yogurt
- 1 tablespoon cinnamon
- 1 large Granny Smith apple, cored, peeled, and finely chopped
- ¼ cup chopped walnuts
- ½ cup powdered sugar
- 1 tablespoon milk

Directions:
1. Preheat the air fryer to 320°F/160°C.
2. In a medium bowl, combine the flour, baking powder, and salt.
3. In a large bowl, add the brown sugar, vanilla, yogurt, cinnamon, apples, and walnuts. Mix the dry ingredients into the wet, using your hands to combine, until all the ingredients are mixed together. Knead the mixture in the bowl about 4 times.
4. Lightly spray the air fryer basket with olive oil spray.
5. Divide the batter into 6 equally sized balls; then lightly flatten them and place inside the basket. Repeat until all the fritters are formed.
6. Place the basket in the air fryer and cook for 6 minutes, flip, and then cook another 6 minutes.
7. While the fritters are cooking, in a small bowl, mix the powdered sugar with the milk. Set aside.
8. When the cooking completes, remove the air fryer basket and allow the fritters to cool on a wire rack. Drizzle with the homemade glaze and serve.

Apple & Turkey Breakfast Sausages

Servings: 4
Cooking Time: 15 Minutes
Ingredients:
- ½ tsp coriander seeds, crushed
- 1 tbsp chopped rosemary
- 1 tbsp chopped thyme
- Salt and pepper to taste
- 1 tsp fennel seeds, crushed
- ¾ tsp smoked paprika
- ½ tsp garlic powder
- ½ tsp shallot powder
- ⅛ tsp red pepper flakes
- 1 pound ground turkey
- ½ cup minced apples

Directions:
1. Combine all of the seasonings in a bowl. Add turkey and apple and blend seasonings in well with your hands. Form patties about 3 inches in diameter and ¼ inch thick.
2. Preheat air fryer to 400°F/205°C. Arrange patties in a single layer on the greased frying basket. Air Fry for 10 minutes, flipping once until brown and cooked through. Serve.

American Biscuits

Servings: 4
Cooking Time: 30 Minutes
Ingredients:
- 2 cups all-purpose flour
- 1 tbsp baking powder
- ½ tsp baking soda
- ½ tsp cornstarch
- ½ tsp salt
- ½ tsp sugar
- 4 tbsp cold butter, cubed
- 1 ¼ cups buttermilk
- 1/2 tsp vanilla extract
- 1 tsp finely crushed walnuts

Directions:
1. Preheat air fryer at 350ºF/175°C. Combine dry ingredients in a bowl. Stir in the remaining ingredients gradually until a sticky dough forms. Using your floured hands, form dough into 8 balls. Place them into a greased pizza pan. Place pizza pan in the frying basket and Bake for 8 minutes. Serve immediately.

Healthy Granola

Servings: 4
Cooking Time: 10 Minutes
Ingredients:
- ¼ cup chocolate hazelnut spread
- 1 cup chopped pecans
- 1 cup quick-cooking oats
- 1 tbsp chia seeds
- 1 tbsp flaxseed
- 1 tbsp sesame seeds
- 1 cup coconut shreds
- ¼ cup maple syrup
- 1 tbsp light brown sugar
- ½ tsp vanilla extract
- ¼ cup hazelnut flour
- 2 tbsp cocoa powder
- Salt to taste

Directions:

1. Preheat air fryer at 350ºF/175°C. Combine the pecans, oats, chia seeds, flaxseed, sesame seeds, coconut shreds, chocolate hazelnut spread, maple syrup, sugar, vanilla extract, hazelnut flour, cocoa powder, and salt in a bowl. Press mixture into a greased cake pan. Place cake pan in the frying basket and Bake for 5 minutes, stirring once. Let cool completely before crumbling. Store it into an airtight container up to 5 days.

Green Strata

Servings: 4
Cooking Time: 35 Minutes
Ingredients:
- 5 asparagus, chopped
- 4 eggs
- 3 tbsp milk
- 1 cup baby spinach, torn
- 2 bread slices, cubed
- ½ cup grated Gruyere cheese
- 2 tbsp chopped parsley
- Salt and pepper to taste

Directions:
1. Preheat air fryer to 340°F/170°C. Add asparagus spears and 1 tbsp water in a baking pan. Place the pan into the air fryer. Bake until crisp and tender, 3-5 minutes. Remove. Wipe to basket clean and spray with cooking spray. Return asparagus to the pan and arrange the bread cubes.
2. Beat the eggs and milk in a bowl. Then mix in baby spinach and Gruyere cheese, parsley, salt, and pepper. Pour over the asparagus and bread. Return to the fryer and Bake until eggs are set, and the tops browned, 12-14 minutes. Serve warm.

Apricot-cheese Mini Pies

Servings: 6
Cooking Time: 35 Minutes
Ingredients:
- 2 refrigerated piecrusts
- 1/3 cup apricot preserves
- 1 tsp cornstarch
- ½ cup vanilla yogurt
- 1 oz cream cheese
- 1 tsp sugar
- Rainbow sprinkles

Directions:
1. Preheat air fryer to 370°F/185°C. Lay out pie crusts on a flat surface. Cut each sheet of pie crust with a knife into three rectangles for a total of 6 rectangles. Mix apricot preserves and cornstarch in a small bowl. Cover the top half of one rectangle with 1 tbsp of the preserve mixture. Repeat for all rectangles. Fold the bottom of the crust over the preserve-covered top. Crimp and seal all edges with a fork.
2. Lightly coat each tart with cooking oil, then place into the air fryer without stacking. Bake for 10 minutes. Meanwhile, prepare the frosting by mixing yogurt, cream cheese, and sugar. When tarts are done, let cool completely in the air fryer. Frost the tarts and top with sprinkles. Serve.

Sweet-hot Pepperoni Pizza

Servings: 2
Cooking Time: 18 Minutes
Ingredients:
- 1 (6- to 8-ounce) pizza dough ball*
- olive oil
- ½ cup pizza sauce
- ¾ cup grated mozzarella cheese

- ½ cup thick sliced pepperoni
- ⅓ cup sliced pickled hot banana peppers
- ¼ teaspoon dried oregano
- 2 teaspoons honey

Directions:
1. Preheat the air fryer to 390°F/200°C.
2. Cut out a piece of aluminum foil the same size as the bottom of the air fryer basket. Brush the foil circle with olive oil. Shape the dough into a circle and place it on top of the foil. Dock the dough by piercing it several times with a fork. Brush the dough lightly with olive oil and transfer it into the air fryer basket with the foil on the bottom.
3. Air-fry the plain pizza dough for 6 minutes. Turn the dough over, remove the aluminum foil and brush again with olive oil. Air-fry for an additional 4 minutes.
4. Spread the pizza sauce on top of the dough and sprinkle the mozzarella cheese over the sauce. Top with the pepperoni, pepper slices and dried oregano. Lower the temperature of the air fryer to 350°F/175°C and cook for 8 minutes, until the cheese has melted and lightly browned. Transfer the pizza to a cutting board and drizzle with the honey. Slice and serve.

Maple-peach And Apple Oatmeal

Servings: 4
Cooking Time: 15 Minutes
Ingredients:
- 2 cups old-fashioned rolled oats
- ½ tsp baking powder
- 1 ½ tsp ground cinnamon
- ¼ tsp ground flaxseeds
- ⅛ tsp salt
- 1 ¼ cups vanilla almond milk
- ¼ cup maple syrup
- 1 tsp vanilla extract
- 1 peeled peach, diced
- 1 peeled apple, diced

Directions:
1. Preheat air fryer to 350°F/175°C. Mix oats, baking powder, cinnamon, flaxseed, and salt in a large bowl. Next, stir in almond milk, maple syrup, vanilla, and ¾ of the diced peaches, and ¾ of the diced apple. Grease 6 ramekins. Divide the batter evenly between the ramekins and transfer the ramekins to the frying basket. Bake in the air fryer for 8-10 minutes until the top is golden and set. Garnish with the rest of the peaches and apples. Serve.

Mini Everything Bagels

Servings: 4
Cooking Time: 6 Minutes
Ingredients:
- 1 cup all-purpose flour
- 2 teaspoons baking powder
- ½ teaspoon salt
- 1 cup plain Greek yogurt
- 1 egg, whisked
- 1 teaspoon sesame seeds
- 1 teaspoon dehydrated onions
- ½ teaspoon poppy seeds
- ½ teaspoon garlic powder
- ½ teaspoon sea salt flakes

Directions:
1. In a large bowl, mix together the flour, baking powder, and salt. Make a well in the dough and add in the Greek yogurt. Mix with a spoon until a dough forms.

2. Place the dough onto a heavily floured surface and knead for 3 minutes. You may use up to 1 cup of additional flour as you knead the dough, if necessary.
3. Cut the dough into 8 pieces and roll each piece into a 6-inch, snakelike piece. Touch the ends of each piece together so it closes the circle and forms a bagel shape. Brush the tops of the bagels with the whisked egg.
4. In a small bowl, combine the sesame seeds, dehydrated onions, poppy seeds, garlic powder, and sea salt flakes. Sprinkle the seasoning on top of the bagels.
5. Preheat the air fryer to 360°F/180°C. Using a bench scraper or flat-edged spatula, carefully place the bagels into the air fryer basket. Spray the bagel tops with cooking spray. Air-fry the bagels for 6 minutes or until golden brown. Allow the bread to cool at least 10 minutes before slicing for serving.

Honey Donuts

Servings: 6
Cooking Time: 25 Minutes + Chilling Time
Ingredients:
- 1 refrigerated puff pastry sheet
- 2 tsp flour
- 2 ½ cups powdered sugar
- 3 tbsp honey
- 2 tbsp milk
- 2 tbsp butter, melted
- ½ tsp vanilla extract
- ½ tsp ground cinnamon
- Pinch of salt

Directions:
1. Preheat the air fryer to 325°F/160°C. Dust a clean work surface with flour and lay the puff pastry on it, then cut crosswise into five 3-inch wide strips. Cut each strip into thirds for 15 squares. Lay round parchment paper in the bottom of the basket, then add the pastry squares in a single layer.
2. Make sure none are touching. Bake for 13-18 minutes or until brown, then leave on a rack to cool. Repeat for all dough. Combine the sugar, honey, milk, butter, vanilla, cinnamon, and salt in a small bowl and mix with a wire whisk until combined. Dip the top half of each donut in the glaze, turn the donut glaze side up, and return to the wire rack. Let cool until the glaze sets, then serve.

Veggie & Feta Scramble Bowls

Servings: 2
Cooking Time: 25 Minutes
Ingredients:
- 1 russet potato, cubed
- 1 bell pepper, cut into strips
- ½ feta, cubed
- 1 tbsp nutritional yeast
- ½ tsp garlic powder
- ½ tsp onion powder
- ¼ tsp ground turmeric
- 1 tbsp apple cider vinegar

Directions:
1. Preheat air fryer to 400°F/205°C. Put in potato cubes and bell pepper strips and Air Fry for 10 minutes. Combine the feta, nutritional yeast, garlic, onion, turmeric, and apple vinegar in a small pan. Fit a trivet in the fryer, lay the pan on top, and Air Fry for 5 more minutes until potatoes are tender and feta cheese cooked. Share potatoes and bell peppers into 2 bowls and top with feta scramble. Serve.

Easy Vanilla Muffins

Servings: 6
Cooking Time: 35 Minutes + Cooling Time
Ingredients:
- 1 1/3 cups flour
- 5 tbsp butter, melted
- ¼ cup brown sugar
- 2 tbsp raisins
- ½ tsp ground cinnamon
- 1/3 cup granulated sugar
- ¼ cup milk
- 1 large egg
- 1 tsp vanilla extract
- 1 tsp baking powder
- Pinch of salt

Directions:
1. Preheat the air fryer to 330°F/165°C. Combine 1/3 cup of flour, 2 ½ tbsp of butter, brown sugar, and cinnamon in a bowl and mix until crumbly. Set aside. In another bowl, combine the remaining butter, granulated sugar, milk, egg, and vanilla and stir well. Add the remaining flour, baking powder, raisins, and salt and stir until combined.
2. Spray 6 silicone muffin cups with baking spray and spoon half the batter into them. Add a tsp of the cinnamon mixture, then add the rest of the batter and sprinkle with the remaining cinnamon mixture, pressing into the batter. Put the muffin cups in the frying basket and Bake for 14-18 minutes or until a toothpick inserted into the center comes out clean. Cool for 10 minutes, then remove the muffins from the cups. Serve and enjoy!

Baked Eggs With Bacon-tomato Sauce

Servings: 1
Cooking Time: 12 Minutes
Ingredients:
- 1 teaspoon olive oil
- 2 tablespoons finely chopped onion
- 1 teaspoon chopped fresh oregano
- pinch crushed red pepper flakes
- 1 (14-ounce) can crushed or diced tomatoes
- salt and freshly ground black pepper
- 2 slices of bacon, chopped
- 2 large eggs
- ¼ cup grated Cheddar cheese
- fresh parsley, chopped

Directions:
1. Start by making the tomato sauce. Preheat a medium saucepan over medium heat on the stovetop. Add the olive oil and sauté the onion, oregano and pepper flakes for 5 minutes. Add the tomatoes and bring to a simmer. Season with salt and freshly ground black pepper and simmer for 10 minutes.
2. Meanwhile, Preheat the air fryer to 400°F/205°C and pour a little water into the bottom of the air fryer drawer. (This will help prevent the grease that drips into the bottom drawer from burning and smoking.) Place the bacon in the air fryer basket and air-fry at 400°F/205°C for 5 minutes, shaking the basket every once in a while.
3. When the bacon is almost crispy, remove it to a paper-towel lined plate and rinse out the air fryer drawer, draining away the bacon grease.
4. Transfer the tomato sauce to a shallow 7-inch pie dish. Crack the eggs on top of the sauce and scatter the cooked bacon back on top. Season with salt and freshly ground black pepper and transfer the pie dish into the air fryer basket. You can use an aluminum foil sling to help with this by taking a long piece of aluminum foil, folding it in half lengthwise twice until it is roughly 26-inches by 3-inches. Place this under the pie dish and hold the ends of the foil to move the pie dish in and out of the air fryer basket. Tuck the ends of the foil beside the pie dish while it cooks in the air fryer.
5. Air-fry at 400°F/205°C for 5 minutes, or until the eggs are almost cooked to your liking. Sprinkle cheese on top and air-fry for an additional 2 minutes. When the cheese has melted, remove the pie dish from the air fryer, sprinkle with a little chopped parsley and let the eggs cool for a few minutes – just enough time to toast some buttered bread in your air fryer!

Effortless Toffee Zucchini Bread

Servings: 6
Cooking Time: 30 Minutes
Ingredients:
- 1 cup flour
- ½ tsp baking soda
- ½ cup granulated sugar
- ¼ tsp ground cinnamon
- ¼ tsp nutmeg
- ¼ tsp salt
- 1/3 cup grated zucchini
- 1 egg
- 1 tbsp olive oil
- 1 tsp vanilla extract
- 2 tbsp English toffee bits
- 2 tbsp mini chocolate chips
- 1/2 cup chopped walnuts

Directions:
1. Preheat air fryer at 375ºF/190°C. Combine the flour, baking soda, toffee bits, sugar, cinnamon, nutmeg, salt, zucchini, egg, olive oil, vanilla and chocolate chips in a bowl. Add the walnuts to the batter and mix until evenly distributed.
2. Pour the mixture into a greased cake pan. Place the pan in the fryer and Bake for 20 minutes. Let sit for 10 minutes until slightly cooled before slicing. Serve immediately.

Cherry Beignets

Servings: 4
Cooking Time: 25 Minutes
Ingredients:
- 2 tsp baking soda
- 1 ½ cups flour
- ¼ tsp salt
- 3 tbsp brown sugar
- 4 tsp chopped dried cherries
- ½ cup buttermilk
- 1 egg
- 3 tbsp melted lard

Directions:
1. Preheat air fryer to 330°F/165°C. Combine baking soda, flour, salt, and brown sugar in a bowl. Then stir in dried cherries. In a small bowl, beat together buttermilk and egg until smooth. Pour in with the dry ingredients and stir until just moistened.
2. On a floured work surface, pat the dough into a square. Divide it by cutting into 16 pieces. Lightly brush with melted lard. Arrange the squares in the frying basket, without overlapping. Air Fry until puffy and golden brown, 5-8 minutes. Serve.

Cherry-apple Oatmeal Cups

Servings: 2
Cooking Time: 20 Minutes
Ingredients:
- 2/3 cup rolled oats
- 1 cored apple, diced
- 4 pitted cherries, diced
- ½ tsp ground cinnamon
- ¾ cup milk

Directions:
1. Preheat air fryer to 350°F/175°C. Mix the oats, apple, cherries, and cinnamon in a heatproof bowl. Add in milk and Bake for 6 minutes, stir well and Bake for 6 more minutes until the fruit are soft. Serve cooled.

Bacon & Egg Quesadillas

Servings: 4
Cooking Time: 30 Minutes
Ingredients:
- 8 flour tortillas
- ½ lb cooked bacon, crumbled
- 6 eggs, scrambled
- 1 ½ cups grated cheddar
- 1 tsp chopped chives
- 1 tsp parsley
- Black pepper on taste

Directions:
1. Preheat air fryer at 350ºF/175°C. Place 1 tortilla in the bottom of a cake pan. Spread ¼ portion of each crumbled bacon, eggs, chives, parsley, pepper and cheese over the tortilla and top with a second tortilla.
2. Place cake pan in the frying basket and Bake for 4 minutes. Set aside on a large plate and repeat the process with the remaining ingredients. Let cool for 3 minutes before slicing. Serve right away.

Country Gravy

Servings: 2
Cooking Time: 7 Minutes
Ingredients:
- ¼ pound pork sausage, casings removed
- 1 tablespoon butter
- 2 tablespoons flour
- 2 cups whole milk
- ½ teaspoon salt
- freshly ground black pepper
- 1 teaspoon fresh thyme leaves

Directions:
1. Preheat a saucepan over medium heat. Add and brown the sausage, crumbling it into small pieces as it cooks. Add the butter and flour, stirring well to combine. Continue to cook for 2 minutes, stirring constantly.
2. Slowly pour in the milk, whisking as you do, and bring the mixture to a boil to thicken. Season with salt and freshly ground black pepper, lower the heat and simmer until the sauce has thickened to your desired consistency – about 5 minutes. Stir in the fresh thyme, season to taste and serve hot.

Orange Rolls

Servings: 8
Cooking Time: 10 Minutes
Ingredients:
- parchment paper
- 3 ounces low-fat cream cheese
- 1 tablespoon low-fat sour cream or plain yogurt (not Greek yogurt)
- 2 teaspoons sugar
- ¼ teaspoon pure vanilla extract
- ¼ teaspoon orange extract
- 1 can (8 count) organic crescent roll dough
- ¼ cup chopped walnuts
- ¼ cup dried cranberries
- ¼ cup shredded, sweetened coconut
- butter-flavored cooking spray
- Orange Glaze
- ½ cup powdered sugar
- 1 tablespoon orange juice
- ¼ teaspoon orange extract
- dash of salt

Directions:
1. Cut a circular piece of parchment paper slightly smaller than the bottom of your air fryer basket. Set aside.
2. In a small bowl, combine the cream cheese, sour cream or yogurt, sugar, and vanilla and orange extracts. Stir until smooth.
3. Preheat air fryer to 300°F/150°C.
4. Separate crescent roll dough into 8 triangles and divide cream cheese mixture among them. Starting at wide end, spread cheese mixture to within 1 inch of point.
5. Sprinkle nuts and cranberries evenly over cheese mixture.
6. Starting at wide end, roll up triangles, then sprinkle with coconut, pressing in lightly to make it stick. Spray tops of rolls with butter-flavored cooking spray.
7. Place parchment paper in air fryer basket, and place 4 rolls on top, spaced evenly.
8. Cook for 10minutes, until rolls are golden brown and cooked through.
9. Repeat steps 7 and 8 to cook remaining 4 rolls. You should be able to use the same piece of parchment paper twice.
10. In a small bowl, stir together ingredients for glaze and drizzle over warm rolls.

Bacon, Broccoli And Swiss Cheese Bread Pudding

Servings: 2
Cooking Time: 48 Minutes
Ingredients:
- ½ pound thick cut bacon, cut into ¼-inch pieces
- 3 cups brioche bread or rolls, cut into ½-inch cubes
- 3 eggs
- 1 cup milk
- ½ teaspoon salt
- freshly ground black pepper
- 1 cup frozen broccoli florets, thawed and chopped
- 1½ cups grated Swiss cheese

Directions:
1. Preheat the air fryer to 400°F/205°C.
2. Air-fry the bacon for 6 minutes until crispy, shaking the basket a few times while it cooks to help it cook evenly. Remove the bacon and set it aside on a paper towel.
3. Air-fry the brioche bread cubes for 2 minutes to dry and toast lightly. (If your brioche is a few days old and slightly stale, you can omit this step.)
4. Butter a 6- or 7-inch cake pan. Combine all the ingredients in a large bowl and toss well. Transfer the mixture to the buttered cake pan, cover with aluminum foil and refrigerate the bread pudding overnight, or for at least 8 hours.
5. Remove the casserole from the refrigerator an hour before you plan to cook, and let it sit on the countertop to come to room temperature.

6. Preheat the air fryer to 330°F/165°C. Transfer the covered cake pan, to the basket of the air fryer, lowering the dish into the basket using a sling made of aluminum foil (fold a piece of aluminum foil into a strip about 2-inches wide by 24-inches long). Fold the ends of the aluminum foil over the top of the dish before returning the basket to the air fryer. Air-fry for 20 minutes. Remove the foil and air-fry for an additional 20 minutes. If the top starts to brown a little too much before the custard has set, simply return the foil to the pan. The bread pudding has cooked through when a skewer inserted into the center comes out clean.

Viking Toast

Servings: 2
Cooking Time: 20 Minutes
Ingredients:
- 2 tbsp minced green chili pepper
- 1 avocado, pressed
- 1 clove garlic, minced
- ¼ tsp lemon juice
- Salt and pepper to taste
- 2 bread slices
- 2 plum tomatoes, sliced
- 4 oz smoked salmon
- ¼ diced peeled red onion

Directions:
1. Preheat air fryer at 350°F/175°C. Combine the avocado, garlic, lemon juice, and salt in a bowl until you reach your desired consistency. Spread avocado mixture on the bread slices.
2. Top with tomato slices and sprinkle with black pepper. Place bread slices in the frying basket and Bake for 5 minutes. Transfer to a plate. Top each bread slice with salmon, green chili pepper, and red onion. Serve.

Pumpkin Empanadas

Servings: 4
Cooking Time: 30 Minutes
Ingredients:
- 1 can pumpkin purée
- ¼ cup white sugar
- 2 tsp cinnamon
- 1 tbsp brown sugar
- ½ tbsp cornstarch
- ¼ tsp vanilla extract
- 2 tbsp butter
- 4 empanada dough shells

Directions:
1. Place the puree in a pot and top with white and brown sugar, cinnamon, cornstarch, vanilla extract, 1 tbsp of water and butter and stir thoroughly. Bring to a boil over medium heat. Simmer for 4-5 minutes. Allow to cool.
2. Preheat air fryer to 360°F/180°C. Lay empanada shells flat on a clean counter. Spoon the pumpkin mixture into each of the shells. Fold the empanada shells over to cover completely. Seal the edges with water and press down with a fork to secure. Place the empanadas on the greased frying basket and Bake for 15 minutes, flipping once halfway through until golden. Serve hot.

Apple French Toast Sandwich

Servings: 1
Cooking Time: 30 Minutes
Ingredients:
- 2 white bread slices
- 2 eggs
- 1 tsp cinnamon
- ½ peeled apple, sliced
- 1 tbsp brown sugar
- ¼ cup whipped cream

Directions:
1. Preheat air fryer to 350°F/175°C. Coat the apple slices with brown sugar in a small bowl. Whisk the eggs and cinnamon into a separate bowl until fluffy and completely blended. Coat the bread slices with the egg mixture, then place them on the greased frying basket. Top with apple slices and Air Fry for 20 minutes, flipping once until the bread is brown nicely and the apple is crispy.
2. Place one French toast slice onto a serving plate, then spoon the whipped cream on top and spread evenly. Scoop the caramelized apple slices onto the whipped cream, and cover with the second toast slice. Serve.

Peppered Maple Bacon Knots

Servings: 6
Cooking Time: 8 Minutes
Ingredients:
- 1 pound maple smoked center-cut bacon
- ¼ cup maple syrup
- ¼ cup brown sugar
- coarsely cracked black peppercorns

Directions:
1. Tie each bacon strip in a loose knot and place them on a baking sheet.
2. Combine the maple syrup and brown sugar in a bowl. Brush each knot generously with this mixture and sprinkle with coarsely cracked black pepper.
3. Preheat the air fryer to 390°F/200°C.
4. Air-fry the bacon knots in batches. Place one layer of knots in the air fryer basket and air-fry for 5 minutes. Turn the bacon knots over and air-fry for an additional 3 minutes.
5. Serve warm.

Garlic Parmesan Bread Ring

Servings: 6
Cooking Time: 30 Minutes
Ingredients:
- ½ cup unsalted butter, melted
- ¼ teaspoon salt (omit if using salted butter)
- ¾ cup grated Parmesan cheese
- 3 to 4 cloves garlic, minced
- 1 tablespoon chopped fresh parsley
- 1 pound frozen bread dough, defrosted
- olive oil
- 1 egg, beaten

Directions:
1. Combine the melted butter, salt, Parmesan cheese, garlic and chopped parsley in a small bowl.
2. Roll the dough out into a rectangle that measures 8 inches by 17 inches. Spread the butter mixture over the dough, leaving a half-inch border un-buttered along one of the long edges. Roll the dough from one long edge to the other, ending with the un-buttered border. Pinch the seam shut tightly. Shape the log into a circle sealing the ends together by pushing one end into the other and stretching the dough around it.
3. Cut out a circle of aluminum foil that is the same size as the air fryer basket. Brush the foil circle with oil and place an oven safe ramekin or glass in the center. Transfer the dough ring to the aluminum foil circle, around the ramekin. This will help you make sure the dough will fit in the basket and maintain its ring shape. Use kitchen shears to cut 8 slits

around the outer edge of the dough ring halfway to the center. Brush the dough ring with egg wash.

4. Preheat the air fryer to 400°F/205°C for 4 minutes. When it has Preheated, brush the sides of the basket with oil and transfer the dough ring, foil circle and ramekin into the basket. Slide the drawer back into the air fryer, but do not turn the air fryer on. Let the dough rise inside the warm air fryer for 30 minutes.

5. After the bread has proofed in the air fryer for 30 minutes, set the temperature to 340°F/170°C and air-fry the bread ring for 15 minutes. Flip the bread over by inverting it onto a plate or cutting board and sliding it back into the air fryer basket. Air-fry for another 15 minutes. Let the bread cool for a few minutes before slicing the bread ring in between the slits and serving warm.

Oat Bran Muffins

Servings: 8
Cooking Time: 12 Minutes
Ingredients:
- ⅔ cup oat bran
- ½ cup flour
- ¼ cup brown sugar
- 1 teaspoon baking powder
- ½ teaspoon baking soda
- ⅛ teaspoon salt
- ½ cup buttermilk
- 1 egg
- 2 tablespoons canola oil
- ½ cup chopped dates, raisins, or dried cranberries
- 24 paper muffin cups
- cooking spray

Directions:
1. Preheat air fryer to 330°F/165°C.
2. In a large bowl, combine the oat bran, flour, brown sugar, baking powder, baking soda, and salt.
3. In a small bowl, beat together the buttermilk, egg, and oil.
4. Pour buttermilk mixture into bowl with dry ingredients and stir just until moistened. Do not beat.
5. Gently stir in dried fruit.
6. Use triple baking cups to help muffins hold shape during baking. Spray them with cooking spray, place 4 sets of cups in air fryer basket at a time, and fill each one ¾ full of batter.
7. Cook for 12minutes, until top springs back when lightly touched and toothpick inserted in center comes out clean.
8. Repeat for remaining muffins.

Easy Corn Dog Cupcakes

Servings: 6
Cooking Time: 30 Minutes
Ingredients:
- 1 cup cornbread Mix
- 2 tsp granulated sugar
- Salt to taste
- 3/4 cup cream cheese
- 3 tbsp butter, melted
- 1 egg
- ¼ cup minced onions
- 1 tsp dried parsley
- 2 beef hot dogs, sliced and cut into half-moons

Directions:
1. Preheat air fryer at 350ºF/175°C. Combine cornbread, sugar, and salt in a bowl. In another bowl, whisk cream cheese, parsley, butter, and egg. Pour wet ingredients to dry ingredients and toss to combine. Fold in onion and hot dog pieces. Transfer it into 8 greased silicone cupcake liners.

Place it in the frying basket and Bake for 8-10 minutes. Serve right away.

Parma Ham & Egg Toast Cups

Servings: 4
Cooking Time: 25 Minutes
Ingredients:
- 4 crusty rolls
- 4 Gouda cheese thin slices
- 5 eggs
- 2 tbsp heavy cream
- ½ tsp dried thyme
- 3 Parma ham slices, chopped
- Salt and pepper to taste

Directions:
1. Preheat air fryer to 330°F/165°C. Slice off the top of the rolls, then tear out the insides with your fingers, leaving about ½-inch of bread to make a shell. Press one cheese slice inside the roll shell until it takes the shape of the roll.
2. Beat eggs with heavy cream in a medium bowl. Next, mix in the remaining ingredients. Spoon egg mixture into the rolls lined with cheese. Place rolls in the greased frying basket and Bake until eggs are puffy and brown, 8-12 minutes. Serve warm.

Orange Trail Oatmeal

Servings: 4
Cooking Time: 20 Minutes
Ingredients:
- 1 ½ cups quick-cooking oats
- 1/3 cup light brown sugar
- 1 egg
- 1 tsp orange zest
- 1 tbsp orange juice
- 2 tbsp whole milk
- 2 tbsp honey
- 2 tbsp butter, melted
- 2 tsp dried cranberries
- 1 tsp dried blueberries
- 1/8 tsp ground nutmeg
- Salt to taste
- ¼ cup pecan pieces

Directions:
1. Preheat air fryer at 325°F/160°C. Combine the oats, sugar, egg, orange zest, orange juice, milk, honey, butter, dried cranberries, dried blueberries, nutmeg, salt, and pecan in a bowl. Press mixture into a greased cake pan. Place cake pan in the frying basket and Roast for 8 minutes. Let cool onto for 5 minutes before slicing. Serve.

Ham And Cheddar Gritters

Servings: 6
Cooking Time: 12 Minutes
Ingredients:
- 4 cups water
- 1 cup quick-cooking grits
- ¼ teaspoon salt
- 2 tablespoons butter
- 2 cups grated Cheddar cheese, divided
- 1 cup finely diced ham
- 1 tablespoon chopped chives
- salt and freshly ground black pepper
- 1 egg, beaten
- 2 cups panko breadcrumbs
- vegetable oil

Directions:

1. Bring the water to a boil in a saucepan. Whisk in the grits and ¼ teaspoon of salt, and cook for 7 minutes until the grits are soft. Remove the pan from the heat and stir in the butter and 1 cup of the grated Cheddar cheese. Transfer the grits to a bowl and let them cool for just 10 to 15 minutes.
2. Stir the ham, chives and the rest of the cheese into the grits and season with salt and pepper to taste. Add the beaten egg and refrigerate the mixture for 30 minutes. (Try not to chill the grits much longer than 30 minutes, or the mixture will be too firm to shape into patties.)
3. While the grit mixture is chilling, make the country gravy and set it aside.
4. Place the panko breadcrumbs in a shallow dish. Measure out ¼-cup portions of the grits mixture and shape them into patties. Coat all sides of the patties with the panko breadcrumbs, patting them with your hands so the crumbs adhere to the patties. You should have about 16 patties. Spray both sides of the patties with oil.
5. Preheat the air fryer to 400°F/205°C.
6. In batches of 5 or 6, air-fry the fritters for 8 minutes. Using a flat spatula, flip the fritters over and air-fry for another 4 minutes.
7. Serve hot with country gravy.

Thai Turkey Sausage Patties

Servings:4
Cooking Time: 30 Minutes
Ingredients:
- 12 oz turkey sausage
- 1 tsp onion powder
- 1 tsp dried coriander
- ¼ tsp Thai curry paste
- ¼ tsp red pepper flakes
- Salt and pepper to taste

Directions:
1. Preheat air fryer to 350°F/175°C. Place the sausage, onion, coriander, curry paste, red flakes, salt, and black pepper in a large bowl and mix well. Form into eight patties. Arrange the patties on the greased frying basket and Air Fry for 10 minutes, flipping once halfway through. Once the patties are cooked, transfer to a plate and serve hot.

Sweet And Spicy Pumpkin Scones

Servings: 8
Cooking Time: 8 Minutes
Ingredients:
- 2 cups all-purpose flour
- 3 tablespoons packed brown sugar
- ½ teaspoon baking powder
- ¼ teaspoon baking soda
- ½ teaspoon kosher salt
- ½ teaspoon ground cinnamon
- ¼ teaspoon ground ginger
- ¼ teaspoon ground cardamom
- 4 tablespoons cold unsalted butter
- ½ cup plus 2 tablespoons pumpkin puree, divided
- 4 tablespoons milk, divided
- 1 large egg
- 1 cup powdered sugar

Directions:
1. In a large bowl, mix together the flour, brown sugar, baking powder, baking soda, salt, cinnamon, ginger, and cardamom. Using a pastry blender or two knives, cut in the butter until coarse crumbles appear.
2. In a small bowl, whisk together ½ cup of the pumpkin puree, 2 tablespoons of the milk, and the egg until combined.

Pour the wet ingredients into the dry ingredients; stir to combine.
3. Form the dough into a ball and place onto a floured service. Press the dough out or use a rolling pin to roll out the dough until ½ inch thick and in a circle. Cut the dough into 8 wedges.
4. Bake at 360°F/180°C for 8 to 10 minutes or until completely cooked through. Cook in batches as needed.
5. In a medium bowl, whisk together the powdered sugar, the remaining 2 tablespoons of pumpkin puree, and the remaining 2 tablespoons of milk. When the pumpkin scones have cooled, drizzle the pumpkin glaze over the top before serving.

Apple-cinnamon-walnut Muffins

Servings: 8
Cooking Time: 11 Minutes
Ingredients:
- 1 cup flour
- ⅓ cup sugar
- 1 teaspoon baking powder
- ¼ teaspoon baking soda
- ¼ teaspoon salt
- 1 teaspoon cinnamon
- ¼ teaspoon ginger
- ¼ teaspoon nutmeg
- 1 egg
- 2 tablespoons pancake syrup, plus 2 teaspoons
- 2 tablespoons melted butter, plus 2 teaspoons
- ¾ cup unsweetened applesauce
- ½ teaspoon vanilla extract
- ¼ cup chopped walnuts
- ¼ cup diced apple
- 8 foil muffin cups, liners removed and sprayed with cooking spray

Directions:
1. Preheat air fryer to 330°F/165°C.
2. In a large bowl, stir together flour, sugar, baking powder, baking soda, salt, cinnamon, ginger, and nutmeg.
3. In a small bowl, beat egg until frothy. Add syrup, butter, applesauce, and vanilla and mix well.
4. Pour egg mixture into dry ingredients and stir just until moistened.
5. Gently stir in nuts and diced apple.
6. Divide batter among the 8 muffin cups.
7. Place 4 muffin cups in air fryer basket and cook at 330°F/165°C for 11minutes.
8. Repeat with remaining 4 muffins or until toothpick inserted in center comes out clean.

Classic Cinnamon Rolls

Servings: 4
Cooking Time: 6 Minutes
Ingredients:
- 1½ cups all-purpose flour
- 1 tablespoon granulated sugar
- 2 teaspoons baking powder
- ½ teaspoon salt
- 4 tablespoons butter, divided
- ½ cup buttermilk
- 2 tablespoons brown sugar
- 1 teaspoon cinnamon
- 1 cup powdered sugar
- 2 tablespoons milk

Directions:
1. Preheat the air fryer to 360°F/180°C.

2. In a large bowl, stir together the flour, sugar, baking powder, and salt. Cut in 3 tablespoons of the butter with a pastry blender or two knives until coarse crumbs remain. Stir in the buttermilk until a dough forms.
3. Place the dough onto a floured surface and roll out into a square shape about ½ inch thick.
4. Melt the remaining 1 tablespoon of butter in the microwave for 20 seconds. Using a pastry brush or your fingers, spread the melted butter onto the dough.
5. In a small bowl, mix together the brown sugar and cinnamon. Sprinkle the mixture across the surface of the dough. Roll the dough up, forming a long log. Using a pastry cutter or sharp knife, cut 10 cinnamon rolls.
6. Carefully place the cinnamon rolls into the air fryer basket. Then bake at 360°F/180°C for 6 minutes or until golden brown.
7. Meanwhile, in a small bowl, whisk together the powdered sugar and milk.
8. Plate the cinnamon rolls and drizzle the glaze over the surface before serving.

Soft Pretzels

Servings: 12
Cooking Time: 6 Minutes
Ingredients:
- 2 teaspoons yeast
- 1 cup water, warm
- 1 teaspoon sugar
- 1 teaspoon salt
- 2½ cups all-purpose flour
- 2 tablespoons butter, melted
- 1 cup boiling water
- 1 tablespoon baking soda
- coarse sea salt
- melted butter

Directions:
1. Combine the yeast and water in a small bowl. Combine the sugar, salt and flour in the bowl of a stand mixer. With the mixer running and using the dough hook, drizzle in the yeast mixture and melted butter and knead dough until smooth and elastic – about 10 minutes. Shape into a ball and let the dough rise for 1 hour.
2. Punch the dough down to release any air and decide what size pretzels you want to make.
3. a. To make large pretzels, divide the dough into 12 portions.
4. b. To make medium sized pretzels, divide the dough into 24 portions.
5. c. To make mini pretzel knots, divide the dough into 48 portions.
6. Roll each portion into a skinny rope using both hands on the counter and rolling from the center to the ends of the rope. Spin the rope into a pretzel shape (or tie the rope into a knot) and place the tied pretzels on a parchment lined baking sheet.
7. Preheat the air fryer to 350°F/175°C.
8. Combine the boiling water and baking soda in a shallow bowl and whisk to dissolve (this mixture will bubble, but it will settle down). Let the water cool so that you can put your hands in it. Working in batches, dip the pretzels (top side down) into the baking soda-water mixture and let them soak for 30 seconds to a minute. (This step is what gives pretzels their texture and helps them to brown faster.) Then, remove the pretzels carefully and return them (top side up) to the baking sheet. Sprinkle the coarse salt on the top.
9. Air-fry in batches for 3 minutes per side. When the pretzels are finished, brush them generously with the melted butter and enjoy them warm with some spicy mustard.

Filled French Toast

Servings: 4
Cooking Time: 25 Minutes
Ingredients:
- 4 French bread slices
- 2 tbsp blueberry jam
- 1/3 cup fresh blueberries
- 2 egg yolks
- 1/3 cup milk
- 1 tbsp sugar
- ½ tsp vanilla extract
- 3 tbsp sour cream

Directions:
1. Preheat the air fryer to 370°F/185°C. Cut a pocket into the side of each slice of bread. Don't cut all the way through. Combine the blueberry jam and blueberries and crush the blueberries into the jam with a fork. In a separate bowl, beat the egg yolks with milk, sugar, and vanilla until well combined. Smear some sour cream in the pocket of each bread slice and add the blueberry mix on top. Squeeze the edges of the bread to close the opening. Dip the bread in the egg mixture, soak for 3 minutes per side. In a single layer, put the bread in the greased frying basket and Air Fry for 5 minutes. Flip the bread and cook for 3-6 more minutes or until golden.

Pumpkin Loaf

Servings: 6
Cooking Time: 22 Minutes
Ingredients:
- cooking spray
- 1 large egg
- ½ cup granulated sugar
- ⅓ cup oil
- ½ cup canned pumpkin (not pie filling)
- ½ teaspoon vanilla
- ⅔ cup flour plus 1 tablespoon
- ½ teaspoon baking powder
- ½ teaspoon baking soda
- ½ teaspoon salt
- 1 teaspoon pumpkin pie spice
- ¼ teaspoon cinnamon

Directions:
1. Spray 6 x 6-inch baking dish lightly with cooking spray.
2. Place baking dish in air fryer basket and preheat air fryer to 330°F/165°C.
3. In a large bowl, beat eggs and sugar together with a hand mixer.
4. Add oil, pumpkin, and vanilla and mix well.
5. Sift together all dry ingredients. Add to pumpkin mixture and beat well, about 1 minute.
6. Pour batter in baking dish and cook at 330°F/165°C for 22 minutes or until toothpick inserted in center of loaf comes out clean.

White Wheat Walnut Bread

Servings: 8
Cooking Time: 25 Minutes
Ingredients:
- 1 cup lukewarm water (105–115°F)
- 1 packet RapidRise yeast
- 1 tablespoon light brown sugar
- 2 cups whole-grain white wheat flour
- 1 egg, room temperature, beaten with a fork
- 2 teaspoons olive oil

- ½ teaspoon salt
- ½ cup chopped walnuts
- cooking spray

Directions:
1. In a small bowl, mix the water, yeast, and brown sugar.
2. Pour yeast mixture over flour and mix until smooth.
3. Add the egg, olive oil, and salt and beat with a wooden spoon for 2minutes.
4. Stir in chopped walnuts. You will have very thick batter rather than stiff bread dough.
5. Spray air fryer baking pan with cooking spray and pour in batter, smoothing the top.
6. Let batter rise for 15minutes.
7. Preheat air fryer to 360°F/180°C.
8. Cook bread for 25 minutes, until toothpick pushed into center comes out with crumbs clinging. Let bread rest for 10minutes before removing from pan.

Orange-glazed Cinnamon Rolls

Servings:
Cooking Time: 30 Minutes
Ingredients:
- ½ cup + 1 tbsp evaporated cane sugar
- 1 cup Greek yogurt
- 2 cups flour
- 2 tsp baking powder
- ½ tsp salt
- 4 tbsp butter, softened
- 2 tsp ground cinnamon
- 4 oz cream cheese
- ¼ cup orange juice
- 1 tbsp orange zest
- 1 tbsp lemon juice

Directions:
1. Preheat air fryer to 350°F/175°C. Grease a baking dish. Combine yogurt, 1 ¾ cups flour, baking powder, salt, and ¼ cup sugar in a large bowl until dough forms. Dust the rest of the flour onto a flat work surface. Transfer the dough on the flour and roll into a ¼-inch thick rectangle. If the dough continues to stick to the rolling pin, add 1 tablespoon of flour and continue to roll.
2. Mix the butter, cinnamon, orange zest and 1 tbsp of sugar in a bowl. Spread the butter mixture evenly over the dough. Roll the dough into a log, starting with the long side. Tuck in the end. Cut the log into 6 equal pieces. Place in the baking dish swirl-side up. The rolls can touch each other. Bake in the air fryer for 10-12 minutes until the rolls are cooked through, and the tops are golden. Let cool for 10 minutes. While the rolls are cooling, combine cream cheese, the rest of the sugar, lemon juice, and orange juice in a small bowl. When the rolls are cool enough, top with glaze and serve.

Baked Eggs

Servings: 4
Cooking Time: 6 Minutes
Ingredients:
- 4 large eggs
- ⅛ teaspoon black pepper
- ⅛ teaspoon salt

Directions:
1. Preheat the air fryer to 330°F/165°C. Place 4 silicone muffin liners into the air fryer basket.
2. Crack 1 egg at a time into each silicone muffin liner. Sprinkle with black pepper and salt.
3. Bake for 6 minutes. Remove and let cool 2 minutes prior to serving.

Pancake Muffins

Servings: 4
Cooking Time: 8 Minutes
Ingredients:
- 1 cup flour
- 2 tablespoons sugar (optional)
- ½ teaspoon baking soda
- 1 teaspoon baking powder
- ¼ teaspoon salt
- 1 egg, beaten
- 1 cup buttermilk
- 2 tablespoons melted butter
- 1 teaspoon pure vanilla extract
- 24 foil muffin cups
- cooking spray
- Suggested Fillings
- 1 teaspoon of jelly or fruit preserves
- 1 tablespoon or less fresh blueberries; chopped fresh strawberries; chopped frozen cherries; dark chocolate chips; chopped walnuts, pecans, or other nuts; cooked, crumbled bacon or sausage

Directions:
1. In a large bowl, stir together flour, optional sugar, baking soda, baking powder, and salt.
2. In a small bowl, combine egg, buttermilk, butter, and vanilla. Mix well.
3. Pour egg mixture into dry ingredients and stir to mix well but don't overbeat.
4. Double up the muffin cups and remove the paper liners from the top cups. Spray the foil cups lightly with cooking spray.
5. Place 6 sets of muffin cups in air fryer basket. Pour just enough batter into each cup to cover the bottom. Sprinkle with desired filling. Pour in more batter to cover the filling and fill the cups about ¾ full.
6. Cook at 330°F/165°C for 8minutes.
7. Repeat steps 5 and 6 for the remaining 6 pancake muffins.

Crispy Bacon

Servings: 6
Cooking Time: 20 Minutes
Ingredients:
- 12 ounces bacon

Directions:
1. Preheat the air fryer to 350°F/175°C for 3 minutes.
2. Lay out the bacon in a single layer, slightly overlapping the strips of bacon.
3. Air fry for 10 minutes or until desired crispness.
4. Repeat until all the bacon has been cooked.

Scones

Servings: 9
Cooking Time: 8 Minutes Per Batch
Ingredients:
- 2 cups self-rising flour, plus ¼ cup for kneading
- ⅓ cup granulated sugar
- ¼ cup butter, cold
- 1 cup milk

Directions:
1. Preheat air fryer at 360°F/180°C.
2. In large bowl, stir together flour and sugar.
3. Cut cold butter into tiny cubes, and stir into flour mixture with fork.
4. Stir in milk until soft dough forms.

5. Sprinkle ¼ cup of flour onto wax paper and place dough on top. Knead lightly by folding and turning the dough about 6 to 8 times.
6. Pat dough into a 6 x 6-inch square.
7. Cut into 9 equal squares.
8. Place all squares in air fryer basket or as many as will fit in a single layer, close together but not touching.
9. Cook at 360°F/180°C for 8minutes. When done, scones will be lightly browned on top and will spring back when pressed gently with a dull knife.
10. Repeat steps 8 and 9 to cook remaining scones.

Coconut & Peanut Rice Cereal

Servings: 4
Cooking Time: 15 Minutes
Ingredients:
- 4 cups rice cereal
- 1 cup coconut shreds
- 2 tbsp peanut butter
- 1 tsp vanilla extract
- ¼ cup honey
- 1 tbsp light brown sugar
- 2 tsp ground cinnamon
- ¼ cup hazelnut flour
- Salt to taste

Directions:
1. Preheat air fryer at 350°F/175°C. Combine the rice cereal, coconut shreds, peanut butter, vanilla extract, honey, brown sugar, cinnamon, hazelnut flour, and salt in a bowl. Press mixture into a greased cake pan. Place cake pan in the frying basket and Air Fry for 5 minutes, stirring once. Let cool completely for 10 minutes before crumbling. Store it into an airtight container up to 5 days.

Almond Cranberry Granola

Servings: 12
Cooking Time: 9 Minutes
Ingredients:
- 2 tablespoons sesame seeds
- ¼ cup chopped almonds
- ¼ cup sunflower seeds
- ½ cup unsweetened shredded coconut
- 2 tablespoons unsalted butter, melted or at least softened
- 2 tablespoons coconut oil
- ⅓ cup honey
- 2½ cups oats
- ¼ teaspoon sea salt
- ½ cup dried cranberries

Directions:
1. In a large mixing bowl, stir together the sesame seeds, almonds, sunflower seeds, coconut, butter, coconut oil, honey, oats, and salt.
2. Line the air fryer basket with parchment paper. Punch 8 to 10 holes into the parchment paper with a fork so air can circulate. Pour the granola mixture onto the parchment paper.
3. Air fry the granola at 350°F/175°C for 9 minutes, stirring every 3 minutes.
4. When cooking is complete, stir in the dried cranberries and allow the mixture to cool. Store in an airtight container up to 2 weeks or freeze for 6 months.

Spinach And Artichoke White Pizza

Servings: 2

Cooking Time: 18 Minutes
Ingredients:
- olive oil
- 3 cups fresh spinach
- 2 cloves garlic, minced, divided
- 1 (6- to 8-ounce) pizza dough ball*
- ½ cup grated mozzarella cheese
- ¼ cup grated Fontina cheese
- ¼ cup artichoke hearts, coarsely chopped
- 2 tablespoons grated Parmesan cheese
- ¼ teaspoon dried oregano
- salt and freshly ground black pepper

Directions:
1. Heat the oil in a medium sauté pan on the stovetop. Add the spinach and half the minced garlic to the pan and sauté for a few minutes, until the spinach has wilted. Remove the sautéed spinach from the pan and set it aside.
2. Preheat the air fryer to 390°F/200°C.
3. Cut out a piece of aluminum foil the same size as the bottom of the air fryer basket. Brush the foil circle with olive oil. Shape the dough into a circle and place it on top of the foil. Dock the dough by piercing it several times with a fork. Brush the dough lightly with olive oil and transfer it into the air fryer basket with the foil on the bottom.
4. Air-fry the plain pizza dough for 6 minutes. Turn the dough over, remove the aluminum foil and brush again with olive oil. Air-fry for an additional 4 minutes.
5. Sprinkle the mozzarella and Fontina cheeses over the dough. Top with the spinach and artichoke hearts. Sprinkle the Parmesan cheese and dried oregano on top and drizzle with olive oil. Lower the temperature of the air fryer to 350°F/175°C and cook for 8 minutes, until the cheese has melted and is lightly browned. Season to taste with salt and freshly ground black pepper.

Matcha Granola

Servings:4
Cooking Time: 15 Minutes
Ingredients:
- 2 tsp matcha green tea
- ½ cup slivered almonds
- ½ cup pecan pieces
- ½ cup sunflower seeds
- ½ cup pumpkin seeds
- 1 cup coconut flakes
- ¼ cup coconut sugar
- ⅛ cup flour
- ⅛ cup almond flour
- 1 tsp vanilla extract
- 2 tbsp melted butter
- 2 tbsp almond butter
- ⅛ tsp salt

Directions:
1. Preheat air fryer to 300°F/150°C. Mix the green tea, almonds, pecan, sunflower seeds, pumpkin seeds, coconut flakes, sugar, and flour, almond flour, vanilla extract, butter, almond butter, and salt in a bowl. Spoon the mixture into an ungreased round 4-cup baking dish. Place it in the fryer and Bake for 6 minutes, stirring once. Transfer to an airtight container, let cool for 10 minutes, then cover and store at room temperature until ready to serve.

Vegetarians Recipes

Quinoa Green Pizza

Servings: 2
Cooking Time: 25 Minutes
Ingredients:
- ¾ cup quinoa flour
- ½ tsp dried basil
- ½ tsp dried oregano
- 1 tbsp apple cider vinegar
- 1/3 cup ricotta cheese
- 2/3 cup chopped broccoli
- ½ tsp garlic powder

Directions:
1. Preheat air fryer to 350°F/175°C. Whisk quinoa flour, basil, oregano, apple cider vinegar, and ½ cup of water until smooth. Set aside. Cut 2 pieces of parchment paper. Place the quinoa mixture on one paper, top with another piece, and flatten to create a crust. Discard the top piece of paper. Bake for 5 minutes, turn and discard the other piece of paper. Spread the ricotta cheese over the crust, scatter with broccoli, and sprinkle with garlic. Grill at 400°F/205°C for 5 minutes until golden brown. Serve warm.

Green Bean Sautée

Servings: 4
Cooking Time: 25 Minutes
Ingredients:
- 1 ½ lb green beans, trimmed
- 1 tbsp olive oil
- ½ tsp garlic powder
- Salt and pepper to taste
- 4 garlic cloves, thinly sliced
- 1 tbsp fresh basil, chopped

Directions:
1. Preheat the air fryer to 375°F/190°C. Toss the beans with the olive oil, garlic powder, salt, and pepper in a bowl, then add to the frying basket. Air Fry for 6 minutes, shaking the basket halfway through the cooking time. Add garlic to the air fryer and cook for 3-6 minutes or until the green beans are tender and the garlic slices start to brown. Sprinkle with basil and serve warm.

Lentil Burritos With Cilantro Chutney

Servings: 4
Cooking Time: 30 Minutes
Ingredients:
- 1 cup cilantro chutney
- 1 lb cooked potatoes, mashed
- 2 tsp sunflower oil
- 3 garlic cloves, minced
- 1 ½ tbsp fresh lime juice
- 1 ½ tsp cumin powder
- 1 tsp onion powder
- 1 tsp coriander powder
- Salt to taste
- ½ tsp turmeric
- ¼ tsp cayenne powder
- 4 large flour tortillas
- 1 cup cooked lentils
- ½ cup shredded cabbage
- ¼ cup minced red onions

Directions:
1. Preheat air fryer to 390°F/200°C. Place the mashed potatoes, sunflower oil, garlic, lime, cumin, onion powder, coriander, salt, turmeric, and cayenne in a large bowl. Stir well until combined. Lay the tortillas out flat on the counter. In the middle of each, distribute the potato filling. Add some of the lentils, cabbage, and red onions on top of the potatoes. Close the wraps by folding the bottom of the tortillas up and over the filling, then folding the sides in, then roll the bottom up to form a burrito. Place the wraps in the greased frying basket, seam side down. Air Fry for 6-8 minutes, flipping once until golden and crispy. Serve topped with cilantro chutney.

Veggie Burgers

Servings: 4
Cooking Time: 15 Minutes
Ingredients:
- 2 cans black beans, rinsed and drained
- ½ cup cooked quinoa
- ½ cup shredded raw sweet potato
- ¼ cup diced red onion
- 2 teaspoons ground cumin
- 1 teaspoon coriander powder
- ½ teaspoon salt
- oil for misting or cooking spray
- 8 slices bread
- suggested toppings: lettuce, tomato, red onion, Pepper Jack cheese, guacamole

Directions:
1. In a medium bowl, mash the beans with a fork.
2. Add the quinoa, sweet potato, onion, cumin, coriander, and salt and mix well with the fork.
3. Shape into 4 patties, each ¾-inch thick.
4. Mist both sides with oil or cooking spray and also mist the basket.
5. Cook at 390°F/200°C for 15minutes.
6. Follow the recipe for Toast, Plain & Simple.
7. Pop the veggie burgers back in the air fryer for a minute or two to reheat if necessary.
8. Serve on the toast with your favorite burger toppings.

Black Bean Stuffed Potato Boats

Servings: 4
Cooking Time: 55 Minutes
Ingredients:
- 4 russets potatoes
- 1 cup chipotle mayonnaise
- 1 cup canned black beans
- 2 tomatoes, chopped
- 1 scallion, chopped
- 1/3 cup chopped cilantro
- 1 poblano chile, minced
- 1 avocado, diced

Directions:

1. Preheat air fryer to 390°F/200°C. Clean the potatoes, poke with a fork, and spray with oil. Put in the air fryer and Bake for 30 minutes or until softened.
2. Heat the beans in a pan over medium heat. Put the potatoes on a plate and cut them across the top. Open them with a fork so you can stuff them. Top each potato with chipotle mayonnaise, beans, tomatoes, scallions, cilantro, poblano chile, and avocado. Serve immediately.

Creamy Broccoli & Mushroom Casserole

Servings:4
Cooking Time: 30 Minutes
Ingredients:
*   4 cups broccoli florets, chopped
*   1 cup crushed cheddar cheese crisps
*   ¼ cup diced onion
*   ¼ tsp dried thyme
*   ¼ tsp dried marjoram
*   ¼ tsp dried oregano
*   ½ cup diced mushrooms
*   1 egg
*   2 tbsp sour cream
*   ¼ cup mayonnaise
*   Salt and pepper to taste

Directions:
1. Preheat air fryer to 350°F/175°C. Combine all ingredients, except for the cheese crisps, in a bowl. Spoon mixture into a round cake pan. Place cake pan in the frying basket and Bake for 14 minutes. Let sit for 10 minutes. Distribute crushed cheddar cheese crisps over the top and serve.

Italian Stuffed Bell Peppers

Servings: 4
Cooking Time: 75 Minutes
Ingredients:
*   4 green and red bell peppers, tops and insides discarded
*   2 russet potatoes, scrubbed and perforated with a fork
*   2 tsp olive oil
*   2 Italian sausages, cubed
*   2 tbsp milk
*   2 tbsp yogurt
*   1 tsp olive oil
*   1 tbsp Italian seasoning
*   Salt and pepper to taste
*   ¼ cup canned corn kernels
*   ½ cup mozzarella shreds
*   2 tsp chopped parsley
*   1 cup bechamel sauce

Directions:
1. Preheat air fryer at 400°F/205°C. Rub olive oil over both potatoes and sprinkle with salt and pepper. Place them in the frying basket and Bake for 45 minutes, flipping at 30 minutes mark. Let cool onto a cutting board for 5 minutes until cool enough to handle. Scoop out cooled potato into a bowl. Discard skins.
2. Place Italian sausages in the frying basket and Air Fry for 2 minutes. Using the back of a fork, mash cooked potatoes, yogurt, milk, olive oil, Italian seasoning, salt, and pepper until smooth. Toss in cooked sausages, corn, and mozzarella cheese. Stuff bell peppers with the potato mixture. Place bell peppers in the frying basket and Bake for 10 minutes. Serve immediately sprinkled with parsley and bechamel sauce on side.

Mushroom, Zucchini And Black Bean Burgers

Servings: 4
Cooking Time: 18 Minutes
Ingredients:
*   1 cup diced zucchini, (about ½ medium zucchini)
*   1 tablespoon olive oil
*   salt and freshly ground black pepper
*   1 cup chopped brown mushrooms (about 3 ounces)
*   1 small clove garlic
*   1 (15-ounce) can black beans, drained and rinsed
*   1 teaspoon lemon zest
*   1 tablespoon chopped fresh cilantro
*   ½ cup plain breadcrumbs
*   1 egg, beaten
*   ½ teaspoon salt
*   freshly ground black pepper
*   whole-wheat pita bread, burger buns or brioche buns
*   mayonnaise, tomato, avocado and lettuce, for serving

Directions:
1. Preheat the air fryer to 400°F/205°C.
2. Toss the zucchini with the olive oil, season with salt and freshly ground black pepper and air-fry for 6 minutes, shaking the basket once or twice while it cooks.
3. Transfer the zucchini to a food processor with the mushrooms, garlic and black beans and process until still a little chunky but broken down and pasty. Transfer the mixture to a bowl. Add the lemon zest, cilantro, breadcrumbs and egg and mix well. Season again with salt and freshly ground black pepper. Shape the mixture into four burger patties and refrigerate for at least 15 minutes.
4. Preheat the air fryer to 370°F/185°C. Transfer two of the veggie burgers to the air fryer basket and air-fry for 12 minutes, flipping the burgers gently halfway through the cooking time. Keep the burgers warm by loosely tenting them with foil while you cook the remaining two burgers. Return the first batch of burgers back into the air fryer with the second batch for the last two minutes of cooking to re-heat.
5. Serve on toasted whole-wheat pita bread, burger buns or brioche buns with some mayonnaise, tomato, avocado and lettuce.

Easy Cheese & Spinach Lasagna

Servings: 6
Cooking Time: 50 Minutes
Ingredients:
*   1 zucchini, cut into strips
*   1 tbsp butter
*   4 garlic cloves, minced
*   ½ yellow onion, diced
*   1 tsp dried oregano
*   ¼ tsp red pepper flakes
*   1 can diced tomatoes
*   4 oz ricotta
*   3 tbsp grated mozzarella
*   ½ cup grated cheddar
*   3 tsp grated Parmesan cheese
*   ⅛ cup chopped basil
*   2 tbsp chopped parsley
*   Salt and pepper to taste
*   ¼ tsp ground nutmeg

Directions:
1. Preheat air fryer to 375°F/190°C. Melt butter in a medium skillet over medium heat. Stir in half of the garlic and onion and cook for 2 minutes. Stir in oregano and red

pepper flakes and cook for 1 minute. Reduce the heat to medium-low and pour in crushed tomatoes and their juices. Cover the skillet and simmer for 5 minutes.

2. Mix ricotta, mozzarella, cheddar cheese, rest of the garlic, basil, black pepper, and nutmeg in a large bowl. Arrange a layer of zucchini strips in the baking dish. Scoop 1/3 of the cheese mixture and spread evenly over the zucchini. Spread 1/3 of the tomato sauce over the cheese. Repeat the steps two more times, then top the lasagna with Parmesan cheese. Bake in the frying basket for 25 minutes until the mixture is bubbling and the mozzarella is melted. Allow sitting for 10 minutes before cutting. Serve warm sprinkled with parsley and enjoy!

Spicy Sesame Tempeh Slaw With Peanut Dressing

Servings: 2
Cooking Time: 8 Minutes
Ingredients:
- 2 cups hot water
- 1 teaspoon salt
- 8 ounces tempeh, sliced into 1-inch-long pieces
- 2 tablespoons low-sodium soy sauce
- 2 tablespoons rice vinegar
- 1 tablespoon filtered water
- 2 teaspoons sesame oil
- ½ teaspoon fresh ginger
- 1 clove garlic, minced
- ¼ teaspoon black pepper
- ½ jalapeño, sliced
- 4 cups cabbage slaw
- 4 tablespoons Peanut Dressing (see the following recipe)
- 2 tablespoons fresh chopped cilantro
- 2 tablespoons chopped peanuts

Directions:
1. Mix the hot water with the salt and pour over the tempeh in a glass bowl. Stir and cover with a towel for 10 minutes.
2. Discard the water and leave the tempeh in the bowl.
3. In a medium bowl, mix the soy sauce, rice vinegar, filtered water, sesame oil, ginger, garlic, pepper, and jalapeño. Pour over the tempeh and cover with a towel. Place in the refrigerator to marinate for at least 2 hours.
4. Preheat the air fryer to 370°F/185°C. Remove the tempeh from the bowl and discard the remaining marinade.
5. Liberally spray the metal trivet that goes into the air fryer basket and place the tempeh on top of the trivet.
6. Cook for 4 minutes, flip, and cook another 4 minutes.
7. In a large bowl, mix the cabbage slaw with the Peanut Dressing and toss in the cilantro and chopped peanuts.
8. Portion onto 4 plates and place the cooked tempeh on top when cooking completes. Serve immediately.

Falafels

Servings: 12
Cooking Time: 10 Minutes
Ingredients:
- 1 pouch falafel mix
- 2–3 tablespoons plain breadcrumbs
- oil for misting or cooking spray

Directions:
1. Prepare falafel mix according to package directions.
2. Preheat air fryer to 390°F/200°C.
3. Place breadcrumbs in shallow dish or on wax paper.
4. Shape falafel mixture into 12 balls and flatten slightly. Roll in breadcrumbs to coat all sides and mist with oil or cooking spray.

5. Place falafels in air fryer basket in single layer and cook for 5minutes. Shake basket, and continue cooking for 5minutes, until they brown and are crispy.

Tortilla Pizza Margherita

Servings: 1
Cooking Time: 15 Minutes
Ingredients:
- 1 flour tortilla
- ¼ cup tomato sauce
- 1/3 cup grated mozzarella
- 3 basil leaves

Directions:
1. Preheat air fryer to 350°F/175°C. Put the tortilla in the greased basket and pour the sauce in the center. Spread across the whole tortilla. Sprinkle with cheese and Bake for 8-10 minutes or until crisp. Remove carefully and top with basil leaves. Serve hot.

Smoky Sweet Potato Fries

Servings: 4
Cooking Time: 25 Minutes
Ingredients:
- 2 large sweet potatoes, peeled and sliced
- 1 tbsp olive oil
- Salt and pepper to taste
- ¼ tsp garlic powder
- ¼ tsp smoked paprika
- 1 tbsp pumpkin pie spice
- 1 tbsp chopped parsley

Directions:
1. Preheat air fryer to 375°F/190°C. Toss sweet potato slices, olive oil, salt, pepper, garlic powder, pumpkin pie spice and paprika in a large bowl. Arrange the potatoes in a single layer in the frying basket. Air Fry for 5 minutes, then shake the basket. Air Fry for another 5 minutes and shake the basket again. Air Fry for 2-5 minutes until crispy. Serve sprinkled with parsley and enjoy.

Sweet Corn Bread

Servings: 6
Cooking Time: 35 Minutes
Ingredients:
- 2 eggs, beaten
- ½ cup cornmeal
- ½ cup pastry flour
- 1/3 cup sugar
- 1 tsp lemon zest
- ½ tbsp baking powder
- ¼ tsp salt
- ¼ tsp baking soda
- ½ tbsp lemon juice
- ½ cup milk
- ¼ cup sunflower oil

Directions:
1. Preheat air fryer to 350°F/175°C. Add the cornmeal, flour, sugar, lemon zest, baking powder, salt, and baking soda in a bowl. Stir with a whisk until combined. Add the eggs, lemon juice, milk, and oil to another bowl and stir well. Add the wet mixture to the dry mixture and stir gently until combined. Spray a baking pan with oil. Pour the batter in and Bake in the fryer for 25 minutes or until golden and a knife inserted in the center comes out clean. Cut into wedges and serve.

Roasted Vegetable Pita Pizza

Servings: 4
Cooking Time: 20 Minutes
Ingredients:
- 1 medium red bell pepper, seeded and cut into quarters
- 1 teaspoon extra-virgin olive oil
- ⅛ teaspoon black pepper
- ⅛ teaspoon salt
- Two 6-inch whole-grain pita breads
- 6 tablespoons pesto sauce
- ¼ small red onion, thinly sliced
- ½ cup shredded part-skim mozzarella cheese

Directions:
1. Preheat the air fryer to 400°F/205°C.
2. In a small bowl, toss the bell peppers with the olive oil, pepper, and salt.
3. Place the bell peppers in the air fryer and cook for 15 minutes, shaking every 5 minutes to prevent burning.
4. Remove the peppers and set aside. Turn the air fryer temperature down to 350°F/175°C.
5. Lay the pita bread on a flat surface. Cover each with half the pesto sauce; then top with even portions of the red bell peppers and onions. Sprinkle cheese over the top. Spray the air fryer basket with olive oil mist.
6. Carefully lift the pita bread into the air fryer basket with a spatula.
7. Cook for 5 to 8 minutes, or until the outer edges begin to brown and the cheese is melted.
8. Serve warm with desired sides.

Chili Tofu & Quinoa Bowls

Servings: 2
Cooking Time: 30 Minutes
Ingredients:
- 1 cup diced peeled sweet potatoes
- ¼ cup chopped mixed bell peppers
- 1/8 cup sprouted green lentils
- ½ onion, sliced
- 1 tsp avocado oil
- 1/8 cup chopped carrots
- 8 oz extra-firm tofu, cubed
- ½ tsp smoked paprika
- ½ tsp chili powder
- ¼ tsp salt
- 2 tsp lime zest
- 1 cup cooked quinoa
- 2 lime wedges

Directions:
1. Preheat air fryer at 350°F/175°C. Combine the onion, carrots, bell peppers, green lentils, sweet potato, and avocado oil in a bowl. In another bowl, mix the tofu, paprika, chili powder, and salt. Add veggie mixture to the frying basket and Air Fry for 8 minutes. Stir in tofu mixture and cook for 8 more minutes. Combine lime zest and quinoa. Divide into 2 serving bowls. Top each with the tofu mixture and squeeze a lime wedge over. Serve warm.

Meatless Kimchi Bowls

Servings:4
Cooking Time: 20 Minutes
Ingredients:
- 2 cups canned chickpeas
- 1 carrot, julienned
- 6 scallions, sliced
- 1 zucchini, diced

- 2 tbsp coconut aminos
- 2 tsp sesame oil
- 1 tsp rice vinegar
- 2 tsp granulated sugar
- 1 tbsp gochujang
- ¼ tsp salt
- ½ cup kimchi
- 2 tsp roasted sesame seeds

Directions:
1. Preheat air fryer to 350°F/175°C. Combine all ingredients, except for the kimchi, 2 scallions, and sesame seeds, in a baking pan. Place the pan in the frying basket and Air Fry for 6 minutes. Toss in kimchi and cook for 2 more minutes. Divide between 2 bowls and garnish with the remaining scallions and sesame seeds. Serve immediately.

Spicy Bean Patties

Servings: 4
Cooking Time: 20 Minutes
Ingredients:
- 1 cup canned black beans
- 1 bread slice, torn
- 2 tbsp spicy brown mustard
- 1 tbsp chili powder
- 1 egg white
- 2 tbsp grated carrots
- ¼ diced green bell pepper
- 1-2 jalapeño peppers, diced
- ¼ tsp ground cumin
- ¼ tsp smoked paprika
- 2 tbsp cream cheese
- 1 tbsp olive oil

Directions:
1. Preheat air fryer at 350°F/175°C. Using a fork, mash beans until smooth. Stir in the remaining ingredients, except olive oil. Form mixture into 4 patties. Place bean patties in the greased frying basket and Air Fry for 6 minutes, turning once, and brush with olive oil. Serve immediately.

Spinach And Cheese Calzone

Servings: 2
Cooking Time: 10 Minutes
Ingredients:
- ⅔ cup frozen chopped spinach, thawed
- 1 cup grated mozzarella cheese
- 1 cup ricotta cheese
- ½ teaspoon Italian seasoning
- ½ teaspoon salt
- freshly ground black pepper
- 1 store-bought or homemade pizza dough* (about 12 to 16 ounces)
- 2 tablespoons olive oil
- pizza or marinara sauce (optional)

Directions:
1. Drain and squeeze all the water out of the thawed spinach and set it aside. Mix the mozzarella cheese, ricotta cheese, Italian seasoning, salt and freshly ground black pepper together in a bowl. Stir in the chopped spinach.
2. Divide the dough in half. With floured hands or on a floured surface, stretch or roll one half of the dough into a 10-inch circle. Spread half of the cheese and spinach mixture on half of the dough, leaving about one inch of dough empty around the edge.
3. Fold the other half of the dough over the cheese mixture, almost to the edge of the bottom dough to form a half moon. Fold the bottom edge of dough up over the top edge and

crimp the dough around the edges in order to make the crust and seal the calzone. Brush the dough with olive oil. Repeat with the second half of dough to make the second calzone.

4. Preheat the air fryer to 360°F/180°C.

5. Brush or spray the air fryer basket with olive oil. Air-fry the calzones one at a time for 10 minutes, flipping the calzone over half way through. Serve with warm pizza or marinara sauce if desired.

Authentic Mexican Esquites

Servings: 4
Cooking Time: 25 Minutes
Ingredients:
- 4 ears of corn, husk and silk removed
- 1 tbsp ground coriander
- 1 tbsp smoked paprika
- 1 tsp sea salt
- 1 tsp garlic powder
- 1 tsp onion powder
- 1 tsp dried lime peel
- 1 tsp cayenne pepper
- 3 tbsp mayonnaise
- 3 tbsp grated Cotija cheese
- 1 tbsp butter, melted
- 1 tsp epazote seasoning

Directions:
1. Preheat the air fryer to 400°F/205°C. Combine the coriander, paprika, salt, garlic powder, onion powder, lime peel, epazote and cayenne pepper in a small bowl and mix well. Pour into a small glass jar. Put the corn in the greased frying basket and Bake for 6-8 minutes or until the corn is crispy but tender. Make sure to rearrange the ears halfway through cooking.

2. While the corn is frying, combine the mayonnaise, cheese, and melted butter in a small bowl. Spread the mixture over the cooked corn, return to the fryer, and Bake for 3-5 minutes more or until the corn has brown spots. Remove from the fryer and sprinkle each cob with about ½ tsp of the spice mix.

Bell Pepper & Lentil Tacos

Servings: 2
Cooking Time: 40 Minutes
Ingredients:
- 2 corn tortilla shells
- ½ cup cooked lentils
- ½ white onion, sliced
- ½ red pepper, sliced
- ½ green pepper, sliced
- ½ yellow pepper, sliced
- ½ cup shredded mozzarella
- ½ tsp Tabasco sauce

Directions:
1. Preheat air fryer to 320°F/160°C. Sprinkle half of the mozzarella cheese over one of the tortillas, then top with lentils, Tabasco sauce, onion, and peppers. Scatter the remaining mozzarella cheese, cover with the other tortilla and place in the frying basket. Bake for 6 minutes, flipping halfway through cooking. Serve and enjoy!

Vegetable Couscous

Servings: 4
Cooking Time: 10 Minutes
Ingredients:
- 4 ounces white mushrooms, sliced
- ½ medium green bell pepper, julienned
- 1 cup cubed zucchini

- ¼ small onion, slivered
- 1 stalk celery, thinly sliced
- ¼ teaspoon ground coriander
- ¼ teaspoon ground cumin
- salt and pepper
- 1 tablespoon olive oil
- Couscous
- ¾ cup uncooked couscous
- 1 cup vegetable broth or water
- ½ teaspoon salt (omit if using salted broth)

Directions:
1. Combine all vegetables in large bowl. Sprinkle with coriander, cumin, and salt and pepper to taste. Stir well, add olive oil, and stir again to coat vegetables evenly.

2. Place vegetables in air fryer basket and cook at 390°F/200°C for 5minutes. Stir and cook for 5 more minutes, until tender.

3. While vegetables are cooking, prepare the couscous: Place broth or water and salt in large saucepan. Heat to boiling, stir in couscous, cover, and remove from heat.

4. Let couscous sit for 5minutes, stir in cooked vegetables, and serve hot.

Powerful Jackfruit Fritters

Servings:4
Cooking Time: 30 Minutes
Ingredients:
- 1 can jackfruit, chopped
- 1 egg, beaten
- 1 tbsp Dijon mustard
- 1 tbsp mayonnaise
- 1 tbsp prepared horseradish
- 2 tbsp grated yellow onion
- 2 tbsp chopped parsley
- 2 tbsp chopped nori
- 2 tbsp flour
- 1 tbsp Cajun seasoning
- ¼ tsp garlic powder
- ¼ tsp salt
- 2 lemon wedges

Directions:
1. In a bowl, combine jackfruit, egg, mustard, mayonnaise, horseradish, onion, parsley, nori, flour, Cajun seasoning, garlic, and salt. Let chill in the fridge for 15 minutes. Preheat air fryer to 350ºF/175°C. Divide the mixture into 12 balls. Place them in the frying basket and Air Fry for 10 minutes. Serve with lemon wedges.

Pinto Bean Casserole

Servings: 2
Cooking Time: 15 Minutes
Ingredients:
- 1 can pinto beans
- ¼ cup tomato sauce
- 2 tbsp cornstarch
- 2 garlic cloves, minced
- ½ tsp dried oregano
- ½ tsp cumin
- 1 tsp smoked paprika
- Salt and pepper to taste

Directions:
1. Preheat air fryer to 390°F/200°C. Stir the beans, tomato sauce, cornstarch, garlic, oregano, cumin, smoked paprika, salt, and pepper in a bowl until combined. Pour the bean mix into a greased baking pan. Bake in the fryer for 4 minutes. Remove, stir, and Bake for 4 minutes or until the mix is thick and heated through. Serve hot.

Vegetarian Stuffed Bell Peppers

Servings: 3
Cooking Time: 40 Minutes
Ingredients:
- 1 cup mushrooms, chopped
- 1 tbsp allspice
- ¾ cup Alfredo sauce
- ½ cup canned diced tomatoes
- 1 cup cooked rice
- 2 tbsp dried parsley
- 2 tbsp hot sauce
- Salt and pepper to taste
- 3 large bell peppers

Directions:
1. Preheat air fryer to 375°F/190°C. Whisk mushrooms, allspice and 1 cup of boiling water until smooth. Stir in Alfredo sauce, tomatoes and juices, rice, parsley, hot sauce, salt, and black pepper. Set aside. Cut the top of each bell pepper, take out the core and seeds without breaking the pepper. Fill each pepper with the rice mixture and cover them with a 6-inch square of aluminum foil, folding the edges. Roast for 30 minutes until tender. Let cool completely before unwrapping. Serve immediately.

Tex-mex Stuffed Sweet Potatoes

Servings: 2
Cooking Time: 40 Minutes
Ingredients:
- 2 medium sweet potatoes
- 1 can black beans
- 2 scallions, finely sliced
- 1 tbsp hot sauce
- 1 tsp taco seasoning
- 2 tbsp lime juice
- ¼ cup Ranch dressing

Directions:
1. Preheat air fryer to 400°F/205°C. Add in sweet potatoes and Roast for 30 minutes. Toss the beans, scallions, hot sauce, taco seasoning, and lime juice. Set aside. Once the potatoes are ready, cut them lengthwise, 2/3 through. Spoon 1/4 of the bean mixture into each half and drizzle Ranch dressing before serving.

Stuffed Portobellos

Servings: 4
Cooking Time: 45 Minutes
Ingredients:
- 1 cup cherry tomatoes
- 2 ¼ tsp olive oil
- 3 tbsp grated mozzarella
- 1 cup chopped baby spinach
- 1 garlic clove, minced
- ¼ tsp dried oregano
- ¼ tsp dried thyme
- Salt and pepper to taste
- ¼ cup bread crumbs
- 4 portobello mushrooms, stemmed and gills removed
- 1 tbsp chopped parsley

Directions:
1. Preheat air fryer to 360°F/180°C. Combine tomatoes, ¼ teaspoon olive oil, and salt in a small bowl. Arrange in a single layer in the parchment-lined frying basket and Air Fry for 10 minutes. Stir and flatten the tomatoes with the back of a spoon, then Air Fry for another 6-8 minutes. Transfer the tomatoes to a medium bowl and combine with spinach, garlic, oregano, thyme, pepper, bread crumbs, and the rest of the olive oil.

2. Place the mushrooms on a work surface with the gills facing up. Spoon tomato mixture and mozzarella cheese equally into the mushroom caps and transfer the mushrooms to the frying basket. Air Fry for 8-10 minutes until the mushrooms have softened and the tops are golden. Garnish with chopped parsley and serve.

Rainbow Quinoa Patties

Servings: 4
Cooking Time: 20 Minutes
Ingredients:
- 1 cup canned tri-bean blend, drained and rinsed
- 2 tbsp olive oil
- ½ tsp ground cumin
- ½ tsp garlic salt
- 1 tbsp paprika
- 1/3 cup uncooked quinoa
- 2 tbsp chopped onion
- ¼ cup shredded carrot
- 2 tbsp chopped cilantro
- 1 tsp chili powder
- ½ tsp salt
- 2 tbsp mascarpone cheese

Directions:
1. Place 1/3 cup of water, 1 tbsp of olive oil, cumin, and salt in a saucepan over medium heat and bring it to a boil. Remove from the heat and stir in quinoa. Let rest covered for 5 minutes.
2. Preheat air fryer at 350ºF/175ºC. Using the back of a fork, mash beans until smooth. Toss in cooked quinoa and the remaining ingredients. Form mixture into 4 patties. Place patties in the greased frying basket and Air Fry for 6 minutes, turning once, and brush with the remaining olive oil. Serve immediately.

Charred Cauliflower Tacos

Servings: 4
Cooking Time: 10 Minutes
Ingredients:
- 1 head cauliflower, washed and cut into florets
- 2 tablespoons avocado oil
- 2 teaspoons taco seasoning
- 1 medium avocado
- ½ teaspoon garlic powder
- ¼ teaspoon black pepper
- ¼ teaspoon salt
- 2 tablespoons chopped red onion
- 2 teaspoons fresh squeezed lime juice
- ¼ cup chopped cilantro
- Eight 6-inch corn tortillas
- ½ cup cooked corn
- ½ cup shredded purple cabbage

Directions:
1. Preheat the air fryer to 390°F/200°C.
2. In a large bowl, toss the cauliflower with the avocado oil and taco seasoning. Set the metal trivet inside the air fryer basket and liberally spray with olive oil.
3. Place the cauliflower onto the trivet and cook for 10 minutes, shaking every 3 minutes to allow for an even char.
4. While the cauliflower is cooking, prepare the avocado sauce. In a medium bowl, mash the avocado; then mix in the garlic powder, pepper, salt, and onion. Stir in the lime juice and cilantro; set aside.
5. Remove the cauliflower from the air fryer basket.
6. Place 1 tablespoon of avocado sauce in the middle of a tortilla, and top with corn, cabbage, and charred cauliflower. Repeat with the remaining tortillas. Serve immediately.

Crispy Avocados With Pico De Gallo

Servings:2
Cooking Time: 15 Minutes
Ingredients:
- 1 cup diced tomatoes
- 1 tbsp lime juice
- 1 tsp lime zest
- 2 tbsp chopped cilantro
- 1 serrano chiles, minced
- 2 cloves garlic, minced
- 1 tbsp diced white onions
- ½ tsp salt
- 2 avocados, halved and pitted
- 4 tbsp cheddar shreds

Directions:
1. Preheat air fryer to 350ºF/175°C. Combine all ingredients, except for avocados and cheddar cheese, in a bowl and let chill covered in the fridge. Place avocado halves, cut sides-up, in the frying basket, scatter cheese shreds over top of avocado halves, and Air Fry for 4 minutes. Top with pico de gallo and serve.

Vegetarian Eggplant "pizzas"

Servings:4
Cooking Time: 25 Minutes
Ingredients:
- ½ cup diced baby bella mushrooms
- 3 tbsp olive oil
- ¼ cup diced onions
- ½ cup pizza sauce
- 1 eggplant, sliced
- 1 tsp salt
- 1 cup shredded mozzarella
- ¼ cup chopped oregano

Directions:
1. Warm 2 tsp of olive oil in a skillet over medium heat. Add in onion and mushrooms and stir-fry for 4 minutes until tender. Stir in pizza sauce. Turn the heat off.
2. Preheat air fryer to 375ºF/190°C. Brush the eggplant slices with the remaining olive oil on both sides. Lay out slices on a large plate and season with salt. Then, top with the sauce mixture and shredded mozzarella. Place the eggplant pizzas in the frying basket and Air Fry for 5 minutes. Garnish with oregano to serve.

Sweet & Spicy Vegetable Stir-fry

Servings: 2
Cooking Time: 45 Minutes
Ingredients:
- ½ pineapple, cut into bite-size chunks
- ¼ cup Tabasco sauce
- ¼ cup lime juice
- 2 tsp allspice
- 5 oz cauliflower florets
- 1 carrot, thinly sliced
- 1 cup frozen peas, thawed
- 2 scallions, chopped

Directions:
1. Preheat air fryer to 400°F/205°C. Whisk Tabasco sauce, lime juice, and allspice in a bowl. Then toss in cauliflower, pineapple, and carrots until coated. Strain the remaining sauce; reserve it. Air Fry the veggies for 12 minutes, shake, and Air Fry for 10-12 more minutes until cooked. Once the veggies are ready, remove to a bowl. Combine peas, scallions, and reserved sauce until coated. Transfer to a pan and Air Fry them for 3 minutes. Remove them to the bowl and serve right away.

Basil Green Beans

Servings: 4
Cooking Time: 15 Minutes
Ingredients:
- 1 ½ lb green beans, trimmed
- 1 tbsp olive oil
- 1 tbsp fresh basil, chopped
- Garlic salt to taste

Directions:
1. Preheat air fryer to 400°F/205°C. Coat the green beans with olive oil in a large bowl. Combine with fresh basil powder and garlic salt. Put the beans in the frying basket and Air Fry for 7-9 minutes, shaking once until the beans begin to brown. Serve warm and enjoy!

Honey Pear Chips

Servings: 4
Cooking Time: 30 Minutes
Ingredients:
- 2 firm pears, thinly sliced
- 1 tbsp lemon juice
- ½ tsp ground cinnamon
- 1 tsp honey

Directions:
1. Preheat air fryer to 380°F/195°C. Arrange the pear slices on the parchment-lined cooking basket. Drizzle with lemon juice and honey and sprinkle with cinnamon. Air Fry for 6-8 minutes, shaking the basket once, until golden. Leave to cool. Serve immediately or save for later in an airtight container. Good for 2 days.

Garlicky Roasted Mushrooms

Servings: 4
Cooking Time: 30 Minutes
Ingredients:
- 16 garlic cloves, peeled
- 2 tsp olive oil
- 16 button mushrooms
- 2 tbsp fresh chives, snipped
- Salt and pepper to taste
- 1 tbsp white wine

Directions:
1. Preheat air fryer to 350°F/175°C. Coat the garlic with some olive oil in a baking pan, then Roast in the air fryer for 12 minutes. When done, take the pan out and stir in the mushrooms, salt, and pepper. Then add the remaining olive oil and white wine. Put the pan back into the fryer and Bake for 10-15 minutes until the mushrooms and garlic soften. Sprinkle with chives and serve warm.

Home-style Cinnamon Rolls

Servings: 4
Cooking Time: 40 Minutes
Ingredients:
- ½ pizza dough
- 1/3 cup dark brown sugar
- ¼ cup butter, softened
- ½ tsp ground cinnamon

Directions:
1. Preheat air fryer to 360°F/180°C. Roll out the dough into a rectangle. Using a knife, spread the brown sugar and butter, covering all the edges, and sprinkle with cinnamon. Fold the long side of the dough into a log, then cut it into 8 equal pieces, avoiding compression. Place the rolls, spiral-side up, onto a parchment-lined sheet. Let rise for 20 minutes. Grease the rolls with cooking spray and Bake for 8 minutes until golden brown. Serve right away.

Arancini With Marinara

Servings: 6
Cooking Time: 15 Minutes
Ingredients:
- 2 cups cooked rice
- 1 cup grated Parmesan cheese
- 1 egg, whisked
- ¼ teaspoon dried thyme
- ½ teaspoon dried oregano
- ½ teaspoon dried basil
- ½ teaspoon dried parsley
- 1 teaspoon salt
- ¼ teaspoon paprika
- 1 cup breadcrumbs
- 4 ounces mozzarella, cut into 24 cubes
- 2 cups marinara sauce

Directions:
1. In a large bowl, mix together the rice, Parmesan cheese, and egg.
2. In another bowl, mix together the thyme, oregano, basil, parsley, salt, paprika, and breadcrumbs.
3. Form 24 rice balls with the rice mixture. Use your thumb to make an indentation in the center and stuff 1 cube of mozzarella in the center of the rice; close the ball around the cheese.
4. Roll the rice balls in the seasoned breadcrumbs until all are coated.
5. Preheat the air fryer to 400°F/205°C.
6. Place the rice balls in the air fryer basket and coat with cooking spray. Cook for 8 minutes, shake the basket, and cook another 7 minutes.
7. Heat the marinara sauce in a saucepan until warm. Serve sauce as a dip for arancini.

Tex-mex Potatoes With Avocado Dressing

Servings: 2
Cooking Time: 60 Minutes
Ingredients:
- ¼ cup chopped parsley, dill, cilantro, chives
- ¼ cup yogurt
- ½ avocado, diced
- 2 tbsp milk
- 2 tsp lemon juice
- ½ tsp lemon zest
- 1 green onion, chopped
- 2 cloves garlic, quartered
- Salt and pepper to taste
- 2 tsp olive oil
- 2 russet potatoes, scrubbed and perforated with a fork
- 1 cup steamed broccoli florets
- ½ cup canned white beans

Directions:
1. In a food processor, blend the yogurt, avocado, milk, lemon juice, lemon zest, green onion, garlic, parsley, dill, cilantro, chives, salt and pepper until smooth. Transfer it to a small bowl and let chill the dressing covered in the fridge until ready to use.
2. Preheat air fryer at 400°F/205°C. Rub olive oil over both potatoes and sprinkle with salt and pepper. Place them in the frying basket and Bake for 45 minutes, flipping at 30 minutes mark. Let cool onto a cutting board for 5 minutes until cool enough to handle. Cut each potato lengthwise into slices and pinch ends together to open up each slice. Stuff broccoli and beans into potatoes and put them back into the basket, and cook for 3 more minutes. Drizzle avocado dressing over and serve.

Spinach & Brie Frittata

Servings:4
Cooking Time: 25 Minutes
Ingredients:
- 5 eggs
- Salt and pepper to taste
- ½ cup baby spinach
- 1 shallot, diced
- 4 oz brie cheese, cubed
- 1 tomato, sliced

Directions:
1. Preheat air fryer to 320ºF/160°C. Whisk all ingredients, except for the tomato slices, in a bowl. Transfer to a baking pan greased with olive oil and top with tomato slices. Place the pan in the frying basket and Bake for 14 minutes. Let cool for 5 minutes before slicing. Serve and enjoy!

Bite-sized Blooming Onions

Servings: 4
Cooking Time: 35 Minutes + Cooling Time
Ingredients:
- 1 lb cipollini onions
- 1 cup flour
- 1 tsp salt
- ½ tsp paprika
- 1 tsp cayenne pepper
- 2 eggs
- 2 tbsp milk

Directions:
1. Preheat the air fryer to 375°F/190°C. Carefully peel the onions and cut a ½ inch off the stem ends and trim the root ends. Place them root-side down on the cutting surface and cut the onions into quarters. Be careful not to cut al the way to the bottom. Cut each quarter into 2 sections and pull the wedges apart without breaking them.
2. In a shallow bowl, add the flour, salt, paprika, and cayenne, and in a separate shallow bowl, beat the eggs with the milk. Dip the onions in the flour, then dip in the egg mix, coating evenly, and then in the flour mix again. Shake off excess flour. Put the onions in the frying basket, cut-side up, and spray with cooking oil. Air Fry for 10-15 minutes until the onions are crispy on the outside, tender on the inside. Let cool for 10 minutes, then serve.

Fried Rice With Curried Tofu

Servings:4
Cooking Time: 25 Minutes
Ingredients:
- 8 oz extra-firm tofu, cubed
- ½ cup canned coconut milk
- 2 tsp red curry paste
- 2 cloves garlic, minced
- 1 tbsp avocado oil
- 1 tbsp coconut oil
- 2 cups cooked rice
- 1 tbsp turmeric powder
- Salt and pepper to taste
- 4 lime wedges
- ¼ cup chopped cilantro

Directions:
1. Preheat air fryer to 350ºF/175°C. Combine tofu, coconut milk, curry paste, garlic, and avocado oil in a bowl. Pour the

mixture into a baking pan. Place the pan in the frying basket and Air Fry for 10 minutes, stirring once.

2.   Melt the coconut oil in a skillet over medium heat. Add in rice, turmeric powder, salt, and black pepper, and cook for 2 minutes or until heated through. Divide the cooked rice between 4 medium bowls and top with tofu mixture and sauce. Top with cilantro and lime wedges to serve.

Smoked Paprika Sweet Potato Fries

Servings: 4
Cooking Time: 35 Minutes
Ingredients:

- 2 sweet potatoes, peeled
- 1 ½ tbsp cornstarch
- 1 tbsp canola oil
- 1 tbsp olive oil
- 1 tsp smoked paprika
- 1 tsp garlic powder
- Salt and pepper to taste
- 1 cup cocktail sauce

Directions:
1.   Cut the potatoes lengthwise to form French fries. Put in a resealable plastic bag and add cornstarch. Seal and shake to coat the fries. Combine the canola oil, olive oil, paprika, garlic powder, salt, and pepper fries in a large bowl. Add the sweet potato fries and mix to combine.
2.   Preheat air fryer to 380°F/195°C. Place fries in the greased basket and fry for 20-25 minutes, shaking the basket once until crisp. Drizzle with Cocktail sauce to serve.

Chicano Rice Bowls

Servings: 4
Cooking Time: 10 Minutes
Ingredients:

- 1 cup sour cream
- 2 tbsp milk
- 1 tsp ground cumin
- 1 tsp chili powder
- 1/8 tsp cayenne pepper
- 1 tbsp tomato paste
- 1 white onion, chopped
- 1 clove garlic, minced
- ½ tsp ground turmeric
- ½ tsp salt
- 1 cup canned black beans
- 1 cup canned corn kernels
- 1 tsp olive oil
- 4 cups cooked brown rice
- 3 tomatoes, diced
- 1 avocado, diced

Directions:
1.   Whisk the sour cream, milk, cumin, ground turmeric, chili powder, cayenne pepper, and salt in a bowl. Let chill covered in the fridge until ready to use.
2.   Preheat air fryer at 350ºF/175°C. Combine beans, white onion, tomato paste, garlic, corn, and olive oil in a bowl. Transfer it into the frying basket and Air Fry for 5 minutes. Divide cooked rice into 4 serving bowls. Top each with bean mixture, tomatoes, and avocado and drizzle with sour cream mixture over. Serve immediately.

Spicy Vegetable And Tofu Shake Fry

Servings: 4
Cooking Time: 17 Minutes
Ingredients:

- 4 teaspoons canola oil, divided

- 2 tablespoons rice wine vinegar
- 1 tablespoon sriracha chili sauce
- ¼ cup soy sauce*
- ½ teaspoon toasted sesame oil
- 1 teaspoon minced garlic
- 1 tablespoon minced fresh ginger
- 8 ounces extra firm tofu
- ½ cup vegetable stock or water
- 1 tablespoon honey
- 1 tablespoon cornstarch
- ½ red onion, chopped
- 1 red or yellow bell pepper, chopped
- 1 cup green beans, cut into 2-inch lengths
- 4 ounces mushrooms, sliced
- 2 scallions, sliced
- 2 tablespoons fresh cilantro leaves
- 2 teaspoons toasted sesame seeds

Directions:
1.   Combine 1 tablespoon of the oil, vinegar, sriracha sauce, soy sauce, sesame oil, garlic and ginger in a small bowl. Cut the tofu into bite-sized cubes and toss the tofu in with the marinade while you prepare the other vegetables. When you are ready to start cooking, remove the tofu from the marinade and set it aside. Add the water, honey and cornstarch to the marinade and bring to a simmer on the stovetop, just until the sauce thickens. Set the sauce aside.
2.   Preheat the air fryer to 400°F/205°C.
3.   Toss the onion, pepper, green beans and mushrooms in a bowl with a little canola oil and season with salt. Air-fry at 400°F/205°C for 11 minutes, shaking the basket and tossing the vegetables every few minutes. When the vegetables are cooked to your preferred doneness, remove them from the air fryer and set aside.
4.   Add the tofu to the air fryer basket and air-fry at 400°F/205°C for 6 minutes, shaking the basket a few times during the cooking process. Add the vegetables back to the basket and air-fry for another minute. Transfer the vegetables and tofu to a large bowl, add the scallions and cilantro leaves and toss with the sauce. Serve over rice with sesame seeds sprinkled on top.

Fake Shepherd´s Pie

Servings:6
Cooking Time: 40 Minutes
Ingredients:

- ½ head cauliflower, cut into florets
- 1 sweet potato, diced
- 1 tbsp olive oil
- ¼ cup cheddar shreds
- 2 tbsp milk
- Salt and pepper to taste
- 2 tsp avocado oil
- 1 cup beefless grounds
- ½ onion, diced
- 2 cloves garlic, minced
- 1 carrot, diced
- ½ cup green peas
- 1 stalk celery, diced
- 2/3 cup tomato sauce
- 1 tsp chopped rosemary
- 1 tsp thyme leaves

Directions:
1.   Place cauliflower and sweet potato in a pot of salted boiling water over medium heat and simmer for 7 minutes until fork tender. Strain and transfer to a bowl. Put in

avocado oil, cheddar, milk, salt and pepper. Mash until smooth.

2. Warm olive oil in a skillet over medium-high heat and stir in beefless grounds and vegetables and stir-fry for 4 minutes until veggies are tender. Stir in tomato sauce, rosemary, thyme, salt, and black pepper. Set aside.

3. Preheat air fryer to 350ºF/175°C. Spoon filling into a round cake pan lightly greased with olive oil and cover with the topping. Using the tines of a fork, run shallow lines in the top of cauliflower for a decorative touch. Place cake pan in the frying basket and Air Fry for 12 minutes. Let sit for 10 minutes before serving.

Balsamic Caprese Hasselback

Servings:4
Cooking Time: 15 Minutes
Ingredients:
- 4 tomatoes
- 12 fresh basil leaves
- 1 ball fresh mozzarella
- Salt and pepper to taste
- 1 tbsp olive oil
- 2 tsp balsamic vinegar
- 1 tbsp basil, torn

Directions:
1. Preheat air fryer to 325ºF/160°C. Remove the bottoms from the tomatoes to create a flat surface. Make 4 even slices on each tomato, 3/4 of the way down. Slice the mozzarella and the cut into 12 pieces. Stuff 1 basil leaf and a piece of mozzarella into each slice. Sprinkle with salt and pepper. Place the stuffed tomatoes in the frying basket and Air Fry for 3 minutes. Transfer to a large serving plate. Drizzle with olive oil and balsamic vinegar and scatter the basil over. Serve and enjoy!

Pine Nut Eggplant Dip

Servings: 4
Cooking Time: 35 Minutes
Ingredients:
- 2 ½ tsp olive oil
- 1 eggplant, halved lengthwise
- 1/2 cup Parmesan cheese
- 2 tsp pine nuts
- 1 tbsp chopped walnuts
- ¼ cup tahini
- 1 tbsp lemon juice
- 2 cloves garlic, minced
- 1/8 tsp ground cumin
- 1 tsp smoked paprika
- Salt and pepper to taste
- 1 tbsp chopped parsley

Directions:
1. Preheat air fryer at 375ºF/190°C. Rub olive oil over eggplant and pierce the eggplant flesh 3 times with a fork. Place eggplant, flat side down, in the frying basket and Bake for 25 minutes. Let cool onto a cutting board for 5 minutes until cool enough to handle. Scoop out eggplant flesh. Add pine nuts and walnuts to the basket and Air Fry for 2 minutes, shaking every 30 seconds to ensure they don´t burn. Set aside in a bowl.

2. In a food processor, blend eggplant flesh, tahini, lemon juice, garlic, smoked paprika, cumin, salt, and pepper until smooth. Transfer to a bowl. Scatter with the roasted pine nuts, Parmesan cheese, and parsley. Drizzle the dip with the remaining olive oil. Serve and enjoy!

Mexican Twice Air-fried Sweet Potatoes

Servings: 2
Cooking Time: 42 Minutes
Ingredients:
- 2 large sweet potatoes
- olive oil
- salt and freshly ground black pepper
- ⅓ cup diced red onion
- ⅓ cup diced red bell pepper
- ½ cup canned black beans, drained and rinsed
- ½ cup corn kernels, fresh or frozen
- ½ teaspoon chili powder
- 1½ cups grated pepper jack cheese, divided
- Jalapeño peppers, sliced

Directions:
1. Preheat the air fryer to 400°F/205°C.
2. Rub the outside of the sweet potatoes with olive oil and season with salt and freshly ground black pepper. Transfer the potatoes into the air fryer basket and air-fry at 400°F/205°C for 30 minutes, rotating the potatoes a few times during the cooking process.
3. While the potatoes are air-frying, start the potato filling. Preheat a large sauté pan over medium heat on the stovetop. Add the onion and pepper and sauté for a few minutes, until the vegetables start to soften. Add the black beans, corn, and chili powder and sauté for another 3 minutes. Set the mixture aside.
4. Remove the sweet potatoes from the air fryer and let them rest for 5 minutes. Slice off one inch of the flattest side of both potatoes. Scrape the potato flesh out of the potatoes, leaving half an inch of potato flesh around the edge of the potato. Place all the potato flesh into a large bowl and mash it with a fork. Add the black bean mixture and 1 cup of the pepper jack cheese to the mashed sweet potatoes. Season with salt and freshly ground black pepper and mix well. Stuff the hollowed out potato shells with the black bean and sweet potato mixture, mounding the filling high in the potatoes.
5. Transfer the stuffed potatoes back into the air fryer basket and air-fry at 370°F/185°C for 10 minutes. Sprinkle the remaining cheese on top of each stuffed potato, lower the heat to 340°F and air-fry for an additional 2 minutes to melt the cheese. Top with a couple slices of Jalapeño pepper and serve warm with a green salad.

Pizza Eggplant Rounds

Servings: 4
Cooking Time: 25 Minutes
Ingredients:
- 3 tsp olive oil
- ¼ cup diced onion
- ½ tsp garlic powder
- ½ tsp dried oregano
- ½ cup diced mushrooms
- ½ cup marinara sauce
- 1 eggplant, sliced
- 1 tsp salt
- 1 cup shredded mozzarella
- 2 tbsp Parmesan cheese
- ¼ cup chopped basil

Directions:
1. Warm 2 tsp of olive oil in a skillet over medium heat. Add in onion and mushrooms and cook for 5 minutes until the onions are translucent. Stir in marinara sauce, then add oregano and garlic powder. Turn the heat off.

2. Preheat air fryer at 375ºF/190°C. Rub the remaining olive oil over both sides of the eggplant circles. Lay circles on a large plate and sprinkle with salt and black pepper. Top each circle with the marinara sauce mixture and shredded mozzarella and Parmesan cheese. Place eggplant circles in the frying basket and Bake for 5 minutes. Scatter with the basil and serve.

Veggie-stuffed Bell Peppers

Servings:4
Cooking Time: 40 Minutes
Ingredients:
- ½ cup canned fire-roasted diced tomatoes, including juice
- 2 red bell peppers
- 4 tsp olive oil
- ½ yellow onion, diced
- 1 zucchini, diced
- ¾ cup chopped mushrooms
- ¼ cup tomato sauce
- 2 tsp Italian seasoning
- ¼ tsp smoked paprika
- Salt and pepper to taste

Directions:
1. Cut bell peppers in half from top to bottom and discard the seeds. Brush inside and tops of the bell peppers with some olive oil. Set aside. Warm the remaining olive oil in a skillet over medium heat. Stir-fry the onion, zucchini, and mushrooms for 5 minutes until the onions are tender. Combine tomatoes and their juice, tomato sauce, Italian seasoning, paprika, salt, and pepper in a bowl.
2. Preheat air fryer to 350ºF/175°C. Divide both mixtures between bell pepper halves. Place bell pepper halves in the frying basket and Air Fry for 8 minutes. Serve immediately.

Effortless Mac `n´ Cheese

Servings: 4
Cooking Time: 15 Minutes
Ingredients:
- 1 cup heavy cream
- 1 cup milk
- ½ cup mozzarella cheese
- 2 tsp grated Parmesan cheese
- 16 oz cooked elbow macaroni

Directions:
1. Preheat air fryer to 400°F/205°C. Whisk the heavy cream, milk, mozzarella cheese, and Parmesan cheese until smooth in a bowl. Stir in the macaroni and pour into a baking dish. Cover with foil and Bake in the air fryer for 6 minutes. Remove foil and Bake until cooked through and bubbly, 3-5 minutes. Serve warm.

Vegetarian Paella

Servings: 3
Cooking Time: 50 Minutes
Ingredients:
- ½ cup chopped artichoke hearts
- ½ sliced red bell peppers
- 4 mushrooms, thinly sliced
- ½ cup canned diced tomatoes
- ½ cup canned chickpeas
- 3 tbsp hot sauce
- 2 tbsp lemon juice
- 1 tbsp allspice
- 1 cup rice

Directions:

1. Preheat air fryer to 400°F/205°C. Combine the artichokes, peppers, mushrooms, tomatoes and their juices, chickpeas, hot sauce, lemon juice, and allspice in a baking pan. Roast for 10 minutes. Pour in rice and 2 cups of boiling water, cover with aluminum foil, and Roast for 22 minutes. Discard the foil and Roast for 3 minutes until the top is crisp. Let cool slightly before stirring. Serve.

Tomato & Squash Stuffed Mushrooms

Servings:2
Cooking Time: 15 Minutes
Ingredients:
- 12 whole white button mushrooms
- 3 tsp olive oil
- 2 tbsp diced zucchini
- 1 tsp soy sauce
- ¼ tsp salt
- 2 tbsp tomato paste
- 1 tbsp chopped parsley

Directions:
1. Preheat air fryer to 350ºF/175°C. Remove the stems from the mushrooms. Chop the stems finely and set in a bowl. Brush 1 tsp of olive oil around the top ridge of mushroom caps. To the bowl of the stem, add all ingredients, except for parsley, and mix. Divide and press mixture into tops of mushroom caps. Place the mushrooms in the frying basket and Air Fry for 5 minutes. Top with parsley. Serve.

Rice & Bean Burritos

Servings: 4
Cooking Time: 20 Minutes
Ingredients:
- 1 bell pepper, sliced
- ½ red onion, thinly sliced
- 2 garlic cloves, peeled
- 1 tbsp olive oil
- 1 cup cooked brown rice
- 1 can pinto beans
- ½ tsp salt
- ¼ tsp chili powder
- ¼ tsp ground cumin
- ¼ tsp smoked paprika
- 1 tbsp lime juice
- 4 tortillas
- 2 tsp grated Parmesan cheese
- 1 avocado, diced
- 4 tbsp salsa
- 2 tbsp chopped cilantro

Directions:
1. Preheat air fryer to 400°F/205°C. Combine bell pepper, onion, garlic, and olive oil. Place in the frying basket and Roast for 5 minutes. Shake and roast for another 5 minutes.
2. Remove the garlic from the basket and mince finely. Add to a large bowl along with brown rice, pinto beans, salt, chili powder, cumin, paprika, and lime juice. Divide the roasted vegetable mixture between the tortillas. Top with rice mixture, Parmesan, avocado, cilantro, and salsa. Fold in the sides, then roll the tortillas over the filling. Serve.

Zucchini & Bell Pepper Stir-fry

Servings: 4
Cooking Time: 25 Minutes
Ingredients:
- 1 zucchini, cut into rounds
- 1 red bell pepper, sliced
- 3 garlic cloves, sliced

- 2 tbsp olive oil
- 1/3 cup vegetable broth
- 1 tbsp lemon juice
- 2 tsp cornstarch
- 1 tsp dried basil
- Salt and pepper to taste

Directions:
1. Preheat the air fryer to 400°F/205°C. Combine the veggies, garlic, and olive oil in a bowl. Put the bowl in the frying basket and Air Fry the zucchini mixture for 5 minutes, stirring once; drain. While the veggies are cooking, whisk the broth, lemon juice, cornstarch, basil, salt, and pepper in a bowl. Pour the broth into the bowl along with the veggies and stir. Air Fry for 5-9 more minutes until the veggies are tender and the sauce is thick. Serve and enjoy!

Quinoa Burgers With Feta Cheese And Dill

Servings: 6
Cooking Time: 10 Minutes
Ingredients:
- 1 cup quinoa (red, white or multi-colored)
- 1½ cups water
- 1 teaspoon salt
- freshly ground black pepper
- 1½ cups rolled oats
- 3 eggs, lightly beaten
- ¼ cup minced white onion
- ½ cup crumbled feta cheese
- ¼ cup chopped fresh dill
- salt and freshly ground black pepper
- vegetable or canola oil, in a spray bottle
- whole-wheat hamburger buns (or gluten-free hamburger buns*)
- arugula
- tomato, sliced
- red onion, sliced
- mayonnaise

Directions:
1. Make the quinoa: Rinse the quinoa in cold water in a saucepan, swirling it with your hand until any dry husks rise to the surface. Drain the quinoa as well as you can and then put the saucepan on the stovetop to dry and toast the quinoa. Turn the heat to medium-high and shake the pan regularly until you see the quinoa moving easily and can hear the seeds moving in the pan, indicating that they are dry. Add the water, salt and pepper. Bring the liquid to a boil and then reduce the heat to low or medium-low. You should see just a few bubbles, not a boil. Cover with a lid, leaving it askew and simmer for 20 minutes. Turn the heat off and fluff the quinoa with a fork. If there's any liquid left in the bottom of the pot, place it back on the burner for another 3 minutes or so. Spread the cooked quinoa out on a sheet pan to cool.
2. Combine the room temperature quinoa in a large bowl with the oats, eggs, onion, cheese and dill. Season with salt and pepper and mix well (remember that feta cheese is salty). Shape the mixture into 6 patties with flat sides (so they fit more easily into the air fryer). Add a little water or a few more rolled oats if necessary to get the mixture to be the right consistency to make patties.
3. Preheat the air-fryer to 400°F/205°C.
4. Spray both sides of the patties generously with oil and transfer them to the air fryer basket in one layer (you will probably have to cook these burgers in batches, depending on the size of your air fryer). Air-fry each batch at 400°F/205°C

for 10 minutes, flipping the burgers over halfway through the cooking time.
5. Build your burger on the whole-wheat hamburger buns with arugula, tomato, red onion and mayonnaise.

Hearty Salad

Servings: 2
Cooking Time: 15 Minutes
Ingredients:
- 5 oz cauliflower, cut into florets
- 2 grated carrots
- 1 tbsp olive oil
- 1 tbsp lemon juice
- 2 tbsp raisins
- 2 tbsp roasted pepitas
- 2 tbsp diced red onion
- ¼ cup mayonnaise
- 1/8 tsp black pepper
- 1 tsp cumin
- ½ tsp chia seeds
- ½ tsp sesame seeds

Directions:
1. Preheat air fryer at 350°F/175°C. Combine the cauliflower, cumin, olive oil, black pepper and lemon juice in a bowl, place it in the frying basket, and Bake for 5 minutes. Transfer it to a serving dish. Toss in the remaining ingredients. Let chill covered in the fridge until ready to use. Serve sprinkled with sesame and chia seeds.

Pinto Taquitos

Servings: 4
Cooking Time: 8 Minutes
Ingredients:
- 12 corn tortillas (6- to 7-inch size)
- Filling
- ½ cup refried pinto beans
- ½ cup grated sharp Cheddar or Pepper Jack cheese
- ¼ cup corn kernels (if frozen, measure after thawing and draining)
- 2 tablespoons chopped green onion
- 2 tablespoons chopped jalapeño pepper (seeds and ribs removed before chopping)
- ½ teaspoon lime juice
- ½ teaspoon chile powder, plus extra for dusting
- ½ teaspoon cumin
- ½ teaspoon garlic powder
- oil for misting or cooking spray
- salsa, sour cream, or guacamole for dipping

Directions:
1. Mix together all filling Ingredients.
2. Warm refrigerated tortillas for easier rolling. (Wrap in damp paper towels and microwave for 30 to 60 seconds.)
3. Working with one at a time, place 1 tablespoon of filling on tortilla and roll up. Spray with oil or cooking spray and dust outside with chile powder to taste.
4. Place 6 taquitos in air fryer basket (4 on bottom layer, 2 stacked crosswise on top). Cook at 390°F/200°C for 8 minutes, until crispy and brown.
5. Repeat step 4 to cook remaining taquitos.
6. Serve plain or with salsa, sour cream, or guacamole for dipping.

Vegetable Hand Pies

Servings: 8
Cooking Time: 10 Minutes Per Batch
Ingredients:
- ¾ cup vegetable broth
- 8 ounces potatoes
- ¾ cup frozen chopped broccoli, thawed
- ¼ cup chopped mushrooms
- 1 tablespoon cornstarch
- 1 tablespoon milk
- 1 can organic flaky biscuits (8 large biscuits)
- oil for misting or cooking spray

Directions:
1. Place broth in medium saucepan over low heat.
2. While broth is heating, grate raw potato into a bowl of water to prevent browning. You will need ¾ cup grated potato.
3. Roughly chop the broccoli.
4. Drain potatoes and put them in the broth along with the broccoli and mushrooms. Cook on low for 5 minutes.
5. Dissolve cornstarch in milk, then stir the mixture into the broth. Cook about a minute, until mixture thickens a little. Remove from heat and cool slightly.
6. Separate each biscuit into 2 rounds. Divide vegetable mixture evenly over half the biscuit rounds, mounding filling in the center of each.
7. Top the four rounds with filling, then the other four rounds and crimp the edges together with a fork.
8. Spray both sides with oil or cooking spray and place 4 pies in a single layer in the air fryer basket.
9. Cook at 330°F/160°C for approximately 10 minutes.
10. Repeat with the remaining biscuits. The second batch may cook more quickly because the fryer will be hot.

Harissa Veggie Fries

Servings: 4
Cooking Time: 55 Minutes
Ingredients:
- 1 pound red potatoes, cut into rounds
- 1 onion, diced
- 1 green bell pepper, diced
- 1 red bell pepper, diced
- 2 tbsp olive oil
- Salt and pepper to taste
- ¾ tsp garlic powder
- ¾ tsp harissa seasoning

Directions:
1. Combine all ingredients in a large bowl and mix until potatoes are well coated and seasoned. Preheat air fryer to 350°F/175°C. Pour all of the contents in the bowl into the frying basket. Bake for 35 minutes, shaking every 10 minutes, until golden brown and soft. Serve hot.

Sushi-style Deviled Eggs

Servings:4
Cooking Time: 20 Minutes
Ingredients:
- ¼ cup crabmeat, shells discarded
- 4 eggs
- 2 tbsp mayonnaise
- ½ tsp soy sauce
- ¼ avocado, diced
- ¼ tsp wasabi powder
- 2 tbsp diced cucumber
- 1 sheet nori, sliced
- 8 jarred pickled ginger slices

- 1 tsp toasted sesame seeds
- 2 spring onions, sliced

Directions:
1. Preheat air fryer to 260ºF/180°C. Place the eggs in muffin cups to avoid bumping around and cracking during the cooking process. Add silicone cups to the frying basket and Air Fry for 15 minutes. Remove and plunge the eggs immediately into an ice bath to cool, about 5 minutes. Carefully peel and slice them in half lengthwise. Spoon yolks into a separate medium bowl and arrange white halves on a large plate. Mash the yolks with a fork. Stir in mayonnaise, soy sauce, avocado, and wasabi powder until smooth. Mix in cucumber and spoon into white halves. Scatter eggs with crabmeat, nori, pickled ginger, spring onions and sesame seeds to serve.

Zucchini Tamale Pie

Servings: 4
Cooking Time: 45 Minutes
Ingredients:
- 1 cup canned diced tomatoes with juice
- 1 zucchini, diced
- 3 tbsp safflower oil
- 1 cup cooked pinto beans
- 3 garlic cloves, minced
- 1 tbsp corn masa flour
- 1 tsp dried oregano
- ½ tsp ground cumin
- 1 tsp onion powder
- Salt to taste
- ½ tsp red chili flakes
- ½ cup ground cornmeal
- 1 tsp nutritional yeast
- 2 tbsp chopped cilantro
- ½ tsp lime zest

Directions:
1. Warm 2 tbsp of the oil in a skillet over medium heat and sauté the zucchini for 3 minutes or until they begin to brown. Add the beans, tomatoes, garlic, flour, oregano, cumin, onion powder, salt, and chili flakes. Cook over medium heat, stirring often, about 5 minutes until the mix is thick and no liquid remains. Remove from heat. Spray a baking pan with oil and pour the mix inside. Smooth out the top and set aside.
2. In a pot over high heat, add the cornmeal, 1 ½ cups of water, and salt. Whisk constantly as the mix begins to boil. Once it boils, reduce the heat to low. Add the yeast and oil and continue to cook, stirring often, for 10 minutes or until the mix is thick and hard to stir. Remove. Preheat air fryer to 325°F/160°C. Add the cilantro and lime zest into the cornmeal mix and thoroughly combine. Using a rubber spatula, spread it evenly over the filling in the baking pan to form a crust topping. Put in the frying basket and Bake for 20 minutes or until the top is golden. Let it cool for 5 to 10 minutes, then cut and serve.

Egg Rolls

Servings: 4
Cooking Time: 8 Minutes
Ingredients:
- 1 clove garlic, minced
- 1 teaspoon sesame oil
- 1 teaspoon olive oil
- ½ cup chopped celery
- ½ cup grated carrots
- 2 green onions, chopped
- 2 ounces mushrooms, chopped

- 2 cups shredded Napa cabbage
- 1 teaspoon low-sodium soy sauce
- 1 teaspoon cornstarch
- salt
- 1 egg
- 1 tablespoon water
- 4 egg roll wraps
- olive oil for misting or cooking spray

Directions:
1. In a large skillet, sauté garlic in sesame and olive oils over medium heat for 1 minute.
2. Add celery, carrots, onions, and mushrooms to skillet. Cook 1 minute, stirring.
3. Stir in cabbage, cover, and cook for 1 minute or just until cabbage slightly wilts.
4. In a small bowl, mix soy sauce and cornstarch. Stir into vegetables to thicken. Remove from heat. Salt to taste if needed.
5. Beat together egg and water in a small bowl.
6. Divide filling into 4 portions and roll up in egg roll wraps. Brush all over with egg wash to seal.
7. Mist egg rolls very lightly with olive oil or cooking spray and place in air fryer basket.
8. Cook at 390°F/200°C for 4minutes. Turn over and cook 4 more minutes, until golden brown and crispy.

Gorgeous Jalapeño Poppers

Servings: 6
Cooking Time: 25 Minutes
Ingredients:
- 6 center-cut bacon slices, halved
- 6 jalapeños, halved lengthwise
- 4 oz cream cheese
- ¼ cup grated Gruyere cheese
- 2 tbsp chives, chopped

Directions:
1. Scoop out seeds and membranes of the jalapeño halves, discard. Combine cream cheese, Gruyere cheese, and chives in a bowl. Fill the jalapeño halves with the cream cheese filling using a small spoon. Wrap each pepper with a slice of bacon and secure with a toothpick.
2. Preheat air fryer to 325°F/160°C. Put the stuffed peppers in a single layer on the greased frying basket and Bake until the peppers are tender, cheese is melted, and the bacon is brown, 11-13minutes. Serve warm and enjoy!

Asparagus, Mushroom And Cheese Soufflés

Servings: 3
Cooking Time: 21 Minutes
Ingredients:
- butter
- grated Parmesan cheese
- 3 button mushrooms, thinly sliced
- 8 spears asparagus, sliced ½-inch long
- 1 teaspoon olive oil
- 1 tablespoon butter
- 4½ teaspoons flour
- pinch paprika
- pinch ground nutmeg
- salt and freshly ground black pepper
- ½ cup milk
- ½ cup grated Gruyère cheese or other Swiss cheese (about 2 ounces)
- 2 eggs, separated

Directions:
1. Butter three 6-ounce ramekins and dust with grated Parmesan cheese. (Butter the ramekins and then coat the butter with Parmesan by shaking it around in the ramekin and dumping out any excess.)
2. Preheat the air fryer to 400°F/205°C.
3. Toss the mushrooms and asparagus in a bowl with the olive oil. Transfer the vegetables to the air fryer and air-fry for 7 minutes, shaking the basket once or twice to redistribute the Ingredients while they cook.
4. While the vegetables are cooking, make the soufflé base. Melt the butter in a saucepan on the stovetop over medium heat. Add the flour, stir and cook for a minute or two. Add the paprika, nutmeg, salt and pepper. Whisk in the milk and bring the mixture to a simmer to thicken. Remove the pan from the heat and add the cheese, stirring to melt. Let the mixture cool for just a few minutes and then whisk the egg yolks in, one at a time. Stir in the cooked mushrooms and asparagus. Let this soufflé base cool.
5. In a separate bowl, whisk the egg whites to soft peak stage (the point at which the whites can almost stand up on the end of your whisk). Fold the whipped egg whites into the soufflé base, adding a little at a time.
6. Preheat the air fryer to 330°F/165°C.
7. Transfer the batter carefully to the buttered ramekins, leaving about ½-inch at the top. Place the ramekins into the air fryer basket and air-fry for 14 minutes. The soufflés should have risen nicely and be brown on top. Serve immediately.

Berbere Eggplant Dip

Servings:4
Cooking Time: 35 Minutes
Ingredients:
- 1 eggplant, halved lengthwise
- 3 tsp olive oil
- 2 tsp pine nuts
- ¼ cup tahini
- 1 tbsp lemon juice
- 2 cloves garlic, minced
- ¼ tsp berbere seasoning
- ⅛ tsp ground cumin
- Salt and pepper to taste
- 1 tbsp chopped parsley

Directions:
1. Preheat air fryer to 370ºF/185°C. Brush the eggplant with some olive oil. With a fork, pierce the eggplant flesh a few times. Place them, flat sides-down, in the frying basket. Air Fry for 25 minutes. Transfer the eggplant to a cutting board and let cool for 3 minutes until easy to handle. Place pine nuts in the frying basket and Air Fry for 2 minutes, shaking every 30 seconds. Set aside in a bowl.
2. Scoop out the eggplant flesh and add to a food processor. Add in tahini, lemon juice, garlic, berbere seasoning, cumin, salt, and black pepper and pulse until smooth. Transfer to a serving bowl. Scatter with toasted pine nuts, parsley, and the remaining olive oil. Serve immediately.

Roasted Vegetable Lasagna

Servings: 6
Cooking Time: 55 Minutes
Ingredients:
- 1 zucchini, sliced
- 1 yellow squash, sliced
- 8 ounces mushrooms, sliced
- 1 red bell pepper, cut into 2-inch strips
- 1 tablespoon olive oil

- 2 cups ricotta cheese
- 2 cups grated mozzarella cheese, divided
- 1 egg
- 1 teaspoon salt
- freshly ground black pepper
- ¼ cup shredded carrots
- ½ cup chopped fresh spinach
- 8 lasagna noodles, cooked
- Béchamel Sauce:
- 3 tablespoons butter
- 3 tablespoons flour
- 2½ cups milk
- ½ cup grated Parmesan cheese
- ½ teaspoon salt
- freshly ground black pepper
- pinch of ground nutmeg

Directions:
1. Preheat the air fryer to 400°F/205°C.
2. Toss the zucchini, yellow squash, mushrooms and red pepper in a large bowl with the olive oil and season with salt and pepper. Air-fry for 10 minutes, shaking the basket once or twice while the vegetables cook.
3. While the vegetables are cooking, make the béchamel sauce and cheese filling. Melt the butter in a medium saucepan over medium-high heat on the stovetop. Add the flour and whisk, cooking for a couple of minutes. Add the milk and whisk vigorously until smooth. Bring the mixture to a boil and simmer until the sauce thickens. Stir in the Parmesan cheese and season with the salt, pepper and nutmeg. Set the sauce aside.
4. Combine the ricotta cheese, 1¼ cups of the mozzarella cheese, egg, salt and pepper in a large bowl and stir until combined. Fold in the carrots and spinach.
5. When the vegetables have finished cooking, build the lasagna. Use a baking dish that is 6 inches in diameter and 4 inches high. Cover the bottom of the baking dish with a little béchamel sauce. Top with two lasagna noodles, cut to fit the dish and overlapping each other a little. Spoon a third of the ricotta cheese mixture and then a third of the roasted veggies on top of the noodles. Pour ½ cup of béchamel sauce on top and then repeat these layers two more times: noodles – cheese mixture – vegetables – béchamel sauce. Sprinkle the remaining mozzarella cheese over the top. Cover the dish with aluminum foil, tenting it loosely so the aluminum doesn't touch the cheese.
6. Lower the dish into the air fryer basket using an aluminum foil sling (fold a piece of aluminum foil into a strip about 2-inches wide by 24-inches long). Fold the ends of the aluminum foil over the top of the dish before returning the basket to the air fryer. Air-fry for 45 minutes, removing the foil for the last 2 minutes, to slightly brown the cheese on top.
7. Let the lasagna rest for at least 20 minutes to set up a little before slicing into it and serving.

Vietnamese Gingered Tofu

Servings: 4
Cooking Time: 25 Minutes
Ingredients:
- 1 package extra-firm tofu, cubed
- 4 tsp shoyu

- 1 tsp onion powder
- ½ tsp garlic powder
- ½ tsp ginger powder
- ½ tsp turmeric powder
- Black pepper to taste
- 2 tbsp nutritional yeast
- 1 tsp dried rosemary
- 1 tsp dried dill
- 2 tsp cornstarch
- 2 tsp sunflower oil

Directions:
1. Sprinkle the tofu with shoyu and toss to coat. Add the onion, garlic, ginger, turmeric, and pepper. Gently toss to coat. Add the yeast, rosemary, dill, and cornstarch. Toss to coat. Dribble with the oil and toss again.
2. Preheat air fryer to 390°F/200°C. Spray the fryer basket with oil, put the tofu in the basket and Bake for 7 minutes. Remove, shake gently, and cook for another 7 minutes or until the tofu is crispy and golden. Serve warm.

Thyme Meatless Patties

Servings: 3
Cooking Time: 25 Minutes
Ingredients:
- ½ cup oat flour
- 1 tsp allspice
- ½ tsp ground thyme
- 1 tsp maple syrup
- ½ tsp liquid smoke
- 1 tsp balsamic vinegar

Directions:
1. Preheat air fryer to 400°F/205°C. Mix the oat flour, allspice, thyme, maple syrup, liquid smoke, balsamic vinegar, and 2 tbsp of water in a bowl. Make 6 patties out of the mixture. Place them onto a parchment paper and flatten them to ½-inch thick. Grease the patties with cooking spray. Grill for 12 minutes until crispy, turning once. Serve warm.

Garlicky Brussel Sprouts With Saffron Aioli

Servings: 4
Cooking Time: 20 Minutes
Ingredients:
- 1 lb Brussels sprouts, halved
- 1 tsp garlic powder
- Salt and pepper to taste
- ½ cup mayonnaise
- ½ tbsp olive oil
- 1 tbsp Dijon mustard
- 1 tsp minced garlic
- Salt and pepper to taste
- ½ tsp liquid saffron

Directions:
1. Preheat air fryer to 380°F/195°C. Combine the Brussels sprouts, garlic powder, salt and pepper in a large bowl. Place in the fryer and spray with cooking oil. Bake for 12-14 minutes, shaking once, until just brown.
2. Meanwhile, in a small bowl, mix mayonnaise, olive oil, mustard, garlic, saffron, salt and pepper. When the Brussels sprouts are slightly cool, serve with aioli. Enjoy!

Poultry Recipes

Chicken Thighs In Salsa Verde

Servings: 4
Cooking Time: 35 Minutes
Ingredients:
- 4 boneless, skinless chicken thighs
- 1 cup salsa verde
- 1 tsp mashed garlic

Directions:
1. Preheat air fryer at 350ºF/175°C. Add chicken thighs to a cake pan and cover with salsa verde and mashed garlic. Place cake pan in the frying basket and Bake for 30 minutes. Let rest for 5 minutes before serving.

Daadi Chicken Salad

Servings: 2
Cooking Time: 30 Minutes
Ingredients:
- ½ cup chopped golden raisins
- 1 Granny Smith apple, grated
- 2 chicken breasts
- Salt and pepper to taste
- ¾ cup mayonnaise
- 1 tbsp lime juice
- 1 tsp curry powder
- ½ sliced avocado
- 1 scallion, minced
- 2 tbsp chopped pecans
- 1 tsp poppy seeds

Directions:
1. Preheat air fryer at 350ºF/175°C. Sprinkle chicken breasts with salt and pepper, place them in the greased frying basket, and Air Fry for 8-10 minutes, tossing once. Let rest for 5 minutes before cutting. In a salad bowl, combine chopped chicken, mayonnaise, lime juice, curry powder, raisins, apple, avocado, scallion, and pecans. Let sit covered in the fridge until ready to eat. Before serve sprinkled with the poppy seeds.

Saucy Chicken Thighs

Servings: 4
Cooking Time: 35 Minutes
Ingredients:
- 8 boneless, skinless chicken thighs
- 1 tbsp Italian seasoning
- Salt and pepper to taste
- 2 garlic cloves, minced
- ½ tsp apple cider vinegar
- ½ cup honey
- ¼ cup Dijon mustard

Directions:
1. Preheat air fryer to 400°F/205°C. Season the chicken with Italian seasoning, salt, and black pepper. Place in the greased frying basket and Bake for 15 minutes, flipping once halfway through cooking.
2. While the chicken is cooking, add garlic, honey, vinegar, and Dijon mustard in a saucepan and stir-fry over medium heat for 4 minutes or until the sauce has thickened and

warmed through. Transfer the thighs to a serving dish and drizzle with honey-mustard sauce. Serve and enjoy!

The Ultimate Chicken Bulgogi

Servings:4
Cooking Time: 30 Minutes
Ingredients:
- 1 ½ lb boneless, skinless chicken thighs, cubed
- 1 cucumber, thinly sliced
- ¼ cup apple cider vinegar
- 4 garlic cloves, minced
- ¼ tsp ground ginger
- ⅛ tsp red pepper flakes
- 2 tsp honey
- ⅛ tsp salt
- 2 tbsp tamari
- 2 tsp sesame oil
- 2 tsp granular honey
- 2 tbsp lemon juice
- ½ tsp lemon zest
- 3 scallions, chopped
- 2 cups cooked white rice
- 2 tsp roasted sesame seeds

Directions:
1. In a bowl, toss the cucumber, vinegar, half of the garlic, half of the ginger, pepper flakes, honey, and salt and store in the fridge covered. Combine the tamari, sesame oil, granular honey, lemon juice, remaining garlic, remaining ginger, and chicken in a large bowl. Toss to coat and marinate in the fridge for 10 minutes.
2. Preheat air fryer to 350ºF/175°C. Place chicken in the frying basket, do not discard excess marinade. Air Fry for 11 minutes, shaking once and pouring excess marinade over. Place the chicken bulgogi over the cooked rice and scatter with scallion greens, pickled cucumbers, and sesame seeds. Serve and enjoy!

Japanese-style Turkey Meatballs

Servings: 4
Cooking Time: 25 Minutes
Ingredients:
- 1 1/3 lb ground turkey
- ¼ cup panko bread crumbs
- 4 chopped scallions
- ¼ cup chopped cilantro
- 1 egg
- 1 tbsp grated ginger
- 1 garlic clove, minced
- 3 tbsp shoyu
- 2 tsp toasted sesame oil
- ¾ tsp salt
- 2 tbsp oyster sauce sauce
- 2 tbsp fresh orange juice

Directions:
1. Add ground turkey, panko, 3 scallions, cilantro, egg, ginger, garlic, 1 tbsp of shoyu sauce, sesame oil, and salt in a bowl. Mix with hands until combined. Divide the mixture into 12 equal parts and roll into balls. Preheat air fryer to 380°F/195°C. Place the meatballs in the greased frying

basket. Bake for about 9-11 minutes, flipping once until browned and cooked through. Repeat for all meatballs.

2.   In a small saucepan over medium heat, add oyster sauce, orange juice and remaining shoyu sauce. Bring to a boil, then reduce the heat to low. Cook until the sauce is slightly reduced, 3 minutes. Serve the meatballs with the oyster sauce drizzled over them and topped with the remaining scallions.

Maple Bacon Wrapped Chicken Breasts

Servings: 2
Cooking Time: 18 Minutes
Ingredients:
- 2 (6-ounce) boneless, skinless chicken breasts
- 2 tablespoons maple syrup, divided
- freshly ground black pepper
- 6 slices thick-sliced bacon
- fresh celery or parsley leaves
- Ranch Dressing:
- ¼ cup mayonnaise
- ¼ cup buttermilk
- ¼ cup Greek yogurt
- 1 tablespoon chopped fresh chives
- 1 tablespoon chopped fresh parsley
- 1 tablespoon chopped fresh dill
- 1 tablespoon lemon juice
- salt and freshly ground black pepper

Directions:
1.   Brush the chicken breasts with half the maple syrup and season with freshly ground black pepper. Wrap three slices of bacon around each chicken breast, securing the ends with toothpicks.
2.   Preheat the air fryer to 380°F/195°C.
3.   Air-fry the chicken for 6 minutes. Then turn the chicken breasts over, pour more maple syrup on top and air-fry for another 6 minutes. Turn the chicken breasts one more time, brush the remaining maple syrup all over and continue to air-fry for a final 6 minutes.
4.   While the chicken is cooking, prepare the dressing by combining all the dressing ingredients together in a bowl.
5.   When the chicken has finished cooking, remove the toothpicks and serve each breast with a little dressing drizzled over each one. Scatter lots of fresh celery or parsley leaves on top.

Granny Pesto Chicken Caprese

Servings: 4
Cooking Time: 30 Minutes
Ingredients:
- 2 tbsp grated Parmesan cheese
- 4 oz fresh mozzarella cheese, thinly sliced
- 16 grape tomatoes, halved
- 4 garlic cloves, minced
- 1 tsp olive oil
- Salt and pepper to taste
- 4 chicken cutlets
- 1 tbsp prepared pesto
- 1 large egg, beaten
- ½ cup bread crumbs
- 2 tbsp Italian seasoning
- 1 tsp balsamic vinegar
- 2 tbsp chopped fresh basil

Directions:

1.   Preheat air fryer to 400°F/205°C. In a bowl, coat the tomatoes with garlic, olive oil, salt and pepper. Air Fry for 5 minutes, shaking them twice. Set aside when soft.
2.   Place the cutlets between two sheets of parchment paper. Pound the chicken to ¼-inch thickness using a meat mallet. Season on both sides with salt and pepper. Spread an even coat of pesto. Put the beaten egg in a shallow bowl. Mix the crumbs, Italian seasoning, and Parmesan in a second shallow bowl. Dip the chicken in the egg bowl, and then in the crumb mix. Press the crumbs so that they stick to the chicken.
3.   Place the chicken in the greased frying basket. Air Fry the chicken for 6-8 minutes, flipping once until golden and cooked through. Put 1 oz of mozzarella and ¼ of the tomatoes on top of each cutlet. When all of the cutlets are cooked, return them to the frying basket and melt the cheese for 2 minutes. Remove from the fryer, drizzle with balsamic vinegar and basil on top.

Buffalo Egg Rolls

Servings: 8
Cooking Time: 9 Minutes Per Batch
Ingredients:
- 1 teaspoon water
- 1 tablespoon cornstarch
- 1 egg
- 2½ cups cooked chicken, diced or shredded (see opposite page)
- ⅓ cup chopped green onion
- ⅓ cup diced celery
- ⅓ cup buffalo wing sauce
- 8 egg roll wraps
- oil for misting or cooking spray
- Blue Cheese Dip
- 3 ounces cream cheese, softened
- ⅓ cup blue cheese, crumbled
- 1 teaspoon Worcestershire sauce
- ¼ teaspoon garlic powder
- ¼ cup buttermilk (or sour cream)

Directions:
1.   Mix water and cornstarch in a small bowl until dissolved. Add egg, beat well, and set aside.
2.   In a medium size bowl, mix together chicken, green onion, celery, and buffalo wing sauce.
3.   Divide chicken mixture evenly among 8 egg roll wraps, spooning ½ inch from one edge.
4.   Moisten all edges of each wrap with beaten egg wash.
5.   Fold the short ends over filling, then roll up tightly and press to seal edges.
6.   Brush outside of wraps with egg wash, then spritz with oil or cooking spray.
7.   Place 4 egg rolls in air fryer basket.
8.   Cook at 390°F/200°C for 9minutes or until outside is brown and crispy.
9.   While the rolls are cooking, prepare the Blue Cheese Dip. With a fork, mash together cream cheese and blue cheese.
10.   Stir in remaining ingredients.
11.   Dip should be just thick enough to slightly cling to egg rolls. If too thick, stir in buttermilk or milk 1 tablespoon at a time until you reach the desired consistency.
12.   Cook remaining 4 egg rolls as in steps 7 and 8.
13.   Serve while hot with Blue Cheese Dip, more buffalo wing sauce, or both.

Sage & Paprika Turkey Cutlets

Servings: 4
Cooking Time: 15 Minutes
Ingredients:
- ½ cup bread crumbs
- ¼ tsp paprika
- Salt and pepper to taste
- ⅛ tsp dried sage
- ⅛ tsp garlic powder
- ¼ tsp ground cumin
- 1 egg
- 4 turkey breast cutlets
- 2 tbsp chopped chervil

Directions:
1. Preheat air fryer to 380°F/195°C. Combine the bread crumbs, paprika, salt, black pepper, sage, cumin, and garlic powder in a bowl and mix well. Beat the egg in another bowl until frothy. Dip the turkey cutlets into the egg mixture, then coat them in the bread crumb mixture. Put the breaded turkey cutlets in the frying basket. Bake for 4 minutes. Turn the cutlets over, then Bake for 4 more minutes. Decorate with chervil and serve.

Chicken Nuggets

Servings: 20
Cooking Time: 14 Minutes Per Batch
Ingredients:
- 1 pound boneless, skinless chicken thighs, cut into 1-inch chunks
- ¾ teaspoon salt
- ½ teaspoon black pepper
- ½ teaspoon garlic powder
- ½ teaspoon onion powder
- ½ cup flour
- 2 eggs, beaten
- ½ cup panko breadcrumbs
- 3 tablespoons plain breadcrumbs
- oil for misting or cooking spray

Directions:
1. In the bowl of a food processor, combine chicken, ½ teaspoon salt, pepper, garlic powder, and onion powder. Process in short pulses until chicken is very finely chopped and well blended.
2. Place flour in one shallow dish and beaten eggs in another. In a third dish or plastic bag, mix together the panko crumbs, plain breadcrumbs, and ¼ teaspoon salt.
3. Shape chicken mixture into small nuggets. Dip nuggets in flour, then eggs, then panko crumb mixture.
4. Spray nuggets on both sides with oil or cooking spray and place in air fryer basket in a single layer, close but not overlapping.
5. Cook at 360°F/180°C for 10minutes. Spray with oil and cook 4 minutes, until chicken is done and coating is golden brown.
6. Repeat step 5 to cook remaining nuggets.

Mexican Chicken Roll-ups

Servings: 4
Cooking Time: 35 Minutes
Ingredients:
- ½ red bell pepper, cut into strips
- ½ green bell pepper, cut into strips
- 2 chicken breasts
- ½ lime, juiced
- 2 tbsp taco seasoning
- 1 spring onion, thinly sliced

Directions:
1. Preheat air fryer to 400°F/205°C. Cut the chicken into cutlets by slicing the chicken breast in half horizontally in order to have 4 thin cutlets. Drizzle with lime juice and season with taco seasoning. Divide the red pepper, green pepper, and spring onion equally between the 4 cutlets. Roll up the cutlets. Secure with toothpicks. Place the chicken roll-ups in the air fryer and lightly spray with cooking oil. Bake for 12 minutes, turning once. Serve warm.

Japanese-inspired Glazed Chicken

Servings: 4
Cooking Time: 25 Minutes
Ingredients:
- 4 chicken breasts
- Chicken seasoning to taste
- Salt and pepper to taste
- 2 tsp grated fresh ginger
- 2 garlic cloves, minced
- ¼ cup molasses
- 2 tbsp tamari sauce

Directions:
1. Preheat air fryer to 400°F/205°C. Season the chicken with seasoning, salt, and pepper. Place the chicken in the greased frying basket and Air Fry for 7 minutes, then flip the chicken. Cook for another 3 minutes.
2. While the chicken is cooking, combine ginger, garlic, molasses, and tamari sauce in a saucepan over medium heat. Cook for 4 minutes or until the sauce thickens. Transfer all of the chicken to a serving dish. Drizzle with ginger-tamari glaze and serve.

Cal-mex Turkey Patties

Servings: 4
Cooking Time: 30 Minutes
Ingredients:
- 1/3 cup crushed corn tortilla chips
- 1/3 cup grated American cheese
- 1 egg, beaten
- ¼ cup salsa
- Salt and pepper to taste
- 1 lb ground turkey
- 1 tbsp olive oil
- 1 tsp chili powder

Directions:
1. Preheat air fryer to 330°F/165°C. Mix together egg, tortilla chips, salsa, cheese, salt, and pepper in a bowl. Using your hands, add the ground turkey and mix gently until just combined. Divide the meat into 4 equal portions and shape into patties about ½ inch thick. Brush the patties with olive oil and sprinkle with chili powder. Air Fry the patties for 14-16 minutes, flipping once until cooked through and golden. Serve and enjoy!

Indian-inspired Chicken Skewers

Servings:4
Cooking Time: 40 Minutes + Chilling Time
Ingredients:
- 1 lb boneless, skinless chicken thighs, cubed
- 1 red onion, diced
- 1 tbsp grated ginger
- 2 tbsp lime juice
- 1 cup canned coconut milk
- 2 tbsp tomato paste
- 2 tbsp olive oil
- 1 tbsp ground cumin
- 1 tbsp ground coriander
- 1 tsp cayenne pepper

- 1 tsp ground turmeric
- ½ tsp red chili powder
- ¼ tsp curry powder
- 2 tsp salt
- 2 tbsp chopped cilantro

Directions:
1. Toss red onion, ginger, lime juice, coconut milk, tomato paste, olive oil, cumin, coriander, cayenne pepper, turmeric, chili powder, curry powder, salt, and chicken until fully coated. Let chill in the fridge for 2 hours.
2. Preheat air fryer to 350°F/175°C. Thread chicken onto 8 skewers and place them on a kebab rack. Place rack in the frying basket and Air Fry for 12 minutes. Discard marinade. Garnish with cilantro to serve.

Chicken Burgers With Blue Cheese Sauce

Servings: 4
Cooking Time: 40 Minutes
Ingredients:
- ¼ cup crumbled blue cheese
- ¼ cup sour cream
- 2 tbsp mayonnaise
- 1 tbsp red hot sauce
- Salt to taste
- 3 tbsp buffalo wing sauce
- 1 lb ground chicken
- 2 tbsp grated carrot
- 2 tbsp diced celery
- 1 egg white

Directions:
1. Whisk the blue cheese, sour cream, mayonnaise, red hot sauce, salt, and 1 tbsp of buffalo sauce in a bowl. Let sit covered in the fridge until ready to use.
2. Preheat air fryer at 350°F/175°C. In another bowl, combine the remaining ingredients. Form mixture into 4 patties, making a slight indentation in the middle of each. Place patties in the greased frying basket and Air Fry for 13 minutes until you reach your desired doneness, flipping once. Serve with the blue cheese sauce.

Parmesan Chicken Meatloaf

Servings: 4
Cooking Time: 45 Minutes
Ingredients:
- 1 ½ tsp evaporated cane sugar
- 1 lb ground chicken
- 4 garlic cloves, minced
- 2 tbsp grated Parmesan
- ¼ cup heavy cream
- ¼ cup minced onion
- 2 tbsp chopped basil
- 2 tbsp chopped parsley
- Salt and pepper to taste
- ½ tsp onion powder
- ½ cup bread crumbs
- ¼ tsp red pepper flakes
- 1 egg
- 1 cup tomato sauce
- ½ tsp garlic powder
- ½ tsp dried thyme
- ½ tsp dried oregano
- 1 tbsp coconut aminos

Directions:
1. Preheat air fryer to 400°F/205°C. Combine chicken, garlic, minced onion, oregano, thyme, basil, salt, pepper, onion powder, Parmesan cheese, red pepper flakes, bread crumbs, egg, and cream in a large bowl. Transfer the chicken mixture to a prepared baking dish. Stir together tomato sauce, garlic powder, coconut aminos, and sugar in a small bowl. Spread over the meatloaf. Loosely cover with foil. Place the pan in the frying basket and bake for 15 minutes. Take the foil off and bake for another 15 minutes. Allow resting for 10 minutes before slicing. Serve sprinkled with parsley.

Mushroom & Turkey Bread Pizza

Servings: 4
Cooking Time: 35 Minutes
Ingredients:
- 10 cooked turkey sausages, sliced
- 1 cup shredded mozzarella cheese
- 1 cup shredded Cheddar cheese
- 1 French loaf bread
- 2 tbsp butter, softened
- 1 tsp garlic powder
- 1 1/3 cups marinara sauce
- 1 tsp Italian seasoning
- 2 scallions, chopped
- 1 cup mushrooms, sliced

Directions:
1. Preheat the air fryer to 370°F/185°C. Cut the bread in half crosswise, then split each half horizontally. Combine butter and garlic powder, then spread on the cut sides of the bread. Bake the halves in the fryer for 3-5 minutes or until the leaves start to brown. Set the toasted bread on a work surface and spread marinara sauce over the top. Sprinkle the Italian seasoning, then top with sausages, scallions, mushrooms, and cheeses. Set the pizzas in the air fryer and Bake for 8-12 minutes or until the cheese is melted and starting to brown. Serve hot.

Chicken Hand Pies

Servings: 8
Cooking Time: 10 Minutes Per Batch
Ingredients:
- ¾ cup chicken broth
- ¾ cup frozen mixed peas and carrots
- 1 cup cooked chicken, chopped
- 1 tablespoon cornstarch
- 1 tablespoon milk
- salt and pepper
- 1 8-count can organic flaky biscuits
- oil for misting or cooking spray

Directions:
1. In a medium saucepan, bring chicken broth to a boil. Stir in the frozen peas and carrots and cook for 5minutes over medium heat. Stir in chicken.
2. Mix the cornstarch into the milk until it dissolves. Stir it into the simmering chicken broth mixture and cook just until thickened.
3. Remove from heat, add salt and pepper to taste, and let cool slightly.
4. Lay biscuits out on wax paper. Peel each biscuit apart in the middle to make 2 rounds so you have 16 rounds total. Using your hands or a rolling pin, flatten each biscuit round slightly to make it larger and thinner.
5. Divide chicken filling among 8 of the biscuit rounds. Place remaining biscuit rounds on top and press edges all around. Use the tines of a fork to crimp biscuit edges and make sure they are sealed well.
6. Spray both sides lightly with oil or cooking spray.
7. Cook in a single layer, 4 at a time, at 330°F/165°C for 10minutes or until biscuit dough is cooked through and golden brown.

Chicken Chimichangas

Servings: 4
Cooking Time: 10 Minutes
Ingredients:
- 2 cups cooked chicken, shredded
- 2 tablespoons chopped green chiles
- ½ teaspoon oregano
- ½ teaspoon cumin
- ½ teaspoon onion powder
- ¼ teaspoon garlic powder
- salt and pepper
- 8 flour tortillas (6- or 7-inch diameter)
- oil for misting or cooking spray
- Chimichanga Sauce
- 2 tablespoons butter
- 2 tablespoons flour
- 1 cup chicken broth
- ¼ cup light sour cream
- ¼ teaspoon salt
- 2 ounces Pepper Jack or Monterey Jack cheese, shredded

Directions:
1. Make the sauce by melting butter in a saucepan over medium-low heat. Stir in flour until smooth and slightly bubbly. Gradually add broth, stirring constantly until smooth. Cook and stir 1 minute, until the mixture slightly thickens. Remove from heat and stir in sour cream and salt. Set aside.
2. In a medium bowl, mix together the chicken, chiles, oregano, cumin, onion powder, garlic, salt, and pepper. Stir in 3 to 4 tablespoons of the sauce, using just enough to make the filling moist but not soupy.
3. Divide filling among the 8 tortillas. Place filling down the center of tortilla, stopping about 1 inch from edges. Fold one side of tortilla over filling, fold the two sides in, and then roll up. Mist all sides with oil or cooking spray.
4. Place chimichangas in air fryer basket seam side down. To fit more into the basket, you can stand them on their sides with the seams against the sides of the basket.
5. Cook at 360°F/180°C for 10 minutes or until heated through and crispy brown outside.
6. Add the shredded cheese to the remaining sauce. Stir over low heat, warming just until the cheese melts. Don't boil or sour cream may curdle.
7. Drizzle the sauce over the chimichangas.

Crispy Cordon Bleu

Servings: 4
Cooking Time: 25 Minutes
Ingredients:
- 4 deli ham slices, halved lengthwise
- 2 tbsp grated Parmesan
- 4 chicken breast halves
- Salt and pepper to taste
- 8 Swiss cheese slices
- 1 egg
- 2 egg whites
- ¾ cup bread crumbs
- 1 tsp garlic powder
- 1 tsp onion powder
- 1 tsp mustard powder

Directions:
1. Preheat air fryer to 400°F/205°C. Season the chicken cutlets with salt and pepper. On one cutlet, put a half slice of ham and cheese on the top. Roll the chicken tightly, then set aside. Beat the eggs and egg whites in a shallow bowl. Put the crumbs, Parmesan, garlic, onion, and mustard powder, in a second bowl. Dip the cutlet in the egg bowl and then in the crumb mix. Press so that they stick to the chicken. Put the rolls of chicken seam side down in the greased frying basket and Air Fry for 12-14 minutes, flipping once until golden and cooked through. Serve.

Chicken Schnitzel Dogs

Servings: 4
Cooking Time: 10 Minutes
Ingredients:
- ½ cup flour
- ½ teaspoon salt
- 1 teaspoon marjoram
- 1 teaspoon dried parsley flakes
- ½ teaspoon thyme
- 1 egg
- 1 teaspoon lemon juice
- 1 teaspoon water
- 1 cup breadcrumbs
- 4 chicken tenders, pounded thin
- oil for misting or cooking spray
- 4 whole-grain hotdog buns
- 4 slices Gouda cheese
- 1 small Granny Smith apple, thinly sliced
- ½ cup shredded Napa cabbage
- coleslaw dressing

Directions:
1. In a shallow dish, mix together the flour, salt, marjoram, parsley, and thyme.
2. In another shallow dish, beat together egg, lemon juice, and water.
3. Place breadcrumbs in a third shallow dish.
4. Cut each of the flattened chicken tenders in half lengthwise.
5. Dip flattened chicken strips in flour mixture, then egg wash. Let excess egg drip off and roll in breadcrumbs. Spray both sides with oil or cooking spray.
6. Cook at 390°F/200°C for 5minutes. Spray with oil, turn over, and spray other side.
7. Cook for 3 to 5minutes more, until well done and crispy brown.
8. To serve, place 2 schnitzel strips on bottom of each hot dog bun. Top with cheese, sliced apple, and cabbage. Drizzle with coleslaw dressing and top with other half of bun.

Thai Turkey And Zucchini Meatballs

Servings: 4
Cooking Time: 12 Minutes
Ingredients:
- 1½ cups grated zucchini,
- squeezed dry in a clean kitchen towel (about 1 large zucchini)
- 3 scallions, finely chopped
- 2 cloves garlic, minced
- 1 tablespoon grated fresh ginger
- 1 tablespoon finely chopped fresh cilantro
- zest of 1 lime
- 1 teaspoon salt
- freshly ground black pepper
- 1½ pounds ground turkey (a mix of light and dark meat)
- 2 eggs, lightly beaten
- 1 cup Thai sweet chili sauce (spring roll sauce)
- lime wedges, for serving

Directions:
1. Combine the zucchini, scallions, garlic, ginger, cilantro, lime zest, salt, pepper, ground turkey and eggs in a bowl and

mix the ingredients together. Gently shape the mixture into 24 balls, about the size of golf balls.

2. Preheat the air fryer to 380°F/195°C.

3. Working in batches, air-fry the meatballs for 12 minutes, turning the meatballs over halfway through the cooking time. As soon as the meatballs have finished cooking, toss them in a bowl with the Thai sweet chili sauce to coat.

4. Serve the meatballs over rice noodles or white rice with the remaining Thai sweet chili sauce and lime wedges to squeeze over the top.

Mom's Chicken Wings

Servings:4
Cooking Time: 35 Minutes
Ingredients:
- 2 lb chicken wings, split at the joint
- 1 tbsp water
- 1 tbsp sesame oil
- 2 tbsp Dijon mustard
- ¼ tsp chili powder
- 1 tbsp tamari
- 1 tsp honey
- 1 tsp white wine vinegar

Directions:
1. Preheat air fryer to 400°F/205°C. Coat the wings with sesame oil. Place them in the frying basket and Air Fry for 16-18 minutes, tossing once or twice. Whisk the remaining ingredients in a bowl. Reserve. When ready, transfer the wings to a serving bowl. Pour the previously prepared sauce over and toss to coat. Serve immediately.

Pecan Turkey Cutlets

Servings: 4
Cooking Time: 12 Minutes
Ingredients:
- ¾ cup panko breadcrumbs
- ¼ teaspoon salt
- ¼ teaspoon pepper
- ¼ teaspoon dry mustard
- ¼ teaspoon poultry seasoning
- ½ cup pecans
- ¼ cup cornstarch
- 1 egg, beaten
- 1 pound turkey cutlets, ½-inch thick
- salt and pepper
- oil for misting or cooking spray

Directions:
1. Place the panko crumbs, ¼ teaspoon salt, ¼ teaspoon pepper, mustard, and poultry seasoning in food processor. Process until crumbs are finely crushed. Add pecans and process in short pulses just until nuts are finely chopped. Go easy so you don't overdo it!

2. Preheat air fryer to 360°F/180°C.

3. Place cornstarch in one shallow dish and beaten egg in another. Transfer coating mixture from food processor into a third shallow dish.

4. Sprinkle turkey cutlets with salt and pepper to taste.

5. Dip cutlets in cornstarch and shake off excess. Then dip in beaten egg and roll in crumbs, pressing to coat well. Spray both sides with oil or cooking spray.

6. Place 2 cutlets in air fryer basket in a single layer and cook for 12 minutes or until juices run clear.

7. Repeat step 6 to cook remaining cutlets.

Chicken Pinchos Morunos

Servings: 4

Cooking Time: 35 Minutes
Ingredients:
- 1 yellow summer squash, sliced
- 3 chicken breasts
- ¼ cup plain yogurt
- 2 tbsp olive oil
- 1 tsp sweet pimentón
- 1 tsp dried thyme
- ½ tsp sea salt
- ½ tsp garlic powder
- ½ tsp ground cumin
- 2 red bell peppers
- 3 scallions
- 16 large green olives

Directions:
1. Preheat the air fryer to 400°F/205°C. Combine yogurt, olive oil, pimentón, thyme, cumin, salt, and garlic in a bowl and add the chicken. Stir to coat. Cut the bell peppers and scallions into 1-inch pieces. Remove the chicken from the marinade; set aside the rest of the marinade. Thread the chicken, peppers, scallions, squash, and olives onto the soaked skewers. Brush the kebabs with marinade. Discard any remaining marinade. Lay the kebabs in the frying basket. Add a raised rack and put the rest of the kebabs on it. Bake for 18-23 minutes, flipping once around minute 10. Serve hot.

Buttered Chicken Thighs

Servings: 4
Cooking Time: 30 Minutes
Ingredients:
- 4 bone-in chicken thighs, skinless
- 2 tbsp butter, melted
- 1 tsp garlic powder
- 1 tsp lemon zest
- Salt and pepper to taste
- 1 lemon, sliced

Directions:
1. Preheat air fryer to 380°F/195°C. Stir the chicken thighs in the butter, lemon zest, garlic powder, and salt. Divide the chicken thighs between 4 pieces of foil and sprinkle with black pepper, and then top with slices of lemon. Bake in the air fryer for 20-22 minutes until golden. Serve.

Southern-fried Chicken Livers

Servings: 4
Cooking Time: 12 Minutes
Ingredients:
- 2 eggs
- 2 tablespoons water
- ¾ cup flour
- 1½ cups panko breadcrumbs
- ½ cup plain breadcrumbs
- 1 teaspoon salt
- ½ teaspoon black pepper
- 20 ounces chicken livers, salted to taste
- oil for misting or cooking spray

Directions:
1. Beat together eggs and water in a shallow dish. Place the flour in a separate shallow dish.

2. In the bowl of a food processor, combine the panko, plain breadcrumbs, salt, and pepper. Process until well mixed and panko crumbs are finely crushed. Place crumbs in a third shallow dish.

3. Dip livers in flour, then egg wash, and then roll in panko mixture to coat well with crumbs.

4. Spray both sides of livers with oil or cooking spray. Cooking in two batches, place livers in air fryer basket in single layer.
5. Cook at 390°F/200°C for 7minutes. Spray livers, turn over, and spray again. Cook for 5 more minutes, until done inside and coating is golden brown.
6. Repeat to cook remaining livers.

Easy Turkey Meatballs

Servings: 4
Cooking Time: 20 Minutes
Ingredients:
- 1 lb ground turkey
- ½ celery stalk, chopped
- 1 egg
- ¼ tsp red pepper flakes
- ¼ cup bread crumbs
- Salt and pepper to taste
- ½ tsp garlic powder
- ½ tsp onion powder
- ½ tsp cayenne pepper

Directions:
1. Preheat air fryer to 360°F/180°C. Add all of the ingredients to a bowl and mix well. Shape the mixture into 12 balls and arrange them on the greased frying basket. Air Fry for 10-12 minutes or until the meatballs are cooked through and browned. Serve and enjoy!

Apricot Glazed Chicken Thighs

Servings: 2
Cooking Time: 22 Minutes
Ingredients:
- 4 bone-in chicken thighs (about 2 pounds)
- olive oil
- 1 teaspoon salt
- ¼ teaspoon freshly ground black pepper
- ½ teaspoon onion powder
- ¾ cup apricot preserves 1½ tablespoons Dijon mustard
- ½ teaspoon dried thyme
- 1 teaspoon soy sauce
- fresh thyme leaves, for garnish

Directions:
1. Preheat the air fryer to 380°F/195°C.
2. Brush or spray both the air fryer basket and the chicken with the olive oil. Combine the salt, pepper and onion powder and season both sides of the chicken with the spice mixture.
3. Place the seasoned chicken thighs, skin side down in the air fryer basket. Air-fry for 10 minutes.
4. While chicken is cooking, make the glaze by combining the apricot preserves, Dijon mustard, thyme and soy sauce in a small bowl.
5. When the time is up on the air fryer, spoon half of the apricot glaze over the chicken thighs and air-fry for 2 minutes. Then flip the chicken thighs over so that the skin side is facing up and air-fry for an additional 8 minutes. Finally, spoon and spread the rest of the glaze evenly over the chicken thighs and air-fry for a final 2 minutes. Transfer the chicken to a serving platter and sprinkle the fresh thyme leaves on top.

Sesame Orange Chicken

Servings: 2
Cooking Time: 9 Minutes
Ingredients:
- 1 pound boneless, skinless chicken breasts, cut into cubes
- salt and freshly ground black pepper
- ¼ cup cornstarch
- 2 eggs, beaten
- 1½ cups panko breadcrumbs
- vegetable or peanut oil, in a spray bottle
- 12 ounces orange marmalade
- 1 tablespoon soy sauce
- 1 teaspoon minced ginger
- 2 tablespoons hoisin sauce
- 1 tablespoon sesame oil
- sesame seeds, toasted

Directions:
1. Season the chicken pieces with salt and pepper. Set up a dredging station. Put the cornstarch in a zipper-sealable plastic bag. Place the beaten eggs in a bowl and put the panko breadcrumbs in a shallow dish. Transfer the seasoned chicken to the bag with the cornstarch and shake well to completely coat the chicken on all sides. Remove the chicken from the bag, shaking off any excess cornstarch and dip the pieces into the egg. Let any excess egg drip from the chicken and transfer into the breadcrumbs, pressing the crumbs onto the chicken pieces with your hands. Spray the chicken pieces with vegetable or peanut oil.
2. Preheat the air fryer to 400°F/205°C.
3. Combine the orange marmalade, soy sauce, ginger, hoisin sauce and sesame oil in a saucepan. Bring the mixture to a boil on the stovetop, lower the heat and simmer for 10 minutes, until the sauce has thickened. Set aside and keep warm.
4. Transfer the coated chicken to the air fryer basket and air-fry at 400°F/205°C for 9 minutes, shaking the basket a few times during the cooking process to help the chicken cook evenly.
5. Right before serving, toss the browned chicken pieces with the sesame orange sauce. Serve over white rice with steamed broccoli. Sprinkle the sesame seeds on top.

Windsor´s Chicken Salad

Servings:4
Cooking Time: 30 Minutes
Ingredients:
- ½ cup halved seedless red grapes
- 2 chicken breasts, cubed
- Salt and pepper to taste
- ¾ cup mayonnaise
- 1 tbsp lemon juice
- 2 tbsp chopped parsley
- ½ cup chopped celery
- 1 shallot, diced

Directions:
1. Preheat air fryer to 350ºF/175°C. Sprinkle chicken with salt and pepper. Place the chicken cubes in the frying basket and Air Fry for 9 minutes, flipping once. In a salad bowl, combine the cooked chicken, mayonnaise, lemon juice, parsley, grapes, celery, and shallot and let chill covered in the fridge for 1 hour up to overnight.

Fiery Chicken Meatballs

Servings: 4
Cooking Time: 20 Minutes + Chilling Time
Ingredients:
- 2 jalapeños, seeded and diced
- 2 tbsp shredded Cheddar cheese
- 1 tsp Quick Pickled Jalapeños
- 2 tbsp white wine vinegar
- ½ tsp granulated sugar

- Salt and pepper to taste
- 1 tbsp ricotta cheese
- ¾ lb ground chicken
- ¼ tsp smoked paprika
- 1 tsp garlic powder
- 1 cup bread crumbs
- ¼ tsp salt

Directions:
1. Combine the jalapeños, white wine vinegar, sugar, black pepper, and salt in a bowl. Let sit the jalapeño mixture in the fridge for 15 minutes. In a bowl, combine ricotta cheese, cheddar cheese, and 1 tsp of the jalapeños. Form mixture into 8 balls. Mix the ground chicken, smoked paprika, garlic powder, and salt in a bowl. Form mixture into 8 meatballs. Form a hole in the chicken meatballs, press a cheese ball into the hole and form chicken around the cheese ball, sealing the cheese ball in meatballs.
2. Preheat air fryer at 350°F/175°C. Mix the breadcrumbs and salt in a bowl. Roll stuffed meatballs in the mixture. Place the meatballs in the greased frying basket. Air Fry for 10 minutes, turning once. Serve immediately.

Teriyaki Chicken Bites

Servings:4
Cooking Time: 30 Minutes
Ingredients:
- 1 lb boneless, skinless chicken thighs, cubed
- 1 green onion, sliced diagonally
- 1 large egg
- 1 tbsp teriyaki sauce
- 4 tbsp flour
- 1 tsp sesame oil
- 2 tsp balsamic vinegar
- 2 tbsp tamari
- 3 cloves garlic, minced
- 2 tsp grated fresh ginger
- 2 tsp chili garlic sauce
- 2 tsp granular honey
- Salt and pepper to taste

Directions:
1. Preheat air fryer to 400°F/205°C. Beat the egg, teriyaki sauce, and flour in a bowl. Stir in chicken pieces until fully coated. In another bowl, combine the remaining ingredients, except for the green onion. Reserve. Place chicken pieces in the frying basket lightly greased with olive oil and Air Fry for 15 minutes, tossing every 5 minutes. Remove them to the bowl with the sauce and toss to coat. Scatter with green onions to serve. Enjoy!

Sticky Drumsticks

Servings: 4
Cooking Time: 45 Minutes
Ingredients:
- 1 lb chicken drumsticks
- 1 tbsp chicken seasoning
- 1 tsp dried chili flakes
- Salt and pepper to taste
- ¼ cup honey
- 1 cup barbecue sauce

Directions:
1. Preheat air fryer to 390°F/200°C. Season drumsticks with chicken seasoning, chili flakes, salt, and pepper. Place one batch of drumsticks in the greased frying basket and Air Fry for 18-20 minutes, flipping once until golden.

2. While the chicken is cooking, combine honey and barbecue sauce in a small bowl. Remove the drumsticks to a serving dish. Drizzle honey-barbecue sauce over and serve.

Turkey-hummus Wraps

Servings: 4
Cooking Time: 7 Minutes Per Batch
Ingredients:
- 4 large whole wheat wraps
- ½ cup hummus
- 16 thin slices deli turkey
- 8 slices provolone cheese
- 1 cup fresh baby spinach (or more to taste)

Directions:
1. To assemble, place 2 tablespoons of hummus on each wrap and spread to within about a half inch from edges. Top with 4 slices of turkey and 2 slices of provolone. Finish with ¼ cup of baby spinach—or pile on as much as you like.
2. Roll up each wrap. You don't need to fold or seal the ends.
3. Place 2 wraps in air fryer basket, seam side down.
4. Cook at 360°F/180°C for 4minutes to warm filling and melt cheese. If you like, you can continue cooking for 3 more minutes, until the wrap is slightly crispy.
5. Repeat step 4 to cook remaining wraps.

Classic Chicken Cobb Salad

Servings:4
Cooking Time: 30 Minutes
Ingredients:
- 4 oz cooked bacon, crumbled
- 2 chicken breasts, cubed
- 1 tbsp sesame oil
- Salt and pepper to taste
- 4 cups torn romaine lettuce
- 2 tbsp olive oil
- 1 tbsp white wine vinegar
- 2 hard-boiled eggs, sliced
- 2 tomatoes, diced
- 6 radishes, finely sliced
- ¼ cup blue cheese crumbles
- ¼ cup diced red onions
- 1 avocado, diced

Directions:
1. Preheat air fryer to 350°F/175°C. Combine chicken cubes, sesame oil, salt, and black pepper in a bowl. Place chicken cubes in the frying basket and Air Fry for 9 minutes, flipping once. Reserve. In a bowl, combine the lettuce, olive oil, and vinegar. Divide between 4 bowls. Add in the cooked chicken, hard-boiled egg slices, bacon, tomato cubes, radishes, blue cheese, onion, and avocado cubes. Serve.

Farmer's Fried Chicken

Servings: 4
Cooking Time: 55 Minutes
Ingredients:
- 3 lb whole chicken, cut into breasts, drumsticks, and thighs
- 2 cups flour
- 4 tsp salt
- 4 tsp dried basil
- 4 tsp dried thyme
- 2 tsp dried shallot powder
- 2 tsp smoked paprika
- 1 tsp mustard powder
- 1 tsp celery salt

- 1 cup kefir
- ¼ cup honey

Directions:
1. Preheat the air fryer to 370°F/185°C. Combine the flour, salt, basil, thyme, shallot, paprika, mustard powder, and celery salt in a bowl. Pour into a glass jar. Mix the kefir and honey in a large bowl and add the chicken, stir to coat. Marinate for 15 minutes at room temperature. Remove the chicken from the kefir mixture; discard the rest. Put 2/3 cup of the flour mix onto a plate and dip the chicken. Shake gently and put on a wire rack for 10 minutes. Line the frying basket with round parchment paper with holes punched in it. Place the chicken in a single layer and spray with cooking oil. Air Fry for 18-25 minutes, flipping once around minute 10. Serve hot.

Basic Chicken Breasts(1)

Servings: 4
Cooking Time: 15 Minutes
Ingredients:
- 2 tsp olive oil
- 4 chicken breasts
- Salt and pepper to taste
- 1 tbsp Italian seasoning

Directions:
1. Preheat air fryer at 350ºF/175°C. Rub olive oil over chicken breasts and sprinkle with salt, Italian seasoning and black pepper. Place them in the frying basket and Air Fry for 8-10 minutes. Let rest for 5 minutes before cutting. Store it covered in the fridge for up to 1 week.

Cornflake Chicken Nuggets

Servings: 4
Cooking Time: 25 Minutes
Ingredients:
- 1 egg white
- 1 tbsp lemon juice
- ½ tsp dried basil
- ½ tsp ground paprika
- 1 lb chicken breast fingers
- ½ cup ground cornflakes
- 2 slices bread, crumbled

Directions:
1. Preheat air fryer to 400°F/205°C. Whisk the egg white, lemon juice, basil, and paprika, then add the chicken and stir. Combine the cornflakes and breadcrumbs on a plate, then put the chicken fingers in the mix to coat. Put the nuggets in the frying basket and Air Fry for 10-13 minutes, turning halfway through, until golden, crisp and cooked through. Serve hot!

Thai Chicken Drumsticks

Servings: 4
Cooking Time: 20 Minutes
Ingredients:
- 2 tablespoons soy sauce
- ¼ cup rice wine vinegar
- 2 tablespoons chili garlic sauce
- 2 tablespoons sesame oil
- 1 teaspoon minced fresh ginger
- 2 teaspoons sugar
- ½ teaspoon ground coriander
- juice of 1 lime
- 8 chicken drumsticks (about 2½ pounds)
- ¼ cup chopped peanuts
- chopped fresh cilantro
- lime wedges

Directions:
1. Combine the soy sauce, rice wine vinegar, chili sauce, sesame oil, ginger, sugar, coriander and lime juice in a large bowl and mix together. Add the chicken drumsticks and marinate for 30 minutes.
2. Preheat the air fryer to 370°F/185°C.
3. Place the chicken in the air fryer basket. It's ok if the ends of the drumsticks overlap a little. Spoon half of the marinade over the chicken, and reserve the other half.
4. Air-fry for 10 minutes. Turn the chicken over and pour the rest of the marinade over the chicken. Air-fry for an additional 10 minutes.
5. Transfer the chicken to a plate to rest and cool to an edible temperature. Pour the marinade from the bottom of the air fryer into a small saucepan and bring it to a simmer over medium-high heat. Simmer the liquid for 2 minutes so that it thickens enough to coat the back of a spoon.
6. Transfer the chicken to a serving platter, pour the sauce over the chicken and sprinkle the chopped peanuts on top. Garnish with chopped cilantro and lime wedges.

Pickle Brined Fried Chicken

Servings: 4
Cooking Time: 47 Minutes
Ingredients:
- 4 bone-in, skin-on chicken legs, cut into drumsticks and thighs (about 3½ pounds)
- pickle juice from a 24-ounce jar of kosher dill pickles
- ½ cup flour
- salt and freshly ground black pepper
- 2 eggs
- 1 cup fine breadcrumbs
- 1 teaspoon salt
- 1 teaspoon freshly ground black pepper
- ½ teaspoon ground paprika
- ⅛ teaspoon ground cayenne pepper
- vegetable or canola oil in a spray bottle

Directions:
1. Place the chicken in a shallow dish and pour the pickle juice over the top. Cover and transfer the chicken to the refrigerator to brine in the pickle juice for 3 to 8 hours.
2. When you are ready to cook, remove the chicken from the refrigerator to let it come to room temperature while you set up a dredging station. Place the flour in a shallow dish and season well with salt and freshly ground black pepper. Whisk the eggs in a second shallow dish. In a third shallow dish, combine the breadcrumbs, salt, pepper, paprika and cayenne pepper.
3. Preheat the air fryer to 370°F/185°C.
4. Remove the chicken from the pickle brine and gently dry it with a clean kitchen towel. Dredge each piece of chicken in the flour, then dip it into the egg mixture, and finally press it into the breadcrumb mixture to coat all sides of the chicken. Place the breaded chicken on a plate or baking sheet and spray each piece all over with vegetable oil.
5. Air-fry the chicken in two batches. Place two chicken thighs and two drumsticks into the air fryer basket. Air-fry for 10 minutes. Then, gently turn the chicken pieces over and air-fry for another 10 minutes. Remove the chicken pieces and let them rest on plate – do not cover. Repeat with the second batch of chicken, air-frying for 20 minutes, turning the chicken over halfway through.
6. Lower the temperature of the air fryer to 340°F. Place the first batch of chicken on top of the second batch already in the basket and air-fry for an additional 7 minutes. Serve warm and enjoy.

Tortilla Crusted Chicken Breast

Servings: 2
Cooking Time: 12 Minutes
Ingredients:
- ⅓ cup flour
- 1 teaspoon salt
- 1½ teaspoons chili powder
- 1 teaspoon ground cumin
- freshly ground black pepper
- 1 egg, beaten
- ¾ cup coarsely crushed yellow corn tortilla chips
- 2 (3- to 4-ounce) boneless chicken breasts
- vegetable oil
- ½ cup salsa
- ½ cup crumbled queso fresco
- fresh cilantro leaves
- sour cream or guacamole (optional)

Directions:
1. Set up a dredging station with three shallow dishes. Combine the flour, salt, chili powder, cumin and black pepper in the first shallow dish. Beat the egg in the second shallow dish. Place the crushed tortilla chips in the third shallow dish.
2. Dredge the chicken in the spiced flour, covering all sides of the breast. Then dip the chicken into the egg, coating the chicken completely. Finally, place the chicken into the tortilla chips and press the chips onto the chicken to make sure they adhere to all sides of the breast. Spray the coated chicken breasts on both sides with vegetable oil.
3. Preheat the air fryer to 380°F/195°C.
4. Air-fry the chicken for 6 minutes. Then turn the chicken breasts over and air-fry for another 6 minutes. (Increase the cooking time if you are using chicken breasts larger than 3 to 4 ounces.)
5. When the chicken has finished cooking, serve each breast with a little salsa, the crumbled queso fresco and cilantro as the finishing touch. Serve some sour cream and/or guacamole at the table, if desired.

Maewoon Chicken Legs

Servings: 4
Cooking Time: 30 Minutes + Chilling Time
Ingredients:
- 4 scallions, sliced, whites and greens separated
- ¼ cup tamari
- 2 tbsp sesame oil
- 1 tsp sesame seeds
- ¼ cup honey
- 2 tbsp gochujang
- 2 tbsp ketchup
- 4 cloves garlic, minced
- ½ tsp ground ginger
- Salt and pepper to taste
- 1 tbsp parsley
- 1 ½ lb chicken legs

Directions:
1. Whisk all ingredients, except chicken and scallion greens, in a bowl. Reserve ¼ cup of marinade. Toss chicken legs in the remaining marinade and chill for 30 minutes.
2. Preheat air fryer at 400°F/205°C. Place chicken legs in the greased frying basket and Air Fry for 10 minutes. Turn chicken. Cook for 8 more minutes. Let sit in a serving dish for 5 minutes. Coat the cooked chicken with the reserved marinade and scatter with scallion greens, sesame seeds and parsley to serve.

Fantasy Sweet Chili Chicken Strips

Servings: 2
Cooking Time: 20 Minutes
Ingredients:
- 1 lb chicken strips
- 1 cup sweet chili sauce
- ½ cup bread crumbs
- ½ cup cornmeal

Directions:
1. Preheat air fryer at 350°F/175°C. Combine chicken strips and sweet chili sauce in a bowl until fully coated. In another bowl, mix the remaining ingredients. Dredge strips in the mixture. Shake off any excess. Place chicken strips in the greased frying basket and Air Fry for 10 minutes, tossing once. Serve right away.

Turkey Tenderloin With A Lemon Touch

Servings: 4
Cooking Time: 45 Minutes
Ingredients:
- 1 lb boneless, skinless turkey breast tenderloin
- Salt and pepper to taste
- ½ tsp garlic powder
- ½ tsp chili powder
- ½ tsp dried thyme
- 1 lemon, juiced
- 1 tbsp chopped cilantro

Directions:
1. Preheat air fryer to 350°F/175°C. Dry the turkey completely with a paper towel, then season with salt, pepper, garlic powder, chili powder, and thyme. Place the turkey in the frying basket. Squeeze the lemon juice over the turkey and bake for 10 minutes. Turn the turkey and bake for another 10 to 15 minutes. Allow to rest for 10 minutes before slicing. Serve sprinkled with cilantro and enjoy.

Chicken Fried Steak With Gravy

Servings: 4
Cooking Time: 10 Minutes Per Batch
Ingredients:
- ½ cup flour
- 2 teaspoons salt, divided
- freshly ground black pepper
- ¼ teaspoon garlic powder
- 1 cup buttermilk
- 1 cup fine breadcrumbs
- 4 tenderized top round steaks (about 6 to 8 ounces each; ½-inch thick)
- vegetable or canola oil
- For the Gravy:
- 2 tablespoons butter or bacon drippings
- ¼ onion, minced (about ¼ cup)
- 1 clove garlic, smashed
- ¼ teaspoon dried thyme
- 3 tablespoons flour
- 1 cup milk
- salt and lots of freshly ground black pepper
- a few dashes of Worcestershire sauce

Directions:
1. Set up a dredging station. Combine the flour, 1 teaspoon of salt, black pepper and garlic powder in a shallow bowl. Pour the buttermilk into a second shallow bowl. Finally, put the breadcrumbs and 1 teaspoon of salt in a third shallow bowl.

2. Dip the tenderized steaks into the flour, then the buttermilk, and then the breadcrumb mixture, pressing the crumbs onto the steak. Place them on a baking sheet and spray both sides generously with vegetable or canola oil.
3. Preheat the air fryer to 400°F/205°C.
4. Transfer the steaks to the air fryer basket, two at a time, and air-fry for 10 minutes, flipping the steaks over halfway through the cooking time. This will cook your steaks to medium. If you want the steaks cooked a little more or less, add or subtract a minute or two. Hold the first batch of steaks warm in a 170°F/75°C oven while you cook the second batch.
5. While the steaks are cooking, make the gravy. Melt the butter in a small saucepan over medium heat on the stovetop. Add the onion, garlic and thyme and cook for five minutes, until the onion is soft and just starting to brown. Stir in the flour and cook for another five minutes, stirring regularly, until the mixture starts to brown. Whisk in the milk and bring the mixture to a boil to thicken. Season to taste with salt, lots of freshly ground black pepper and a few dashes of Worcestershire sauce.
6. Plate the chicken fried steaks with mashed potatoes and vegetables and serve the gravy at the table to pour over the top.

Restaurant-style Chicken Thighs

Servings: 4
Cooking Time: 30 Minutes
Ingredients:
- 1 lb boneless, skinless chicken thighs
- ¼ cup barbecue sauce
- 2 cloves garlic, minced
- 1 tsp lemon zest
- 2 tbsp parsley, chopped
- 2 tbsp lemon juice

Directions:
1. Coat the chicken with barbecue sauce, garlic, and lemon juice in a medium bowl. leave to marinate for 10 minutes.
2. Preheat air fryer to 380°F/195°C. When ready to cook, remove the chicken from the bowl and shake off any drips. Arrange the chicken in the air fryer and Bake for 16-18 minutes, until golden and cooked through. Serve topped with lemon zest and parsley. Enjoy!

Simple Salsa Chicken Thighs

Servings:2
Cooking Time: 35 Minutes
Ingredients:
- 1 lb boneless, skinless chicken thighs
- 1 cup mild chunky salsa
- ½ tsp taco seasoning
- 2 lime wedges for serving

Directions:
1. Preheat air fryer to 350°F/175°C. Add chicken thighs into a baking pan and pour salsa and taco seasoning over. Place the pan in the frying basket and Air Fry for 30 minutes until golden brown. Serve with lime wedges.

Cajun Fried Chicken

Servings: 3
Cooking Time: 35 Minutes
Ingredients:
- 1 cup Cajun seasoning
- ½ tsp mango powder
- 6 chicken legs, bone-in

Directions:
1. Preheat air fryer to 360°F/180°C. Place half of the Cajun seasoning and 3/4 cup of water in a bowl and mix well to dissolve any lumps. Add the remaining Cajun seasoning and mango powder to a shallow bowl and stir to combine. Dip the chicken in the batter, then coat it in the mango seasoning. Lightly spritz the chicken with cooking spray. Place the chicken in the air fryer and Air Fry for 14-16 minutes, turning once until the chicken is cooked and the coating is brown. Serve and enjoy!

Chicken Wings Al Ajillo

Servings:4
Cooking Time: 35 Minutes
Ingredients:
- 2 lb chicken wings, split at the joint
- 2 tbsp melted butter
- 2 tbsp grated Cotija cheese
- 4 cloves garlic, minced
- ½ tbsp hot paprika
- ¼ tsp salt

Directions:
1. Preheat air fryer to 250ºF/120°C. Coat the chicken wings with 1 tbsp of butter. Place them in the basket and Air Fry for 12 minutes, tossing once. In another bowl, whisk 1 tbsp of butter, Cotija cheese, garlic, hot paprika, and salt. Reserve. Increase temperature to 400°F/205°C. Air Fry wings for 10 more minutes, tossing twice. Transfer them to the bowl with the sauce, and toss to coat. Serve immediately.

Italian-inspired Chicken Pizzadillas

Servings: 4
Cooking Time: 25 Minutes
Ingredients:
- 2 cups cooked boneless, skinless chicken, shredded
- 1 cup grated provolone cheese
- 8 basil and menta leaves, julienned
- ½ tsp salt
- 1 tsp garlic powder
- 3 tbsp butter, melted
- 8 flour tortillas
- 1 cup marinara sauce
- 1 cup grated cheddar cheese

Directions:
1. Preheat air fryer at 350ºF/175°C. Sprinkle chicken with salt and garlic powder. Brush on one side of a tortilla lightly with melted butter. Spread ¼ cup of marinara sauce, then top with ½ cup of chicken, ¼ cup of cheddar cheese, ¼ cup of provolone, and finally, ¼ of basil and menta leaves. Top with a second tortilla and lightly brush with butter on top. Repeat with the remaining ingredients. Place quesadillas, butter side down, in the frying basket and Bake for 3 minutes. Cut them into 6 sections and serve.

Asian Sweet Chili Chicken

Servings: 4
Cooking Time: 30 Minutes
Ingredients:
- 2 chicken breasts, cut into 1-inch pieces
- 1 cup cornstarch
- 1 tsp chicken seasoning
- Salt and pepper to taste
- 2 eggs
- 1 ½ cups sweet chili sauce

Directions:
1. Preheat air fryer to 360°F/180°C. Mix cornstarch, chicken seasoning, salt and pepper in a large bowl. In another bowl, beat the eggs. Dip the chicken in the cornstarch

mixture to coat. Next, dip the chicken into the egg, then return to the cornstarch. Transfer chicken to the air fryer.

2.   Lightly spray all of the chicken with cooking oil. Air Fry for 15-16 minutes, shaking the basket once or until golden. Transfer chicken to a serving dish and drizzle with sweet-and-sour sauce. Serve immediately.

Chicken Parmigiana

Servings: 2
Cooking Time: 35 Minutes
Ingredients:
- 2 chicken breasts
- 1 cup breadcrumbs
- 2 eggs, beaten
- Salt and pepper to taste
- 1 tbsp dried basil
- 1 cup passata
- 2 provolone cheese slices
- 1 tbsp Parmesan cheese

Directions:
1.   Preheat air fryer to 350°F/175°C. Mix the breadcrumbs, basil, salt, and pepper in a mixing bowl. Coat the chicken breasts with the crumb mixture, then dip in the beaten eggs. Finally, coat again with the dry ingredients. Arrange the coated chicken breasts on the greased frying basket and Air Fry for 20 minutes. At the 10-minutes mark, turn the breasts over and cook for the remaining 10 minutes.

2.   Pour half of the passata into a baking pan. When the chicken is ready, remove it to the passata-covered pan. Pour the remaining passata over the fried chicken and arrange the provolone cheese slices on top and sprinkle with Parmesan cheese. Bake for 5 minutes until the chicken is crisped and the cheese melted and lightly toasted. Serve.

Asian-style Orange Chicken

Servings: 4
Cooking Time: 25 Minutes
Ingredients:
- 1 lb chicken breasts, cubed
- Salt and pepper to taste
- 6 tbsp cornstarch
- 1 cup orange juice
- ¼ cup orange marmalade
- ¼ cup ketchup
- ½ tsp ground ginger
- 2 tbsp soy sauce
- 1 1/3 cups edamame beans

Directions:
1.   Preheat the air fryer to 375°F/190°C. Sprinkle the cubes with salt and pepper. Coat with 4 tbsp of cornstarch and set aside on a wire rack. Mix the orange juice, marmalade, ketchup, ginger, soy sauce, and the remaining cornstarch in a cake pan, then stir in the beans. Set the pan in the frying basket and Bake for 5-8 minutes, stirring once during cooking until the sauce is thick and bubbling. Remove from the fryer and set aside. Put the chicken in the frying basket and fry for 10-12 minutes, shaking the basket once. Stir the chicken into the sauce and beans in the pan. Return to the fryer and reheat for 2 minutes.

Goat Cheese Stuffed Turkey Roulade

Servings: 4
Cooking Time: 55 Minutes
Ingredients:
- 1 boneless turkey breast, skinless
- Salt and pepper to taste
- 4 oz goat cheese

- 1 tbsp marjoram
- 1 tbsp sage
- 2 garlic cloves, minced
- 2 tbsp olive oil
- 2 tbsp chopped cilantro

Directions:
1.   Preheat air fryer to 380°F/195°C. Butterfly the turkey breast with a sharp knife and season with salt and pepper. Mix together the goat cheese, marjoram, sage, and garlic in a bowl. Spread the cheese mixture over the turkey breast, then roll it up tightly, tucking the ends underneath.

2.   Put the turkey breast roulade onto a piece of aluminum foil, wrap it up, and place it into the air fryer. Bake for 30 minutes. Turn the turkey breast, brush the top with oil, and then continue to cook for another 10-15 minutes. Slice and serve sprinkled with cilantro.

Chicken Chunks

Servings: 4
Cooking Time: 10 Minutes
Ingredients:
- 1 pound chicken tenders cut in large chunks, about 1½ inches
- salt and pepper
- ½ cup cornstarch
- 2 eggs, beaten
- 1 cup panko breadcrumbs
- oil for misting or cooking spray

Directions:
1.   Season chicken chunks to your liking with salt and pepper.
2.   Dip chicken chunks in cornstarch. Then dip in egg and shake off excess. Then roll in panko crumbs to coat well.
3.   Spray all sides of chicken chunks with oil or cooking spray.
4.   Place chicken in air fryer basket in single layer and cook at 390°F/200°C for 5minutes. Spray with oil, turn chunks over, and spray other side.
5.   Cook for an additional 5minutes or until chicken juices run clear and outside is golden brown.
6.   Repeat steps 4 and 5 to cook remaining chicken.

Jerk Turkey Meatballs

Servings: 7
Cooking Time: 8 Minutes
Ingredients:
- 1 pound lean ground turkey
- ¼ cup chopped onion
- 1 teaspoon minced garlic
- ½ teaspoon dried thyme
- ¼ teaspoon ground cinnamon
- 1 teaspoon cayenne pepper
- ½ teaspoon paprika
- ½ teaspoon salt
- ⅛ teaspoon black pepper
- ¼ teaspoon red pepper flakes
- 2 teaspoons brown sugar
- 1 large egg, whisked
- ⅓ cup panko breadcrumbs
- 2⅓ cups cooked brown Jasmine rice
- 2 green onions, chopped
- ¾ cup sweet onion dressing

Directions:
1.   Preheat the air fryer to 350°F/175°C.
2.   In a medium bowl, mix the ground turkey with the onion, garlic, thyme, cinnamon, cayenne pepper, paprika, salt, pepper, red pepper flakes, and brown sugar. Add the whisked

egg and stir in the breadcrumbs until the turkey starts to hold together.

3. Using a 1-ounce scoop, portion the turkey into meatballs. You should get about 28 meatballs.

4. Spray the air fryer basket with olive oil spray.

5. Place the meatballs into the air fryer basket and cook for 5 minutes, shake the basket, and cook another 2 to 4 minutes (or until the internal temperature of the meatballs reaches 165°F/75°C).

6. Remove the meatballs from the basket and repeat for the remaining meatballs.

7. Serve warm over a bed of rice with chopped green onions and spicy Caribbean jerk dressing.

Turkey Scotch Eggs

Servings: 4
Cooking Time: 30 Minutes
Ingredients:
- 1 ½ lb ground turkey
- 1 tbsp ground cumin
- 1 tsp ground coriander
- 2 garlic cloves, minced
- 3 raw eggs
- 1 ½ cups bread crumbs
- 6 hard-cooked eggs, peeled
- ½ cup flour

Directions:
1. Preheat air fryer to 370°F/185°C. Place the ground turkey, cumin, coriander, garlic, one egg, and ½ cup of bread crumbs in a large bowl and mix until well incorporated.

2. Divide into 6 equal portions, then flatten each into long ovals. Set aside. In a shallow bowl, beat the remaining raw eggs. In another shallow bowl, add flour. Do the same with another plate for bread crumbs. Roll each cooked egg in flour, then wrap with one oval of chicken sausage until completely covered.

3. Roll again in flour, then coat in the beaten egg before rolling in bread crumbs. Arrange the eggs in the greased frying basket. Air Fry for 12-14 minutes, flipping once until the sausage is cooked and the eggs are brown. Serve.

Basic Chicken Breasts(2)

Servings:4
Cooking Time: 15 Minutes
Ingredients:
- 2 tsp olive oil
- 2 chicken breasts
- Salt and pepper to taste
- ½ tsp garlic powder
- ½ tsp rosemary

Directions:
1. Preheat air fryer to 350°F/175°C. Rub the chicken breasts with olive oil over tops and bottom and sprinkle with garlic powder, rosemary, salt, and pepper. Place the chicken in the frying basket and Air Fry for 9 minutes, flipping once. Let rest onto a serving plate for 5 minutes before cutting into cubes. Serve and enjoy!

Chicken Meatballs With A Surprise

Servings:4
Cooking Time: 35 Minutes
Ingredients:
- 1/3 cup cottage cheese crumbles
- 1 lb ground chicken
- ½ tsp onion powder
- ¼ cup chopped basil
- ½ cup bread crumbs
- ½ tsp garlic powder

Directions:
1. Preheat air fryer to 350ºF/175°C. Combine the ground chicken, onion, basil, cottage cheese, bread crumbs, and garlic powder in a bowl. Form into 18 meatballs, about 2 tbsp each. Place the chicken meatballs in the greased frying basket and Air Fry for 12 minutes, shaking once. Serve.

Sweet Chili Spiced Chicken

Servings: 4
Cooking Time: 43 Minutes
Ingredients:
- Spice Rub:
- 2 tablespoons brown sugar
- 2 tablespoons paprika
- 1 teaspoon dry mustard powder
- 1 teaspoon chili powder
- 2 tablespoons coarse sea salt or kosher salt
- 2 teaspoons coarsely ground black pepper
- 1 tablespoon vegetable oil
- 1 (3½-pound) chicken, cut into 8 pieces

Directions:
1. Prepare the spice rub by combining the brown sugar, paprika, mustard powder, chili powder, salt and pepper. Rub the oil all over the chicken pieces and then rub the spice mix onto the chicken, covering completely. This is done very easily in a zipper sealable bag. You can do this ahead of time and let the chicken marinate in the refrigerator, or just proceed with cooking right away.

2. Preheat the air fryer to 370°F/185°C.

3. Air-fry the chicken in two batches. Place the two chicken thighs and two drumsticks into the air fryer basket. Air-fry at 370°F for 10 minutes. Then, gently turn the chicken pieces over and air-fry for another 10 minutes. Remove the chicken pieces and let them rest on a plate while you cook the chicken breasts. Air-fry the chicken breasts, skin side down for 8 minutes. Turn the chicken breasts over and air-fry for another 12 minutes.

4. Lower the temperature of the air fryer to 340°F/170°C. Place the first batch of chicken on top of the second batch already in the basket and air-fry for a final 3 minutes.

5. Let the chicken rest for 5 minutes and serve warm with some mashed potatoes and a green salad or vegetables.

Fennel & Chicken Ratatouille

Servings:4
Cooking Time: 30 Minutes
Ingredients:
- 1 lb boneless, skinless chicken thighs, cubed
- 2 tbsp grated Parmesan cheese
- 1 eggplant, cubed
- 1 zucchini, cubed
- 1 bell pepper, diced
- 1 fennel bulb, sliced
- 1 tsp salt
- 1 tsp Italian seasoning
- 2 tbsp olive oil
- 1 can diced tomatoes
- 1 tsp pasta sauce
- 2 tbsp basil leaves

Directions:
1. Preheat air fryer to 400ºF/205°C. Mix the chicken, eggplant, zucchini, bell pepper, fennel, salt, Italian seasoning, and oil in a bowl. Place the chicken mixture in the frying basket and Air Fry for 7 minutes. Transfer it to a cake pan. Mix in tomatoes along with juices and pasta sauce. Air Fry for 8 minutes. Scatter with Parmesan and basil.Serve.

Spiced Mexican Stir-fried Chicken

Servings: 4
Cooking Time: 30 Minutes
Ingredients:
- 1 lb chicken breasts, cubed
- 2 green onions, chopped
- 1 red bell pepper, chopped
- 1 jalapeño pepper, minced
- 2 tsp olive oil
- 2/3 cup canned black beans
- ½ cup salsa
- 2 tsp Mexican chili powder

Directions:
1. Preheat air fryer to 400°F/2055°C. Combine the chicken, green onions, bell pepper, jalapeño, and olive oil in a bowl. Transfer to a bowl to the frying basket and Air Fry for 10 minutes, stirring once during cooking. When done, stir in the black beans, salsa, and chili powder. Air Fry for 7-10 minutes or until cooked through. Serve.

Buttermilk-fried Drumsticks

Servings: 2
Cooking Time: 25 Minutes
Ingredients:
- 1 egg
- ½ cup buttermilk
- ¾ cup self-rising flour
- ¾ cup seasoned panko breadcrumbs
- 1 teaspoon salt
- ¼ teaspoon ground black pepper (to mix into coating)
- 4 chicken drumsticks, skin on
- oil for misting or cooking spray

Directions:
1. Beat together egg and buttermilk in shallow dish.
2. In a second shallow dish, combine the flour, panko crumbs, salt, and pepper.
3. Sprinkle chicken legs with additional salt and pepper to taste.
4. Dip legs in buttermilk mixture, then roll in panko mixture, pressing in crumbs to make coating stick. Mist with oil or cooking spray.
5. Spray air fryer basket with cooking spray.
6. Cook drumsticks at 360°F/180°C for 10minutes. Turn pieces over and cook an additional 10minutes.
7. Turn pieces to check for browning. If you have any white spots that haven't begun to brown, spritz them with oil or cooking spray. Continue cooking for 5 more minutes or until crust is golden brown and juices run clear. Larger, meatier drumsticks will take longer to cook than small ones.

Chicken Pigs In Blankets

Servings: 4
Cooking Time: 40 Minutes
Ingredients:
- 8 chicken drumsticks, boneless, skinless
- 2 tbsp light brown sugar
- 2 tbsp ketchup
- 1 tbsp grainy mustard
- 8 smoked bacon slices
- 1 tsp chopped fresh sage

Directions:
1. Preheat the air fryer to 350°F/175°C. Mix brown sugar, sage, ketchup, and mustard in a bowl and brush the chicken with it. Wrap slices of bacon around the drumsticks and brush with the remaining mix. Line the frying basket with round parchment paper with holes. Set 4 drumsticks on the paper, add a raised rack and set the other drumsticks on it. Bake for 25-35 minutes, moving the bottom drumsticks to the top, top to the bottom, and flipping at about 14-16 minutes. Sprinkle with sage and serve.

Parmesan Chicken Fingers

Servings: 2
Cooking Time: 19 Minutes
Ingredients:
- ½ cup flour
- 1 teaspoon salt
- freshly ground black pepper
- 2 eggs, beaten
- ¾ cup seasoned panko breadcrumbs
- ¾ cup grated Parmesan cheese
- 8 chicken tenders (about 1 pound)
- OR
- 2 to 3 boneless, skinless chicken breasts, cut into strips
- vegetable oil
- marinara sauce

Directions:
1. Set up a dredging station. Combine the flour, salt and pepper in a shallow dish. Place the beaten eggs in second shallow dish, and combine the panko breadcrumbs and Parmesan cheese in a third shallow dish.
2. Dredge the chicken tenders in the flour mixture. Then dip them into the egg, and finally place the chicken in the breadcrumb mixture. Press the coating onto both sides of the chicken tenders. Place the coated chicken tenders on a baking sheet until they are all coated. Spray both sides of the chicken fingers with vegetable oil.
3. Preheat the air fryer to 360°F/180°C.
4. Air-fry the chicken fingers in two batches. Transfer half the chicken fingers to the air fryer basket and air-fry for 9 minutes, turning the chicken over halfway through the cooking time. When the second batch of chicken fingers has finished cooking, return the first batch to the air fryer with the second batch and air-fry for one minute to heat everything through.
5. Serve immediately with marinara sauce, honey-mustard, ketchup or your favorite dipping sauce.

Intense Buffalo Chicken Wings

Servings: 2
Cooking Time: 40 Minutes
Ingredients:
- 8 chicken wings
- ½ cup melted butter
- 2 tbsp Tabasco sauce
- ½ tbsp lemon juice
- 1 tbsp Worcestershire sauce
- 2 tsp cayenne pepper
- 1 tsp garlic powder
- 1 tsp lemon zest
- Salt and pepper to taste

Directions:
1. Preheat air fryer to 350°F/175°C. Place the melted butter, Tabasco, lemon juice, Worcestershire sauce, cayenne, garlic powder, lemon zest, salt, and pepper in a bowl and stir to combine. Dip the chicken wings into the mixture, coating thoroughly. Lay the coated chicken wings on the foil-lined frying basket in an even layer. Air Fry for 16-18 minutes. Shake the basket several times during cooking until the chicken wings are crispy brown. Serve.

Pulled Turkey Quesadillas

Servings: 4
Cooking Time: 15 Minutes
Ingredients:
- ¾ cup pulled cooked turkey breast
- 6 tortilla wraps
- 1/3 cup grated Swiss cheese
- 1 small red onion, sliced
- 2 tbsp Mexican chili sauce

Directions:
1.   Preheat air fryer to 400°F/205°C. Lay 3 tortilla wraps on a clean workspace, then spoon equal amounts of Swiss cheese, turkey, Mexican chili sauce, and red onion on the tortillas. Spritz the exterior of the tortillas with cooking spray. Air Fry the quesadillas, one at a time, for 5-8 minutes. The cheese should be melted and the outsides crispy. Serve.

Hazelnut Chicken Salad With Strawberries

Servings:4
Cooking Time: 30 Minutes
Ingredients:
- 2 chicken breasts, cubed
- Salt and pepper to taste
- ¾ cup mayonnaise
- 1 tbsp lime juice
- ½ cup chopped hazelnuts
- ½ cup chopped celery
- ½ cup diced strawberries

Directions:
1.   Preheat air fryer to 350ºF/175°C. Sprinkle chicken cubes with salt and pepper. Place them in the frying basket and Air Fry for 9 minutes, shaking once. Remove to a bowl and leave it to cool. Add the mayonnaise, lime juice, hazelnuts, celery, and strawberries. Serve.

Mexican Turkey Meatloaves

Servings: 4
Cooking Time: 30 Minutes
Ingredients:
- ¼ cup jarred chunky mild salsa
- 1 lb ground turkey
- 1/3 cup bread crumbs
- 1/3 cup canned black beans
- 1/3 cup frozen corn
- ¼ cup minced onion
- ¼ cup chopped scallions
- 2 tbsp chopped cilantro
- 1 egg, beaten
- 1 tbsp tomato puree
- 1 tsp salt
- ½ tsp ground cumin
- 1 tsp Mulato chile powder
- ½ tsp ground aniseed
- ¼ tsp ground cloves
- 2 tbsp ketchup
- 2 tbsp jarred mild salsa

Directions:
1.   In a bowl, use your hands to mix the turkey, bread crumbs, beans, corn, salsa, onion, scallions, cilantro, egg, tomato puree, salt, chile powder, aniseed, cloves, and cumin. Shape into 4 patties about 1-inch in thickness.
2.   Preheat air fryer to 350°F/175°C. Put the meatloaves in the greased frying basket and Bake for about 18-20 minutes, flipping once until cooked through. Stir together the ketchup and salsa in a small bowl. When all loaves are cooked, brush them with the glaze and return to the fryer to heat up for 2 minutes. Serve immediately.

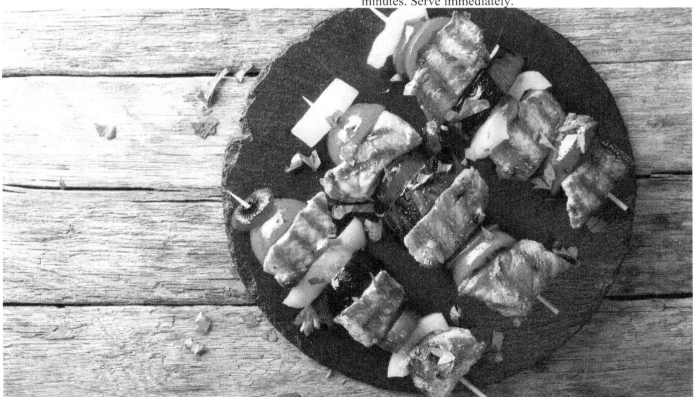

Fish And Seafood Recipes

Coconut-shrimp Po' Boys

Servings: 4
Cooking Time: 5 Minutes
Ingredients:
- ½ cup cornstarch
- 2 eggs
- 2 tablespoons milk
- ¾ cup shredded coconut
- ½ cup panko breadcrumbs
- 1 pound (31–35 count) shrimp, peeled and deveined
- Old Bay Seasoning
- oil for misting or cooking spray
- 2 large hoagie rolls
- honey mustard or light mayonnaise
- 1½ cups shredded lettuce
- 1 large tomato, thinly sliced

Directions:
1. Place cornstarch in a shallow dish or plate.
2. In another shallow dish, beat together eggs and milk.
3. In a third dish mix the coconut and panko crumbs.
4. Sprinkle shrimp with Old Bay Seasoning to taste.
5. Dip shrimp in cornstarch to coat lightly, dip in egg mixture, shake off excess, and roll in coconut mixture to coat well.
6. Spray both sides of coated shrimp with oil or cooking spray.
7. Cook half the shrimp in a single layer at 390°F/200°C for 5minutes.
8. Repeat to cook remaining shrimp.
9. To Assemble
10. Split each hoagie lengthwise, leaving one long edge intact.
11. Place in air fryer basket and cook at 390°F for 1 to 2minutes or until heated through.
12. Remove buns, break apart, and place on 4 plates, cut side up.
13. Spread with honey mustard and/or mayonnaise.
14. Top with shredded lettuce, tomato slices, and coconut shrimp.

Flounder Fillets

Servings: 4
Cooking Time: 8 Minutes
Ingredients:
- 1 egg white
- 1 tablespoon water
- 1 cup panko breadcrumbs
- 2 tablespoons extra-light virgin olive oil
- 4 4-ounce flounder fillets
- salt and pepper
- oil for misting or cooking spray

Directions:
1. Preheat air fryer to 390°F/200°C.
2. Beat together egg white and water in shallow dish.
3. In another shallow dish, mix panko crumbs and oil until well combined and crumbly (best done by hand).
4. Season flounder fillets with salt and pepper to taste. Dip each fillet into egg mixture and then roll in panko crumbs, pressing in crumbs so that fish is nicely coated.
5. Spray air fryer basket with nonstick cooking spray and add fillets. Cook at 390°F/200°C for 3minutes.
6. Spray fish fillets but do not turn. Cook 5 minutes longer or until golden brown and crispy. Using a spatula, carefully remove fish from basket and serve.

Collard Green & Cod Packets

Servings: 4
Cooking Time: 20 Minutes
Ingredients:
- 2 cups collard greens, chopped
- 1 tsp salt
- ½ tsp dried rosemary
- ½ tsp dried thyme
- ½ tsp garlic powder
- 4 cod fillets
- 1 shallot, thinly sliced
- ¼ cup olive oil
- 1 lemon, juiced

Directions:
1. Preheat air fryer to 380°F/195°C. Mix together the salt, rosemary, thyme, and garlic powder in a small bowl. Rub the spice mixture onto the cod fillets. Divide the fish fillets among 4 sheets of foil. Top with shallot slices and collard greens. Drizzle with olive oil and lemon juice. Fold and seal the sides of the foil packets and then place them into the frying basket. Steam in the fryer for 11-13 minutes until the cod is cooked through. Serve and enjoy!

Coconut Shrimp With Plum Sauce

Servings: 2
Cooking Time: 30 Minutes
Ingredients:
- ½ lb raw shrimp, peeled
- 2 eggs
- ½ cup breadcrumbs
- 1 tsp red chili powder
- 2 tbsp dried coconut flakes
- Salt and pepper to taste
- ½ cup plum sauce

Directions:
1. Preheat air fryer to 350°F/175°C. Whisk the eggs with salt and pepper in a bowl. Dip in the shrimp, fully submerging. Combine the bread crumbs, coconut flakes, chili powder, salt, and pepper in another bowl until evenly blended. Coat the shrimp in the crumb mixture and place them in the foil-lined frying basket. Air Fry for 14-16 minutes. Halfway through the cooking time, shake the basket. Serve with plum sauce for dipping and enjoy!

Salmon Patties With Lemon-dill Sauce

Servings: 4
Cooking Time: 40 Minutes
Ingredients:
- 2 tbsp diced red bell peppers

- ¼ cup sour cream
- 6 tbsp mayonnaise
- 2 cloves garlic, minced
- 2 tbsp cup onion
- 2 tbsp chopped dill
- 2 tsp lime juice
- 1 tsp honey
- 1 can salmon
- 1 egg
- ½ cup bread crumbs
- Salt and pepper to taste

Directions:
1. Mix the sour cream, 2 tbsp of mayonnaise, honey, onion, garlic, dill, lime juice, salt and pepper in a bowl. Let chill the resulting dill sauce in the fridge until ready to use.
2. Preheat air fryer at 400°F/205°C. Combine the salmon, remaining mayonnaise, egg, bell peppers, breadcrumbs, and salt in a bowl. Form mixture into patties. Place salmon cakes in the greased frying basket and Air Fry for 10 minutes, flipping once. Let rest for 5 minutes before serving with dill sauce on the side.

Herby Prawn & Zucchini Bake

Servings: 4
Cooking Time: 30 Minutes
Ingredients:
- 1 ¼ lb prawns, peeled and deveined
- 2 zucchini, sliced
- 2 tbsp butter, melted
- ½ tsp garlic salt
- 1 ½ tsp dried oregano
- ⅛ tsp red pepper flakes
- ½ lemon, juiced
- 1 tbsp chopped mint
- 1 tbsp chopped dill

Directions:
1. Preheat air fryer to 350°F/175°C. Combine prawns, zucchini, butter, garlic salt, oregano, and pepper flakes in a large bowl. Toss to coat. Put the prawns and zucchini in the greased frying basket and Air Fry for about 6-8 minutes, shaking the basket once until the zucchini is golden and the shrimp are cooked. Remove the shrimp to a serving plate and cover with foil. Serve hot topped with lemon juice, mint, and dill. Enjoy!

Maple-crusted Salmon

Servings: 2
Cooking Time: 8 Minutes
Ingredients:
- 12 ounces salmon filets
- ⅓ cup maple syrup
- 1 teaspoon Worcestershire sauce
- 2 teaspoons Dijon mustard or brown mustard
- ½ cup finely chopped walnuts
- ½ teaspoon sea salt
- ½ lemon
- 1 tablespoon chopped parsley, for garnish

Directions:
1. Place the salmon in a shallow baking dish. Top with maple syrup, Worcestershire sauce, and mustard. Refrigerate for 30 minutes.
2. Preheat the air fryer to 350°F/175°C.
3. Remove the salmon from the marinade and discard the marinade.
4. Place the chopped nuts on top of the salmon filets, and sprinkle salt on top of the nuts. Place the salmon, skin side down, in the air fryer basket. Cook for 6 to 8 minutes or until the fish flakes in the center.
5. Remove the salmon and plate on a serving platter. Squeeze fresh lemon over the top of the salmon and top with chopped parsley. Serve immediately.

Stuffed Shrimp

Servings: 4
Cooking Time: 12 Minutes Per Batch
Ingredients:
- 16 tail-on shrimp, peeled and deveined (last tail section intact)
- ¾ cup crushed panko breadcrumbs
- oil for misting or cooking spray
- Stuffing
- 2 6-ounce cans lump crabmeat
- 2 tablespoons chopped shallots
- 2 tablespoons chopped green onions
- 2 tablespoons chopped celery
- 2 tablespoons chopped green bell pepper
- ½ cup crushed saltine crackers
- 1 teaspoon Old Bay Seasoning
- 1 teaspoon garlic powder
- ¼ teaspoon ground thyme
- 2 teaspoons dried parsley flakes
- 2 teaspoons fresh lemon juice
- 2 teaspoons Worcestershire sauce
- 1 egg, beaten

Directions:
1. Rinse shrimp. Remove tail section (shell) from 4 shrimp, discard, and chop the meat finely.
2. To prepare the remaining 12 shrimp, cut a deep slit down the back side so that the meat lies open flat. Do not cut all the way through.
3. Preheat air fryer to 360°F/180°C.
4. Place chopped shrimp in a large bowl with all of the stuffing ingredients and stir to combine.
5. Divide stuffing into 12 portions, about 2 tablespoons each.
6. Place one stuffing portion onto the back of each shrimp and form into a ball or oblong shape. Press firmly so that stuffing sticks together and adheres to shrimp.
7. Gently roll each stuffed shrimp in panko crumbs and mist with oil or cooking spray.
8. Place 6 shrimp in air fryer basket and cook at 360°F/180°C for 10minutes. Mist with oil or spray and cook 2 minutes longer or until stuffing cooks through inside and is crispy outside.
9. Repeat step 8 to cook remaining shrimp.

Feta & Shrimp Pita

Servings: 4
Cooking Time: 15 Minutes
Ingredients:
- 1 lb peeled shrimp, deveined
- 2 tbsp olive oil
- 1 tsp dried oregano
- ½ tsp dried thyme
- ½ tsp garlic powder
- ¼ tsp shallot powder
- ¼ tsp tarragon powder
- Salt and pepper to taste
- 4 whole-wheat pitas
- 4 oz feta cheese, crumbled
- 1 cup grated lettuce
- 1 tomato, diced

- ¼ cup black olives, sliced
- 1 lemon

Directions:
1. Preheat the oven to 380°F/195°C. Mix the shrimp with olive oil, oregano, thyme, garlic powder, shallot powder, tarragon powder salt, and pepper in a bowl. Pour shrimp in a single layer in the frying basket and Bake for 6-8 minutes or until no longer pink and cooked through. Divide the shrimp into warmed pitas with feta, lettuce, tomato, olives, and a squeeze of lemon. Serve and enjoy!

Crab Cakes

Servings: 2
Cooking Time: 10 Minutes
Ingredients:
- 1 teaspoon butter
- ⅓ cup finely diced onion
- ⅓ cup finely diced celery
- ¼ cup mayonnaise
- 1 teaspoon Dijon mustard
- 1 egg
- pinch ground cayenne pepper
- 1 teaspoon salt
- freshly ground black pepper
- 16 ounces lump crabmeat
- ½ cup + 2 tablespoons panko breadcrumbs, divided

Directions:
1. Melt the butter in a skillet over medium heat. Sauté the onion and celery until it starts to soften, but not brown – about 4 minutes. Transfer the cooked vegetables to a large bowl. Add the mayonnaise, Dijon mustard, egg, cayenne pepper, salt and freshly ground black pepper to the bowl. Gently fold in the lump crabmeat and 2 tablespoons of panko breadcrumbs. Stir carefully so you don't break up all the crab pieces.
2. Preheat the air fryer to 400°F/205°C.
3. Place the remaining panko breadcrumbs in a shallow dish. Divide the crab mixture into 4 portions and shape each portion into a round patty. Dredge the crab patties in the breadcrumbs, coating both sides as well as the edges with the crumbs.
4. Air-fry the crab cakes for 5 minutes. Using a flat spatula, gently turn the cakes over and air-fry for another 5 minutes. Serve the crab cakes with tartar sauce or cocktail sauce, or dress it up with the suggestion below.

King Prawns Al Ajillo

Servings: 4
Cooking Time: 15 Minutes
Ingredients:
- 1 ¼ lb peeled king prawns, deveined
- ½ cup grated Parmesan
- 1 tbsp olive oil
- 1 tbsp lemon juice
- ½ tsp garlic powder
- 2 garlic cloves, minced

Directions:
1. Preheat the air fryer to 350°F/175°C. In a large bowl, add the prawns and sprinkle with olive oil, lemon juice, and garlic powder. Toss in the minced garlic and Parmesan, then toss to coat. Put the prawns in the frying basket and Air Fry for 10-15 minutes or until the prawns cook through. Shake the basket once while cooking. Serve immediately.

Basil Mushroom & Shrimp Spaghetti

Servings: 6

Cooking Time: 20 Minutes
Ingredients:
- 8 oz baby Bella mushrooms, sliced
- ½ cup grated Parmesan
- 1 lb peeled shrimp, deveined
- 3 tbsp olive oil
- ¼ tsp garlic powder
- ¼ tsp shallot powder
- ¼ tsp cayenne
- 1 lb cooked pasta spaghetti
- 5 garlic cloves, minced
- Salt and pepper to taste
- ½ cup dill

Directions:
1. Preheat air fryer to 380°F/195°C. Toss the shrimp, 1 tbsp of olive oil, garlic powder, shallot powder and cayenne in a bowl. Put the shrimp into the frying basket and Roast for 5 minutes. Remove and set aside.
2. Warm the remaining olive oil in a large skillet over medium heat. Add the garlic and mushrooms and cook for 5 minutes. Pour in the pasta, ½ cup of water, Parmesan, salt, pepper, and dill and stir to coat the pasta. Stir in the shrimp. Remove from heat, then let the mixture rest for 5 minutes. Serve and enjoy!

Peanut-crusted Salmon

Servings: 4
Cooking Time: 30 Minutes
Ingredients:
- 4 salmon fillets
- 2 eggs, beaten
- 3 oz melted butter
- 1 garlic clove, minced
- 1 tsp lemon zest
- 1 lemon
- 1 tsp celery salt
- 1 tbsp parsley, chopped
- 1 tsp dill, chopped
- ½ cup peanuts, crushed

Directions:
1. Preheat air fryer to 350°F/175°C. Put the beaten eggs, melted butter, lemon juice, lemon zest, garlic, parsley, celery salt, and dill and in a bowl and stir thoroughly. Dip in the salmon fillets, then roll them in the crushed peanuts, coating completely. Place the coated salmon fillets in the frying basket. Air Fry for 14-16 minutes, flipping once halfway through cooking, until the salmon is cooked through and the crust is toasted and crispy. Serve.

Southern Shrimp With Cocktail Sauce

Servings: 2
Cooking Time: 20 Minutes
Ingredients:
- ½ lb raw shrimp, tail on, deveined and shelled
- 1 cup ketchup
- 2 tbsp prepared horseradish
- 1 tbsp lemon juice
- ½ tsp Worcestershire sauce
- 1/8 tsp chili powder
- Salt and pepper to taste
- 1/3 cup flour
- 2 tbsp cornstarch
- ¼ cup milk
- 1 egg
- ½ cup bread crumbs

- 1 tbsp Cajun seasoning
- 1 lemon, cut into pieces

Directions:
1. In a small bowl, whisk the ketchup, horseradish, lemon juice, Worcestershire sauce, chili powder, salt, and pepper. Let chill covered in the fridge until ready to use. Preheat air fryer at 375ºF/190°C. In a bowl, mix the flour, cornstarch, and salt. In another bowl, beat the milk and egg and in a third bowl, combine breadcrumbs and Cajun seasoning.
2. Roll the shrimp in the flour mixture, shake off excess flour. Then, dip in the egg, shake off excess egg. Finally, dredge in the breadcrumbs mixture. Place shrimp in the greased frying basket and Air Fry for 8 minutes, flipping once. Serve with cocktail sauce and lemon slices.

Fish Nuggets With Broccoli Dip

Servings: 4
Cooking Time: 40 Minutes
Ingredients:
- 1 lb cod fillets, cut into chunks
- 1 ½ cups broccoli florets
- ¼ cup grated Parmesan
- 3 garlic cloves, peeled
- 3 tbsp sour cream
- 2 tbsp lemon juice
- 2 tbsp olive oil
- 2 egg whites
- 1 cup panko bread crumbs
- 1 tsp dried dill
- Salt and pepper to taste

Directions:
1. Preheat the air fryer to 400°F/205°C. Put the broccoli and garlic in the greased frying basket and Air Fry for 5-7 minutes or until tender. Remove to a blender and add sour cream, lemon juice, olive oil, and ½ tsp of salt and process until smooth. Set the sauce aside. Beat the egg whites until frothy in a shallow bowl. On a plate, combine the panko, Parmesan, dill, pepper, and the remaining ½ tsp of salt. Dip the cod fillets in the egg whites, then the breadcrumbs, pressing to coat. Put half the cubes in the frying basket and spray with cooking oil. Air Fry for 6-8 minutes or until the fish is cooked through. Serve the fish with the sauce and enjoy!

Fish And "chips"

Servings: 2
Cooking Time: 10 Minutes
Ingredients:
- ½ cup flour
- ½ teaspoon paprika
- ¼ teaspoon ground white pepper (or freshly ground black pepper)
- 1 egg
- ¼ cup mayonnaise
- 2 cups salt & vinegar kettle cooked potato chips, coarsely crushed
- 12 ounces cod
- tartar sauce
- lemon wedges

Directions:
1. Set up a dredging station. Combine the flour, paprika and pepper in a shallow dish. Combine the egg and mayonnaise in a second shallow dish. Place the crushed potato chips in a third shallow dish.

2. Cut the cod into 6 pieces. Dredge each piece of fish in the flour, then dip it into the egg mixture and then place it into the crushed potato chips. Make sure all sides of the fish are covered and pat the chips gently onto the fish so they stick well.
3. Preheat the air fryer to 370°F/185°C.
4. Place the coated fish fillets into the air fry basket. (It is ok if a couple of pieces slightly overlap or rest on top of other fillets in order to fit everything in the basket.)
5. Air-fry for 10 minutes, gently turning the fish over halfway through the cooking time.
6. Transfer the fish to a platter and serve with tartar sauce and lemon wedges.

Beer-breaded Halibut Fish Tacos

Servings: 4
Cooking Time: 10 Minutes
Ingredients:
- 1 pound halibut, cut into 1-inch strips
- 1 cup light beer
- 1 jalapeño, minced and divided
- 1 clove garlic, minced
- ¼ teaspoon ground cumin
- ½ cup cornmeal
- ¼ cup all-purpose flour
- 1¼ teaspoons sea salt, divided
- 2 cups shredded cabbage
- 1 lime, juiced and divided
- ¼ cup Greek yogurt
- ¼ cup mayonnaise
- 1 cup grape tomatoes, quartered
- ½ cup chopped cilantro
- ¼ cup chopped onion
- 1 egg, whisked
- 8 corn tortillas

Directions:
1. In a shallow baking dish, place the fish, the beer, 1 teaspoon of the minced jalapeño, the garlic, and the cumin. Cover and refrigerate for 30 minutes.
2. Meanwhile, in a medium bowl, mix together the cornmeal, flour, and ½ teaspoon of the salt.
3. In large bowl, mix together the shredded cabbage, 1 tablespoon of the lime juice, the Greek yogurt, the mayonnaise, and ½ teaspoon of the salt.
4. In a small bowl, make the pico de gallo by mixing together the tomatoes, cilantro, onion, ¼ teaspoon of the salt, the remaining jalapeño, and the remaining lime juice.
5. Remove the fish from the refrigerator and discard the marinade. Dredge the fish in the whisked egg; then dredge the fish in the cornmeal flour mixture, until all pieces of fish have been breaded.
6. Preheat the air fryer to 350°F/175°C.
7. Place the fish in the air fryer basket and spray liberally with cooking spray. Cook for 6 minutes, flip and shake the fish, and cook another 4 minutes.
8. While the fish is cooking, heat the tortillas in a heavy skillet for 1 to 2 minutes over high heat.
9. To assemble the tacos, place the battered fish on the heated tortillas, and top with slaw and pico de gallo. Serve immediately.

Chinese Firecracker Shrimp

Servings: 4
Cooking Time: 20 Minutes
Ingredients:
- 1 lb peeled shrimp, deveined
- 2 green onions, chopped
- 2 tbsp sesame seeds
- Salt and pepper to taste
- 1 egg
- ½ cup all-purpose flour
- ¾ cup panko bread crumbs
- 1/3 cup sour cream
- 2 tbsp Sriracha sauce
- ¼ cup sweet chili sauce

Directions:
1. Preheat air fryer to 400°F/205°C. Set out three small bowls. In the first, add flour. In the second, beat the egg. In the third, add the crumbs. Season the shrimp with salt and pepper. Dip the shrimp in the flour, then dredge in the egg, and finally in the bread crumbs. Place the shrimp in the greased frying basket and Air Fry for 8 minutes, flipping once until crispy. Combine sour cream, Sriracha, and sweet chili sauce in a bowl. Top the shrimp with sesame seeds and green onions and serve with the chili sauce.

Buttery Lobster Tails

Servings:4
Cooking Time: 6 Minutes
Ingredients:
- 4 6- to 8-ounce shell-on raw lobster tails
- 2 tablespoons Butter, melted and cooled
- 1 teaspoon Lemon juice
- ½ teaspoon Finely grated lemon zest
- ½ teaspoon Garlic powder
- ½ teaspoon Table salt
- ½ teaspoon Ground black pepper

Directions:
1. Preheat the air fryer to 375°F /190°C.
2. To give the tails that restaurant look, you need to butterfly the meat. To do so, place a tail on a cutting board so that the shell is convex. Use kitchen shears to cut a line down the middle of the shell from the larger end to the smaller, cutting only the shell and not the meat below, and stopping before the back fins. Pry open the shell, leaving it intact. Use your clean fingers to separate the meat from the shell's sides and bottom, keeping it attached to the shell at the back near the fins. Pull the meat up and out of the shell through the cut line, laying the meat on top of the shell and closing the shell (as well as you can) under the meat. Make two equidistant cuts down the meat from the larger end to near the smaller end, each about ¼ inch deep, for the classic restaurant look on the plate. Repeat this procedure with the remaining tail(s).
3. Stir the butter, lemon juice, zest, garlic powder, salt, and pepper in a small bowl until well combined. Brush this mixture over the lobster meat set atop the shells.
4. When the machine is at temperature, place the tails shell side down in the basket with as much air space between them as possible. Air-fry undisturbed for 6 minutes, or until the lobster meat has pink streaks over it and is firm.
5. Use kitchen tongs to transfer the tails to a wire rack. Cool for only a minute or two before serving.

Mojito Fish Tacos

Servings: 4
Cooking Time: 30 Minutes
Ingredients:
- 1 ½ cups chopped red cabbage
- 1 lb cod fillets
- 2 tsp olive oil
- 3 tbsp lemon juice
- 1 large carrot, grated
- 1 tbsp white rum
- ½ cup salsa
- 1/3 cup Greek yogurt
- 4 soft tortillas

Directions:
1. Preheat air fryer to 390°F/200°C. Rub the fish with olive oil, then a splash with a tablespoon of lemon juice. Place in the fryer and Air Fry for 9-12 minutes. The fish should flake when done. Mix the remaining lemon juice, red cabbage, carrots, salsa, rum, and yogurt in a bowl. Take the fish out of the fryer and tear into large pieces. Serve with tortillas and cabbage mixture. Enjoy!

Kid´s Flounder Fingers

Servings: 4
Cooking Time: 45 Minutes
Ingredients:
- 1 lb catfish flounder fillets, cut into 1-inch chunks
- ½ cup seasoned fish fry breading mix

Directions:
1. Preheat air fryer to 400°F/205°C. In a resealable bag, add flounder and breading mix. Seal bag and shake until the fish is coated. Place the nuggets in the greased frying basket and Air Fry for 18-20 minutes, shaking the basket once until crisp. Serve warm and enjoy!

Lobster Tails With Lemon Garlic Butter

Servings: 2
Cooking Time: 5 Minutes
Ingredients:
- 4 ounces unsalted butter
- 1 tablespoon finely chopped lemon zest
- 1 clove garlic, thinly sliced
- 2 (6-ounce) lobster tails
- salt and freshly ground black pepper
- ½ cup white wine
- ½ lemon, sliced
- vegetable oil

Directions:
1. Start by making the lemon garlic butter. Combine the butter, lemon zest and garlic in a small saucepan. Melt and simmer the butter on the stovetop over the lowest possible heat while you prepare the lobster tails.
2. Prepare the lobster tails by cutting down the middle of the top of the shell. Crack the bottom shell by squeezing the sides of the lobster together so that you can access the lobster meat inside. Pull the lobster tail up out of the shell, but leave it attached at the base of the tail. Lay the lobster meat on top of the shell and season with salt and freshly ground black pepper. Pour a little of the lemon garlic butter on top of the lobster meat and transfer the lobster to the refrigerator so that the butter solidifies a little.
3. Pour the white wine into the air fryer drawer and add the lemon slices. Preheat the air fryer to 400°F/205°C for 5 minutes.
4. Transfer the lobster tails to the air fryer basket. Air-fry at 370°F/185°C for 5 minutes, brushing more butter on halfway through cooking. (Add a minute or two if your lobster tail is more than 6-ounces.) Remove and serve with more butter for dipping or drizzling.

Corn & Shrimp Boil

Servings: 4
Cooking Time: 40 Minutes
Ingredients:

- 8 frozen "mini" corn on the cob
- 1 tbsp smoked paprika
- 2 tsp dried thyme
- 1 tsp dried marjoram
- 1 tsp sea salt
- 1 tsp garlic powder
- 1 tsp onion powder
- 1 tsp cayenne pepper
- 1 lb baby potatoes, halved
- 1 tbsp olive oil
- 1 lb peeled shrimp, deveined
- 1 avocado, sliced

Directions:
1. Preheat the air fryer to 370°F/185°C. Combine the paprika, thyme, marjoram, salt, garlic, onion, and cayenne and mix well. Pour into a small glass jar. Add the potatoes, corn, and olive oil to the frying basket and sprinkle with 2 tsp of the spice mix and toss. Air Fry for 15 minutes, shaking the basket once until tender. Remove and set aside. Put the shrimp in the frying basket and sprinkle with 2 tsp of the spice mix. Air Fry for 5-8 minutes, shaking once until shrimp are tender and pink. Combine all the ingredients in the frying basket and sprinkle with 2 tsp of the spice mix. Toss to coat and cook for 1-2 more minutes or until hot. Serve topped with avocado.

Spicy Fish Street Tacos With Sriracha Slaw

Servings: 2
Cooking Time: 5 Minutes
Ingredients:

- Sriracha Slaw:
- ½ cup mayonnaise
- 2 tablespoons rice vinegar
- 1 teaspoon sugar
- 2 tablespoons sriracha chili sauce
- 5 cups shredded green cabbage
- ¼ cup shredded carrots
- 2 scallions, chopped
- salt and freshly ground black pepper
- Tacos:
- ½ cup flour
- 1 teaspoon chili powder
- ½ teaspoon ground cumin
- 1 teaspoon salt
- freshly ground black pepper
- ½ teaspoon baking powder
- 1 egg, beaten
- ¼ cup milk
- 1 cup breadcrumbs
- 1 pound mahi-mahi or snapper fillets
- 1 tablespoon canola or vegetable oil
- 6 (6-inch) flour tortillas
- 1 lime, cut into wedges

Directions:
1. Start by making the sriracha slaw. Combine the mayonnaise, rice vinegar, sugar, and sriracha sauce in a large bowl. Mix well and add the green cabbage, carrots, and scallions. Toss until all the vegetables are coated with the dressing and season with salt and pepper. Refrigerate the slaw until you are ready to serve the tacos.
2. Combine the flour, chili powder, cumin, salt, pepper and baking powder in a bowl. Add the egg and milk and mix until the batter is smooth. Place the breadcrumbs in shallow dish.
3. Cut the fish fillets into 1-inch wide sticks, approximately 4-inches long. You should have about 12 fish sticks total. Dip the fish sticks into the batter, coating all sides. Let the excess batter drip off the fish and then roll them in the breadcrumbs, patting the crumbs onto all sides of the fish sticks. Set the coated fish on a plate or baking sheet until all the fish has been coated.
4. Preheat the air fryer to 400°F/205°C.
5. Spray the coated fish sticks with oil on all sides. Spray or brush the inside of the air fryer basket with oil and transfer the fish to the basket. Place as many sticks as you can in one layer, leaving a little room around each stick. Place any remaining sticks on top, perpendicular to the first layer.
6. Air-fry the fish for 3 minutes. Turn the fish sticks over and air-fry for an additional 2 minutes.
7. While the fish is air-frying, warm the tortilla shells either in a 350°F/175°C oven wrapped in foil or in a skillet with a little oil over medium-high heat for a couple minutes. Fold the tortillas in half and keep them warm until the remaining tortillas and fish are ready.
8. To assemble the tacos, place two pieces of the fish in each tortilla shell and top with the sriracha slaw. Squeeze the lime wedge over top and dig in.

Sweet Potato–wrapped Shrimp

Servings: 3
Cooking Time: 6 Minutes
Ingredients:

- 24 Long spiralized sweet potato strands
- Olive oil spray
- ¼ teaspoon Garlic powder
- ¼ teaspoon Table salt
- Up to a ⅛ teaspoon Cayenne
- 12 Large shrimp (20–25 per pound), peeled and deveined

Directions:
1. Preheat the air fryer to 400°F/205°C.
2. Lay the spiralized sweet potato strands on a large swath of paper towels and straighten out the strands to long ropes. Coat them with olive oil spray, then sprinkle them with the garlic powder, salt, and cayenne.
3. Pick up 2 strands and wrap them around the center of a shrimp, with the ends tucked under what now becomes the bottom side of the shrimp. Continue wrapping the remainder of the shrimp.
4. Set the shrimp bottom side down in the basket with as much air space between them as possible. Air-fry undisturbed for 6 minutes, or until the sweet potato strands are crisp and the shrimp are pink and firm.
5. Use kitchen tongs to transfer the shrimp to a wire rack. Cool for only a minute or two before serving.

Cheesy Salmon-stuffed Avocados

Servings: 2
Cooking Time: 20 Minutes
Ingredients:

- ¼ cup apple cider vinegar
- 1 tsp granular sugar
- ¼ cup sliced red onions
- 2 oz cream cheese, softened
- 1 tbsp capers
- 2 halved avocados, pitted
- 4 oz smoked salmon

- ¼ tsp dried dill
- 2 cherry tomatoes, halved
- 1 tbsp cilantro, chopped

Directions:

1. Warm apple vinegar and sugar in a saucepan over medium heat and simmer for 4 minutes until boiling. Add in onion and turn the heat off. Let sit until ready to use. Drain before using. In a small bowl, combine cream cheese and capers. Let chill in the fridge until ready to use.
2. Preheat air fryer to 350ºF/175°C. Place avocado halves, cut sides-up, in the frying basket, and Air Fry for 4 minutes. Transfer avocado halves to 2 plates. Top with cream cheese mixture, smoked salmon, dill, red onions, tomato halves and cilantro. Serve immediately.

Curried Sweet-and-spicy Scallops

Servings:3
Cooking Time: 5 Minutes

Ingredients:

- 6 tablespoons Thai sweet chili sauce
- 2 cups (from about 5 cups cereal) Crushed Rice Krispies or other rice-puff cereal
- 2 teaspoons Yellow curry powder, purchased or homemade (see here)
- 1 pound Sea scallops
- Vegetable oil spray

Directions:

1. Preheat the air fryer to 400°F/205°C.
2. Set up and fill two shallow soup plates or small pie plates on your counter: one for the chili sauce and one for crumbs, mixed with the curry powder.
3. Dip a scallop into the chili sauce, coating it on all sides. Set it in the cereal mixture and turn several times to coat evenly. Gently shake off any excess and set the scallop on a cutting board. Continue dipping and coating the remaining scallops. Coat them all on all sides with the vegetable oil spray.
4. Set the scallops in the basket with as much air space between them as possible. Air-fry undisturbed for 5 minutes, or until lightly browned and crunchy.
5. Remove the basket. Set aside for 2 minutes to let the coating set up. Then gently pour the contents of the basket onto a platter and serve at once.

Tuna Nuggets In Hoisin Sauce

Servings: 4
Cooking Time: 7 Minutes

Ingredients:

- ½ cup hoisin sauce
- 2 tablespoons rice wine vinegar
- 2 teaspoons sesame oil
- 1 teaspoon garlic powder
- 2 teaspoons dried lemongrass
- ¼ teaspoon red pepper flakes
- ½ small onion, quartered and thinly sliced
- 8 ounces fresh tuna, cut into 1-inch cubes
- cooking spray
- 3 cups cooked jasmine rice

Directions:

1. Mix the hoisin sauce, vinegar, sesame oil, and seasonings together.
2. Stir in the onions and tuna nuggets.
3. Spray air fryer baking pan with nonstick spray and pour in tuna mixture.
4. Cook at 390°F/200°C for 3minutes. Stir gently.
5. Cook 2minutes and stir again, checking for doneness. Tuna should be barely cooked through, just beginning to

flake and still very moist. If necessary, continue cooking and stirring in 1-minute intervals until done.
6. Serve warm over hot jasmine rice.

Old Bay Lobster Tails

Servings: 2
Cooking Time: 20 Minutes

Ingredients:

- ¼ cup green onions, sliced
- 2 uncooked lobster tails
- 1 tbsp butter, melted
- ½ tsp Old Bay Seasoning
- 1 tbsp chopped parsley
- 1 tsp dried sage
- 1 tsp dried thyme
- 1 garlic clove, chopped
- 1 tbsp basil paste
- 2 lemon wedges

Directions:

1. Preheat air fryer at 400ºF/205°C. Using kitchen shears, cut down the middle of each lobster tail on the softer side. Carefully run your finger between lobster meat and shell to loosen the meat. Place lobster tails, cut side-up, in the frying basket and Air Fry for 4 minutes. Brush the tail meat with butter and season with old bay seasoning, sage, thyme, garlic, green onions, basil paste and cook for another 4 minutes. Scatter with parsley and serve with lemon wedges. Enjoy!

Halibut Quesadillas

Servings: 2
Cooking Time: 30 Minutes

Ingredients:

- ¼ cup shredded cheddar
- ¼ cup shredded mozzarella
- 1 tsp olive oil
- 2 tortilla shells
- 1 halibut fillet
- ½ peeled avocado, sliced
- 1 garlic clove, minced
- Salt and pepper to taste
- ½ tsp lemon juice

Directions:

1. Preheat air fryer to 350°F/175°C. Brush the halibut fillet with olive oil and sprinkle with salt and pepper. Bake in the air fryer for 12-14 minutes, flipping once until cooked through. Combine the avocado, garlic, salt, pepper, and lemon juice in a bowl and, using a fork, mash lightly until the avocado is slightly chunky. Add and spread the resulting guacamole on one tortilla. Top with the cooked fish and cheeses, and cover with the second tortilla. Bake in the air fryer 6-8, flipping once until the cheese is melted. Serve immediately.

Malaysian Shrimp With Sambal Mayo

Servings: 4
Cooking Time: 30 Minutes

Ingredients:

- 24 jumbo shrimp, peeled and deveined
- 2/3 cup panko bread crumbs
- 3 tbsp mayonnaise
- 1 tbsp sambal oelek paste
- 2/3 cup shredded coconut
- 1 lime, zested
- ½ tsp ground coriander
- Salt to taste
- 2 tbsp flour

- 2 eggs

Directions:

1. Mix together mayonnaise and sambal oelek in a bowl. Set aside. In another bowl, stir together coconut, lime, coriander, panko bread crumbs, and salt. In a shallow bowl, add flour. In another shallow bowl, whisk eggs until blended. Season shrimp with salt. First, dip the shrimp into the flour, shake, and dip into the egg mix. Dip again in the coconut mix. Gently press the coconut and panko to the shrimp. Preheat air fryer to 360°F/180°C. Put the shrimp in the greased frying basket and Air Fry for 8 minutes, flipping once until the crust is golden and the shrimp is cooked. Serve alongside the sweet chili mayo.

Old Bay Crab Cake Burgers

Servings: 4
Cooking Time: 30 Minutes
Ingredients:

- ½ cup panko bread crumbs
- 1 egg, beaten
- 1 tbsp hummus
- 1 tsp Dijon mustard
- ¼ cup minced parsley
- 2 spring onions, chopped
- ½ tsp red chili powder
- 1 tbsp lemon juice
- ½ tsp Old Bay seasoning
- ⅛ tsp sweet paprika
- Salt and pepper to taste
- 10 oz lump crabmeat
- ¼ cup mayonnaise
- 2 tbsp minced dill pickle
- 1 tsp fresh lemon juice
- ¾ tsp Cajun seasoning
- 4 Boston lettuce leaves
- 4 buns, split

Directions:

1. Mix the crumbs, egg, hummus, mustard, parsley, lemon juice, red chili, spring onions, Old Bay seasoning, paprika, salt, and pepper in a large bowl. Fold in crabmeat until just coated without overmixing. Divide into 4 equal parts, about ½ cup each, and shape into patties, about ¾-inch thick. Preheat air fryer to 400°F/205°C.

2. Place the cakes in the greased frying basket and Air Fry for 10 minutes, flipping them once until the edges are golden. Meanwhile, mix mayonnaise, lemon juice and Cajun seasoning in a small bowl until well blended. Set aside. When you are ready to serve, start with the bottom of the bun. Add a lettuce leaf, then a crab cake. Top with a heaping tbsp of Cajun mayo, minced pickles, and top with the bun and enjoy.

Teriyaki Salmon

Servings: 4
Cooking Time: 20 Minutes
Ingredients:

- ¼ cup raw honey
- 4 garlic cloves, minced
- 1 tbsp olive oil
- ½ tsp salt
- ½ tsp soy sauce
- ¼ tsp blackening seasoning
- 4 salmon fillets

Directions:

1. Preheat air fryer to 380°F/195°C. Combine together the honey, garlic, olive oil, soy sauce, blackening seasoning and salt in a bowl. Put the salmon in a single layer on the greased frying basket. Brush the top of each fillet with the honey-garlic mixture. Roast for 10-12 minutes. Serve and enjoy!

Garlic-butter Lobster Tails

Servings:2
Cooking Time: 20 Minutes
Ingredients:

- 2 lobster tails
- 1 tbsp butter, melted
- ½ tsp Old Bay Seasoning
- ½ tsp garlic powder
- 1 tbsp chopped parsley
- 2 lemon wedges

Directions:

1. Preheat air fryer to 400ºF/205°C. Using kitchen shears, cut down the middle of each lobster tail on the softer side. Carefully run your finger between the lobster meat and the shell to loosen the meat. Place lobster tails in the frying basket, cut sides up, and Air Fry for 4 minutes. Rub with butter, garlic powder and Old Bay seasoning and cook for 4 more minutes. Garnish with parsley and lemon wedges. Serve and enjoy!

Butternut Squash–wrapped Halibut Fillets

Servings:3
Cooking Time: 11 Minutes
Ingredients:

- 15 Long spiralized peeled and seeded butternut squash strands
- 3 5- to 6-ounce skinless halibut fillets
- 3 tablespoons Butter, melted
- ¾ teaspoon Mild paprika
- ¾ teaspoon Table salt
- ¾ teaspoon Ground black pepper

Directions:

1. Preheat the air fryer to 375°F/190°C .
2. Hold 5 long butternut squash strands together and wrap them around a fillet. Set it aside and wrap any remaining fillet(s).
3. Mix the melted butter, paprika, salt, and pepper in a small bowl. Brush this mixture over the squash-wrapped fillets on all sides.
4. When the machine is at temperature, set the fillets in the basket with as much air space between them as possible. Air-fry undisturbed for 10 minutes, or until the squash strands have browned but not burned. If the machine is at 360°F, you may need to add 1 minute to the cooking time. In any event, watch the fish carefully after the 8-minute mark.
5. Use a nonstick-safe spatula to gently transfer the fillets to a serving platter or plates. Cool for only a minute or so before serving.

Fish Piccata With Crispy Potatoes

Servings: 4
Cooking Time: 30 Minutes
Ingredients:

- 4 cod fillets
- 1 tbsp butter
- 2 tsp capers
- 1 garlic clove, minced
- 2 tbsp lemon juice
- ½ lb asparagus, trimmed
- 2 large potatoes, cubed
- 1 tbsp olive oil
- Salt and pepper to taste

- ¼ tsp garlic powder
- 1 tsp dried rosemary
- 1 tsp dried parsley
- 1 tsp chopped dill

Directions:
1. Preheat air fryer to 380°F/195°C. Place each fillet on a large piece of foil. Top each fillet with butter, capers, dill, garlic, and lemon juice. Fold the foil over the fish and seal the edges to make a pouch. Mix asparagus, parsley, potatoes, olive oil, salt, rosemary, garlic powder, and pepper in a large bowl. Place asparagus in the frying basket. Roast for 4 minutes, then shake the basket. Top vegetable with foil packets and Roast for another 8 minutes. Turn off air fryer and let it stand for 5 minutes. Serve warm and enjoy.

Shrimp Patties

Servings: 4
Cooking Time: 10 Minutes
Ingredients:
- ½ pound shelled and deveined raw shrimp
- ¼ cup chopped red bell pepper
- ¼ cup chopped green onion
- ¼ cup chopped celery
- 2 cups cooked sushi rice
- ½ teaspoon garlic powder
- ½ teaspoon Old Bay Seasoning
- ½ teaspoon salt
- 2 teaspoons Worcestershire sauce
- ½ cup plain breadcrumbs
- oil for misting or cooking spray

Directions:
1. Finely chop the shrimp. You can do this in a food processor, but it takes only a few pulses. Be careful not to overprocess into mush.
2. Place shrimp in a large bowl and add all other ingredients except the breadcrumbs and oil. Stir until well combined.
3. Preheat air fryer to 390°F/200°C.
4. Shape shrimp mixture into 8 patties, no more than ½-inch thick. Roll patties in breadcrumbs and mist with oil or cooking spray.
5. Place 4 shrimp patties in air fryer basket and cook at 390°F/200°C for 10 minutes, until shrimp cooks through and outside is crispy.
6. Repeat step 5 to cook remaining shrimp patties.

Sriracha Salmon Melt Sandwiches

Servings: 4
Cooking Time: 20 Minutes
Ingredients:
- 2 tbsp butter, softened
- 2 cans pink salmon
- 2 English muffins
- 1/3 cup mayonnaise
- 2 tbsp Dijon mustard
- 1 tbsp fresh lemon juice
- 1/3 cup chopped celery
- ½ tsp sriracha sauce
- 4 slices tomato
- 4 slices Swiss cheese

Directions:
1. Preheat the air fryer to 370°F/185°C. Split the English muffins with a fork and spread butter on the 4 halves. Put the halves in the basket and Bake for 3-5 minutes, or until toasted. Remove and set aside. Combine the salmon, mayonnaise, mustard, lemon juice, celery, and sriracha in a bowl. Divide among the English muffin halves. Top each sandwich with tomato and cheese and put in the frying basket. Bake for 4-6 minutes or until the cheese is melted and starts to brown. Serve hot.

Creole Tilapia With Garlic Mayo

Servings: 4
Cooking Time: 20 Minutes
Ingredients:
- 4 tilapia fillets
- 2 tbsp olive oil
- 1 tsp paprika
- 1 tsp garlic powder
- 1 tsp dried basil
- ½ tsp Creole seasoning
- ½ tsp chili powder
- 2 garlic cloves, minced
- 1 tbsp mayonnaise
- 1 tsp olive oil
- ½ lemon, juiced
- Salt and pepper to taste

Directions:
1. Preheat air fryer to 400°F/205°C. Coat the tilapia with some olive oil, then season with paprika, garlic powder, basil, and Creole seasoning. Bake in the greased frying basket for 15 minutes, flipping once during cooking.
2. While the fish is cooking, whisk together garlic, mayonnaise, olive oil, lemon juice, chili powder, salt and pepper in a bowl. Serve the cooked fish with the aioli.

Halibut With Coleslaw

Servings: 4
Cooking Time: 30 Minutes
Ingredients:
- 1 bag coleslaw mix
- ¼ cup mayonnaise
- 1 tsp lemon zest
- 1 tbsp lemon juice
- 1 shredded carrot
- ½ cup buttermilk
- 1 tsp grated onion
- 4 halibut fillets
- Salt and pepper to taste

Directions:
1. Combine coleslaw mix, mayonnaise, carrot, buttermilk, onion, lemon zest, lemon juice, and salt in a bowl. Let chill the coleslaw covered in the fridge until ready to use. Preheat air fryer at 350°F/175°C. Sprinkle halibut with salt and pepper. Place them in the greased frying basket and Air Fry for 10 minutes until the fillets are opaque and flake easily with a fork. Serve with chilled coleslaw.

Rich Salmon Burgers With Broccoli Slaw

Servings: 4
Cooking Time: 25 Minutes
Ingredients:
- 1 lb salmon fillets
- 1 egg
- ¼ cup dill, chopped
- 1 cup bread crumbs
- Salt to taste
- ½ tsp cayenne pepper
- 1 lime, zested
- 1 tsp fish sauce

- 4 buns
- 3 cups chopped broccoli
- ½ cup shredded carrots
- ¼ cup sunflower seeds
- 2 garlic cloves, minced
- 1 cup Greek yogurt

Directions:
1. Preheat air fryer to 360°F/180°C. Blitz the salmon fillets in your food processor until they are finely chopped. Remove to a large bowl and add egg, dill, bread crumbs, salt, and cayenne. Stir to combine. Form the mixture into 4 patties. Put them into the frying basket and Bake for 10 minutes, flipping once. Combine broccoli, carrots, sunflower seeds, garlic, salt, lime, fish sauce, and Greek yogurt in a bowl. Serve the salmon burgers onto buns with broccoli slaw. Enjoy!

Lime Halibut Parcels

Servings: 4
Cooking Time: 45 Minutes
Ingredients:
- 1 lime, sliced
- 4 halibut fillets
- 1 tsp dried thyme
- Salt and pepper to taste
- 1 shredded carrot
- 1 red bell pepper, sliced
- ½ cup sliced celery
- 2 tbsp butter

Directions:
1. Preheat the air fryer to 400°F/205°C. Tear off four 14-inch lengths of parchment paper and fold each piece in half crosswise. Put the lime slices in the center of half of each piece of paper, then top with halibut. Sprinkle each filet with thyme, salt, and pepper, then top each with ¼ of the carrots, bell pepper, and celery. Add a dab of butter. Fold the parchment paper in half and crimp the edges all around to enclose the halibut and vegetables. Put one parchment bundle in the basket, add a raised rack, and add another bundle. Bake for 12-14 minutes or until the bundle puff up. The fish should flake with a fork; put the bundles in the oven to keep warm. Repeat for the second batch of parchment bundles. Hot steam will be released when the bundles are opened.

Cajun-seasoned Shrimp

Servings: 2
Cooking Time: 15 Minutes
Ingredients:
- 1 lb shelled tail on shrimp, deveined
- 2 tsp grated Parmesan cheese
- 2 tbsp butter, melted
- 1 tsp cayenne pepper
- 1 tsp garlic powder
- 2 tsp Cajun seasoning
- 1 tbsp lemon juice

Directions:
1. Preheat air fryer at 350°F/175°C. Toss the shrimp, melted butter, cayenne pepper, garlic powder and cajun seasoning in a bowl, place them in the greased frying basket, and Air Fry for 6 minutes, flipping once. Transfer it to a plate. Squeeze lemon juice over shrimp and stir in Parmesan cheese. Serve immediately.

Lemon-roasted Salmon Fillets

Servings:3
Cooking Time: 7 Minutes
Ingredients:

- 3 6-ounce skin-on salmon fillets
- Olive oil spray
- 9 Very thin lemon slices
- ¾ teaspoon Ground black pepper
- ¼ teaspoon Table salt

Directions:
1. Preheat the air fryer to 400°F/205°C.
2. Generously coat the skin of each of the fillets with olive oil spray. Set the fillets skin side down on your work surface. Place three overlapping lemon slices down the length of each salmon fillet. Sprinkle them with the pepper and salt. Coat lightly with olive oil spray.
3. Use a nonstick-safe spatula to transfer the fillets one by one to the basket, leaving as much air space between them as possible. Air-fry undisturbed for 7 minutes, or until cooked through.
4. Use a nonstick-safe spatula to transfer the fillets to serving plates. Cool for only a minute or two before serving.

Crabmeat-stuffed Flounder

Servings:3
Cooking Time: 12 Minutes
Ingredients:
- 4½ ounces Purchased backfin or claw crabmeat, picked over for bits of shell and cartilage
- 6 Saltine crackers, crushed into fine crumbs
- 2 tablespoons plus 1 teaspoon Regular or low-fat mayonnaise (not fat-free)
- ¾ teaspoon Yellow prepared mustard
- 1½ teaspoons Worcestershire sauce
- ⅛ teaspoon Celery salt
- 3 5- to 6-ounce skinless flounder fillets
- Vegetable oil spray
- Mild paprika

Directions:
1. Preheat the air fryer to 400°F/205°C.
2. Gently mix the crabmeat, crushed saltines, mayonnaise, mustard, Worcestershire sauce, and celery salt in a bowl until well combined.
3. Generously coat the flat side of a fillet with vegetable oil spray. Set the fillet sprayed side down on your work surface. Cut the fillet in half widthwise, then cut one of the halves in half lengthwise. Set a scant ⅓ cup of the crabmeat mixture on top of the undivided half of the fish fillet, mounding the mixture to make an oval that somewhat fits the shape of the fillet with at least a ¼-inch border of fillet beyond the filling all around.
4. Take the two thin divided quarters (that is, the halves of the half) and lay them lengthwise over the filling, overlapping at each end and leaving a little space in the middle where the filling peeks through. Coat the top of the stuffed flounder piece with vegetable oil spray, then sprinkle paprika over the stuffed flounder fillet. Set aside and use the remaining fillet(s) to make more stuffed flounder "packets," repeating steps 3 and
5. Use a nonstick-safe spatula to transfer the stuffed flounder fillets to the basket. Leave as much space between them as possible. Air-fry undisturbed for 12 minutes, or until lightly brown and firm (but not hard).
6. Use that same spatula, plus perhaps another one, to transfer the fillets to a serving platter or plates. Cool for a minute or two, then serve hot.

Shrimp "scampi"

Servings:4
Cooking Time: 5 Minutes
Ingredients:
* 1½ pounds Large shrimp (20–25 per pound), peeled and deveined
* ¼ cup Olive oil
* 2 tablespoons Minced garlic
* 1 teaspoon Dried oregano
* Up to 1 teaspoon Red pepper flakes
* ½ teaspoon Table salt
* 2 tablespoons White balsamic vinegar (see here)

Directions:
1. Preheat the air fryer to 400°F/205°C.
2. Stir the shrimp, olive oil, garlic, oregano, red pepper flakes, and salt in a large bowl until the shrimp are well coated.
3. When the machine is at temperature, transfer the shrimp to the basket. They will overlap and even sit on top of each other. Air-fry for 5 minutes, tossing and rearranging the shrimp twice to make sure the covered surfaces are exposed, until pink and firm.
4. Pour the contents of the basket into a serving bowl. Pour the vinegar over the shrimp while hot and toss to coat.

Mediterranean Salmon Burgers

Servings: 4
Cooking Time: 30 Minutes
Ingredients:
* 1 lb salmon fillets
* 1 scallion, diced
* 4 tbsp mayonnaise
* 1 egg
* 1 tsp capers, drained
* Salt and pepper to taste
* ¼ tsp paprika
* 1 lemon, zested
* 1 lemon, sliced
* 1 tbsp chopped dill
* ¼ cup bread crumbs
* 4 buns, toasted
* 4 tsp whole-grain mustard
* 4 lettuce leaves
* 1 small tomato, sliced

Directions:
1. Preheat air fryer to 400°F/205°C. Divide salmon in half. Cut one of the halves into chunks and transfer the chunks to the food processor. Also, add scallion, 2 tablespoons mayonnaise, egg, capers, dill, salt, pepper, paprika, and lemon zest. Pulse to puree. Dice the rest of the salmon into ¼-inch chunks. Combine chunks and puree along with bread crumbs in a large bowl. Shape the fish into 4 patties and transfer to the frying basket. Air Fry for 5 minutes, then flip the patties. Air Fry for another 5 to 7 minutes. Place the patties each on a bun along with 1 teaspoon mustard, mayonnaise, lettuce, lemon slices, and a slice of tomato. Serve and enjoy.

Holliday Lobster Salad

Servings:2
Cooking Time: 20 Minutes
Ingredients:
* 2 lobster tails
* ¼ cup mayonnaise
* 2 tsp lemon juice
* 1 stalk celery, sliced
* 2 tsp chopped chives
* 2 tsp chopped tarragon
* Salt and pepper to taste
* 2 tomato slices
* 4 cucumber slices
* 1 avocado, diced

Directions:
1. Preheat air fryer to 400°F/205°C. Using kitchen shears, cut down the middle of each lobster tail on the softer side. Carefully run your finger between the lobster meat and the shell to loosen meat. Place lobster tails, cut sides up, in the frying basket, and Air Fry for 8 minutes. Transfer to a large plate and let cool for 3 minutes until easy to handle, then pull lobster meat from the shell and roughly chop it. Combine chopped lobster, mayonnaise, lemon juice, celery, chives, tarragon, salt, and pepper in a bowl. Divide between 2 medium plates and top with tomato slices, cucumber and avocado cubes. Serve immediately.

Californian Tilapia

Servings: 4
Cooking Time: 15 Minutes
Ingredients:
* Salt and pepper to taste
* ¼ tsp garlic powder
* ¼ tsp chili powder
* ¼ tsp dried oregano
* ¼ tsp smoked paprika
* 1 tbsp butter, melted
* 4 tilapia fillets
* 2 tbsp lime juice
* 1 lemon, sliced

Directions:
1. Preheat air fryer to 400°F/205°C. Combine salt, pepper, oregano, garlic powder, chili powder, and paprika in a small bowl. Place tilapia in a pie pan, then pour lime juice and butter over the fish. Season both sides of the fish with the spice blend. Arrange the tilapia in a single layer of the parchment-lined frying basket without touching each other. Air Fry for 4 minutes, then carefully flip the fish. Air Fry for another 4 to 5 minutes until the fish is cooked and the outside is crispy. Serve immediately with lemon slices on the side and enjoy.

Family Fish Nuggets With Tartar Sauce

Servings:4
Cooking Time: 30 Minutes
Ingredients:
* ½ cup mayonnaise
* 1 tbsp yellow mustard
* ½ cup diced dill pickles
* Salt and pepper to taste
* 1 egg, beaten
* ¼ cup cornstarch
* ¼ cup flour
* 1 lb cod, cut into sticks

Directions:
1. In a bowl, whisk the mayonnaise, mustard, pickles, salt, and pepper. Set aside the resulting tarter sauce.
2. Preheat air fryer to 350°F/175°C. Add the beaten egg to a bowl. In another bowl, combine cornstarch, flour, salt, and pepper. Dip fish nuggets in the egg and roll them in the flour mixture. Place fish nuggets in the lightly greased frying basket and Air Fry for 10 minutes, flipping once. Serve with the sauce on the side.

Pecan-crusted Tilapia

Servings: 4
Cooking Time: 8 Minutes
Ingredients:
- 1 pound skinless, boneless tilapia filets
- ¼ cup butter, melted
- 1 teaspoon minced fresh or dried rosemary
- 1 cup finely chopped pecans
- 1 teaspoon sea salt
- ¼ teaspoon paprika
- 2 tablespoons chopped parsley
- 1 lemon, cut into wedges

Directions:
1. Pat the tilapia filets dry with paper towels.
2. Pour the melted butter over the filets and flip the filets to coat them completely.
3. In a medium bowl, mix together the rosemary, pecans, salt, and paprika.
4. Preheat the air fryer to 350°F/175°C.
5. Place the tilapia filets into the air fryer basket and top with the pecan coating. Cook for 6 to 8 minutes. The fish should be firm to the touch and flake easily when fully cooked.
6. Remove the fish from the air fryer. Top the fish with chopped parsley and serve with lemon wedges.

Stuffed Shrimp Wrapped In Bacon

Servings:4
Cooking Time: 30 Minutes
Ingredients:
- 1 lb shrimp, deveined and shelled
- 3 tbsp crumbled goat cheese
- 2 tbsp panko bread crumbs
- ¼ tsp soy sauce
- ½ tsp prepared horseradish
- ¼ tsp garlic powder
- ½ tsp chili powder
- 2 tsp mayonnaise
- Black pepper to taste
- 5 slices bacon, quartered
- ¼ cup chopped parsley

Directions:
1. Preheat air fryer to 400ºF/205°C. Butterfly shrimp by cutting down the spine of each shrimp without going all the way through. Combine the goat cheese, bread crumbs, soy sauce, horseradish, garlic powder, chili powder, mayonnaise, and black pepper in a bowl. Evenly press goat cheese mixture into shrimp. Wrap a piece of bacon around each piece of shrimp to hold in the cheese mixture. Place them in the frying basket and Air Fry for 8-10 minutes, flipping once. Top with parsley to serve.

Potato-wrapped Salmon Fillets

Servings:3
Cooking Time: 8 Minutes
Ingredients:
- 1 Large 1-pound elongated yellow potato(es), peeled
- 3 6-ounce, 1½-inch-wide, quite thick skinless salmon fillets
- Olive oil spray
- ¼ teaspoon Table salt
- ¼ teaspoon Ground black pepper

Directions:
1. Preheat the air fryer to 400°F/205°C.
2. Use a vegetable peeler or mandoline to make long strips from the potato(es). You'll need anywhere from 8 to 12 strips per fillet, depending on the shape of the potato and of the salmon fillet.

3. Drape potato strips over a salmon fillet, overlapping the strips to create an even "crust." Tuck the potato strips under the fillet, overlapping the strips underneath to create as smooth a bottom as you can. Wrap the remaining fillet(s) in the same way.
4. Gently turn the fillets over. Generously coat the bottoms with olive oil spray. Turn them back seam side down and generously coat the tops with the oil spray. Sprinkle the salt and pepper over the wrapped fillets.
5. Use a nonstick-safe spatula to gently transfer the fillets seam side down to the basket. It helps to remove the basket from the machine and set it on your work surface (keeping in mind that the basket's hot). Leave as much air space as possible between the fillets. Air-fry undisturbed for 8 minutes, or until golden brown and crisp.
6. Use a nonstick-safe spatula to gently transfer the fillets to serving plates. Cool for a couple of minutes before serving.

Buttered Swordfish Steaks

Servings: 4
Cooking Time: 30 Minutes
Ingredients:
- 4 swordfish steaks
- 2 eggs, beaten
- 3 oz melted butter
- ½ cup breadcrumbs
- Black pepper to taste
- 1 tsp dried rosemary
- 1 tsp dried marjoram
- 1 lemon, cut into wedges

Directions:
1. Preheat air fryer to 350°F/175°C. Place the eggs and melted butter in a bowl and stir thoroughly. Combine the breadcrumbs, rosemary, marjoram, and black pepper in a separate bowl. Dip the swordfish steaks in the beaten eggs, then coat with the crumb mixture. Place the coated fish in the frying basket. Air Fry for 12-14 minutes, turning once until the fish is cooked through and the crust is toasted and crispy. Serve with lemon wedges.

Sinaloa Fish Fajitas

Servings: 4
Cooking Time: 30 Minutes
Ingredients:
- 1 lemon, thinly sliced
- 16 oz red snapper filets
- 1 tbsp olive oil
- 1 tbsp cayenne pepper
- ½ tsp salt
- 2 cups shredded coleslaw
- 1 carrot, shredded
- 2 tbsp orange juice
- ½ cup salsa
- 4 flour tortillas
- ½ cup sour cream
- 2 avocados, sliced

Directions:
1. Preheat the air fryer to 350°F/175°C. Lay the lemon slices at the bottom of the basket. Drizzle the fillets with olive oil and sprinkle with cayenne pepper and salt. Lay the fillets on top of the lemons and Bake for 6-9 minutes or until the fish easily flakes. While the fish cooks, toss the coleslaw, carrot, orange juice, and salsa in a bowl. When the fish is done, remove it and cover. Toss the lemons. Air Fry the tortillas for 2-3 minutes to warm up. Add the fish to the tortillas and top with a cabbage mix, sour cream, and avocados. Serve and enjoy!

Catalan-style Crab Samfaina

Servings: 4
Cooking Time: 30 Minutes
Ingredients:
- 1 peeled eggplant, cubed
- 1 zucchini, cubed
- 1 onion, chopped
- 1 red bell pepper, chopped
- 2 large tomatoes, chopped
- 1 tbsp olive oil
- ½ tsp dried thyme
- ½ tsp dried basil
- Salt and pepper to taste
- 1 ½ cups cooked crab meat

Directions:
1. Preheat air fryer to 400°F/205°C. In a pan, mix together all ingredients, except the crabmeat. Place the pan in the air fryer and Bake for 9 minutes. Remove the bowl and stir in the crabmeat. Return to the air fryer and roast for another 2-5 minutes until the vegetables are tender and ratatouille bubbling. Serve hot.

Sardinas Fritas

Servings: 2
Cooking Time: 15 Minutes
Ingredients:
- 2 cans boneless, skinless sardines in mustard sauce
- Salt and pepper to taste
- ½ cup bread crumbs
- 2 lemon wedges
- 1 tsp chopped parsley

Directions:
1. Preheat air fryer at 350°F/175°C. Add breadcrumbs, salt and black pepper to a bowl. Roll sardines in the breadcrumbs to coat. Place them in the greased frying basket and Air Fry for 6 minutes, flipping once. Transfer them to a serving dish. Serve topped with parsley and lemon wedges.

Firecracker Popcorn Shrimp

Servings: 6
Cooking Time: 8 Minutes
Ingredients:
- ½ cup all-purpose flour
- 2 teaspoons ground paprika
- 1 teaspoon garlic powder
- ½ teaspoon black pepper
- ¼ teaspoon salt
- 2 eggs, whisked
- 1½ cups panko breadcrumbs
- 1 pound small shrimp, peeled and deveined

Directions:
1. Preheat the air fryer to 360°F/180°C.
2. In a medium bowl, place the flour and mix in the paprika, garlic powder, pepper, and salt.
3. In a shallow dish, place the eggs.
4. In a third dish, place the breadcrumbs.
5. Assemble the shrimp by covering them in the flour, then dipping them into the egg, and then coating them with the breadcrumbs. Repeat until all the shrimp are covered in the breading.
6. Liberally spray the metal trivet that fits in the air fryer basket with olive oil mist. Place the shrimp onto the trivet, leaving space between the shrimp to flip. Cook for 4 minutes, flip the shrimp, and cook another 4 minutes. Repeat until all the shrimp are cooked.
7. Serve warm with desired dipping sauce.

Beer-battered Cod

Servings:3
Cooking Time: 12 Minutes
Ingredients:
- 1½ cups All-purpose flour
- 3 tablespoons Old Bay seasoning
- 1 Large egg(s)
- ¼ cup Amber beer, pale ale, or IPA
- 3 4-ounce skinless cod fillets
- Vegetable oil spray

Directions:
1. Preheat the air fryer to 400°F/205°C.
2. Set up and fill two shallow soup plates or small pie plates on your counter: one with the flour, whisked with the Old Bay until well combined; and one with the egg(s), whisked with the beer until foamy and uniform.
3. Dip a piece of cod in the flour mixture, turning it to coat on all sides (not just the top and bottom). Gently shake off any excess flour and dip the fish in the egg mixture, turning it to coat. Let any excess egg mixture slip back into the rest, then set the fish back in the flour mixture and coat it again, then back in the egg mixture for a second wash, then back in the flour mixture for a third time. Coat the fish on all sides with vegetable oil spray and set it aside. "Batter" the remaining piece(s) of cod in the same way.
4. Set the coated cod fillets in the basket with as much space between them as possible. They should not touch. Air-fry undisturbed for 12 minutes, or until brown and crisp.
5. Use kitchen tongs to gently transfer the fish to a wire rack. Cool for only a couple of minutes before serving.

Dilly Red Snapper

Servings: 4
Cooking Time: 40 Minutes
Ingredients:
- Salt and pepper to taste
- ½ tsp ground cumin
- ¼ tsp cayenne
- ¼ teaspoon paprika
- 1 whole red snapper
- 2 tbsp butter
- 2 garlic cloves, minced
- ¼ cup dill
- 4 lemon wedges

Directions:
1. Preheat air fryer to 360°F/180°C. Combine salt, pepper, cumin, paprika and cayenne in a bowl. Brush the fish with butter, then rub with the seasoning mix. Stuff the minced garlic and dill inside the cavity of the fish. Put the snapper into the basket of the air fryer and Roast for 20 minutes. Flip the snapper over and Roast for 15 more minutes. Serve with lemon wedges and enjoy!

Shrimp, Chorizo And Fingerling Potatoes

Servings: 4
Cooking Time: 16 Minutes
Ingredients:
- ½ red onion, chopped into 1-inch chunks
- 8 fingerling potatoes, sliced into 1-inch slices or halved lengthwise
- 1 teaspoon olive oil
- salt and freshly ground black pepper
- 8 ounces raw chorizo sausage, sliced into 1-inch chunks
- 16 raw large shrimp, peeled, deveined and tails removed

- 1 lime
- ¼ cup chopped fresh cilantro
- chopped orange zest (optional)

Directions:
1. Preheat the air fryer to 380°F/195°C.
2. Combine the red onion and potato chunks in a bowl and toss with the olive oil, salt and freshly ground black pepper.
3. Transfer the vegetables to the air fryer basket and air-fry for 6 minutes, shaking the basket a few times during the cooking process.
4. Add the chorizo chunks and continue to air-fry for another 5 minutes.
5. Add the shrimp, season with salt and continue to air-fry, shaking the basket every once in a while, for another 5 minutes.
6. Transfer the tossed shrimp, chorizo and potato to a bowl and squeeze some lime juice over the top to taste. Toss in the fresh cilantro, orange zest and a drizzle of olive oil, and season again to taste.
7. Serve with a fresh green salad.

Pecan-orange Crusted Striped Bass

Servings: 2
Cooking Time: 9 Minutes
Ingredients:
- flour, for dredging*
- 2 egg whites, lightly beaten
- 1 cup pecans, chopped
- 1 teaspoon finely chopped orange zest, plus more for garnish
- ½ teaspoon salt
- 2 (6-ounce) fillets striped bass
- salt and freshly ground black pepper
- vegetable or olive oil, in a spray bottle
- Orange Cream Sauce (Optional)
- ½ cup fresh orange juice
- ¼ cup heavy cream
- 1 sprig fresh thyme

Directions:
1. Set up a dredging station with three shallow dishes. Place the flour in one shallow dish. Place the beaten egg whites in a second shallow dish. Finally, combine the chopped pecans, orange zest and salt in a third shallow dish.
2. Coat the fish fillets one at a time. First season with salt and freshly ground black pepper. Then coat each fillet in flour. Shake off any excess flour and then dip the fish into the egg white. Let the excess egg drip off and then immediately press the fish into the pecan-orange mixture. Set the crusted fish fillets aside.
3. Preheat the air fryer to 400°F/205°C.
4. Spray the crusted fish with oil and then transfer the fillets to the air fryer basket. Air-fry for 9 minutes at 400°F, flipping the fish over halfway through the cooking time. The nuts on top should be nice and toasty and the fish should feel firm to the touch.
5. If you'd like to make a sauce to go with the fish while it cooks, combine the freshly squeezed orange juice, heavy cream and sprig of thyme in a small saucepan. Simmer on the stovetop for 5 minutes and then set aside.
6. Remove the fish from the air fryer and serve over a bed of salad, like the one below. Then add a sprinkling of orange zest and a spoonful of the orange cream sauce over the top if desired.

Fish Tacos With Jalapeño-lime Sauce

Servings: 4
Cooking Time: 7 Minutes

Ingredients:
- Fish Tacos
- 1 pound fish fillets
- ¼ teaspoon cumin
- ¼ teaspoon coriander
- ⅛ teaspoon ground red pepper
- 1 tablespoon lime zest
- ¼ teaspoon smoked paprika
- 1 teaspoon oil
- cooking spray
- 6–8 corn or flour tortillas (6-inch size)
- Jalapeño-Lime Sauce
- ½ cup sour cream
- 1 tablespoon lime juice
- ¼ teaspoon grated lime zest
- ½ teaspoon minced jalapeño (flesh only)
- ¼ teaspoon cumin
- Napa Cabbage Garnish
- 1 cup shredded Napa cabbage
- ¼ cup slivered red or green bell pepper
- ¼ cup slivered onion

Directions:
1. Slice the fish fillets into strips approximately ½-inch thick.
2. Put the strips into a sealable plastic bag along with the cumin, coriander, red pepper, lime zest, smoked paprika, and oil. Massage seasonings into the fish until evenly distributed.
3. Spray air fryer basket with nonstick cooking spray and place seasoned fish inside.
4. Cook at 390°F/200°C for approximately 5minutes. Shake basket to distribute fish. Cook an additional 2 minutes, until fish flakes easily.
5. While the fish is cooking, prepare the Jalapeño-Lime Sauce by mixing the sour cream, lime juice, lime zest, jalapeño, and cumin together to make a smooth sauce. Set aside.
6. Mix the cabbage, bell pepper, and onion together and set aside.
7. To warm refrigerated tortillas, wrap in damp paper towels and microwave for 30 to 60 seconds.
8. To serve, spoon some of fish into a warm tortilla. Add one or two tablespoons Napa Cabbage Garnish and drizzle with Jalapeño-Lime Sauce.

Almond Topped Trout

Servings: 4
Cooking Time: 20 Minutes
Ingredients:
- 4 trout fillets
- 2 tbsp olive oil
- Salt and pepper to taste
- 2 garlic cloves, sliced
- 1 lemon, sliced
- 1 tbsp flaked almonds

Directions:
1. Preheat air fryer to 380°F/195°C. Lightly brush each fillet with olive oil on both sides and season with salt and pepper. Put the fillets in a single layer in the frying basket. Put the sliced garlic over the tops of the trout fillets, then top with lemon slices and cook for 12-15 minutes. Serve topped with flaked almonds and enjoy!

Lemon-dill Salmon With Green Beans

Servings: 4
Cooking Time: 20 Minutes
Ingredients:

- 20 halved cherry tomatoes
- 4 tbsp butter
- 4 garlic cloves, minced
- ¼ cup chopped dill
- Salt and pepper to taste
- 4 wild-caught salmon fillets
- ¼ cup white wine
- 1 lemon, thinly sliced
- 1 lb green beans, trimmed
- 2 tbsp chopped parsley

Directions:
1. Preheat air fryer to 390°F/200°C. Combine butter, garlic, dill, wine, salt, and pepper in a small bowl. Spread the seasoned butter over the top of the salmon. Arrange the fish in a single layer in the frying basket. Top with ½ of the lemon slices and surround the fish with green beans and tomatoes. Bake for 12-15 minutes until salmon is cooked and vegetables are tender. Top with parsley and serve with lemon slices on the side.

French Grouper Nicoise

Servings: 4
Cooking Time: 20 Minutes
Ingredients:
- 4 grouper fillets
- Salt to taste
- ½ tsp ground cumin
- 3 garlic cloves, minced
- 1 tomato, sliced
- ¼ cup sliced Nicoise olives
- ¼ cup dill, chopped
- 1 lemon, juiced
- ¼ cup olive oil

Directions:
1. Preheat air fryer to 380°F/195°C. Sprinkle the grouper fillets with salt and cumin. Arrange them on the greased frying basket and top with garlic, tomato slices, olives, and fresh dill. Drizzle with lemon juice and olive oil. Bake for 10-12 minutes. Serve and enjoy!

Super Crunchy Flounder Fillets

Servings:2
Cooking Time: 6 Minutes
Ingredients:
- ½ cup All-purpose flour or tapioca flour
- 1 Large egg white(s)
- 1 tablespoon Water
- ¾ teaspoon Table salt
- 1 cup Plain panko bread crumbs (gluten-free, if a concern)
- 2 4-ounce skinless flounder fillet(s)
- Vegetable oil spray

Directions:
1. Preheat the air fryer to 400°F/205°C.
2. Set up and fill three shallow soup plates or small pie plates on your counter: one for the flour; one for the egg white(s), beaten with the water and salt until foamy; and one for the bread crumbs.
3. Dip one fillet in the flour, turning it to coat both sides. Gently shake off any excess flour, then dip the fillet in the egg white mixture, turning it to coat. Let any excess egg white mixture slip back into the rest, then set the fish in the bread crumbs. Turn it several times, gently pressing it into the crumbs to create an even crust. Generously coat both sides of the fillet with vegetable oil spray. If necessary, set it

aside and continue coating the remaining fillet(s) in the same way.
4. Set the fillet(s) in the basket. If working with more than one fillet, they should not touch, although they may be quite close together, depending on the basket's size. Air-fry undisturbed for 6 minutes, or until lightly browned and crunchy.
5. Use a nonstick-safe spatula to transfer the fillet(s) to a wire rack. Cool for only a minute or two before serving.

Black Olive & Shrimp Salad

Servings: 4
Cooking Time: 15 Minutes
Ingredients:
- 1 lb cleaned shrimp, deveined
- ½ cup olive oil
- 4 garlic cloves, minced
- 1 tbsp balsamic vinegar
- ¼ tsp cayenne pepper
- ¼ tsp dried basil
- ¼ tsp salt
- ¼ tsp onion powder
- 1 tomato, diced
- ¼ cup black olives

Directions:
1. Preheat air fryer to 380°F/195°C. Place the olive oil, garlic, balsamic, cayenne, basil, onion powder and salt in a bowl and stir to combine. Divide the tomatoes and black olives between 4 small ramekins. Top with shrimp and pour a quarter of the oil mixture over the shrimp. Bake for 6-8 minutes until the shrimp are cooked through. Serve.

Classic Shrimp Po'boy Sandwiches

Servings: 4
Cooking Time: 20 Minutes
Ingredients:
- 1 lb peeled shrimp, deveined
- 1 egg
- ½ cup flour
- ¾ cup cornmeal
- Salt and pepper to taste
- ½ cup mayonnaise
- 1 tsp Creole mustard
- 1 tsp Worcestershire sauce
- 1 tsp minced garlic
- 2 tbsp sweet pickle relish
- 1 tsp Louisiana hot sauce
- ½ tsp Creole seasoning
- 4 rolls
- 2 cups shredded lettuce
- 8 tomato slices

Directions:
1. Preheat air fryer to 400°F/205°C. Set up three small bowls. In the first, add flour. In the second, beat the egg. In the third, mix cornmeal with salt and pepper. First dip the shrimp in the flour, then dredge in the egg, then dip in the cornmeal. Place in the greased frying basket. Air Fry for 8 minutes, flipping once until crisp. Let cool slightly.
2. While the shrimp is cooking, mix mayonnaise, mustard, Worcestershire, garlic, pickle relish juice, hot sauce, and Creole seasoning in a small bowl. Set aside. To assemble the po'boys, split rolls along the crease and spread the inside with remoulade. Layer ¼ of the shrimp, ½ cup shredded lettuce, and 2 slices of tomato. Serve and enjoy!

Tilapia Teriyaki

Servings: 3
Cooking Time: 10 Minutes
Ingredients:
- 4 tablespoons teriyaki sauce
- 1 tablespoon pineapple juice
- 1 pound tilapia fillets
- cooking spray
- 6 ounces frozen mixed peppers with onions, thawed and drained
- 2 cups cooked rice

Directions:

1. Mix the teriyaki sauce and pineapple juice together in a small bowl.
2. Split tilapia fillets down the center lengthwise.
3. Brush all sides of fish with the sauce, spray air fryer basket with nonstick cooking spray, and place fish in the basket.
4. Stir the peppers and onions into the remaining sauce and spoon over the fish. Save any leftover sauce for drizzling over the fish when serving.
5. Cook at 360°F/1805°C for 10 minutes, until fish flakes easily with a fork and is done in center.
6. Divide into 3 or 4 servings and serve each with approximately ½ cup cooked rice.

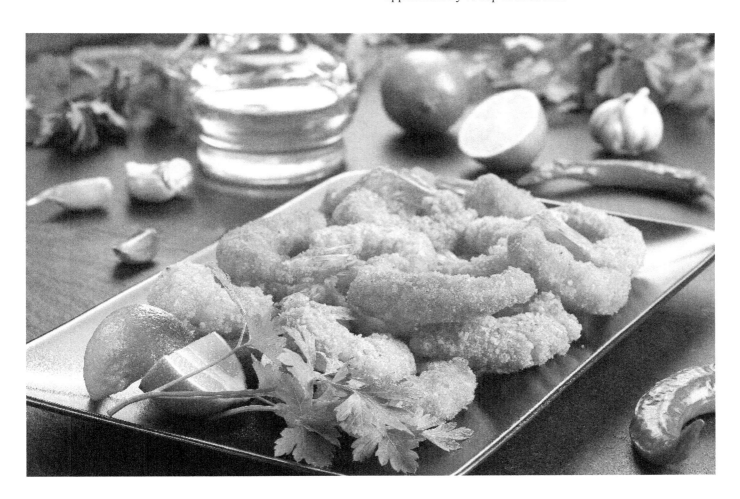

Beef, pork & Lamb Recipes

Pork Chops With Cereal Crust

Servings: 2
Cooking Time: 20 Minutes
Ingredients:
- ¼ cup grated Parmesan
- 1 egg
- 1 tbsp Dijon mustard
- ¼ cup crushed bran cereal
- ¼ tsp black pepper
- ¼ tsp cumin powder
- ¼ tsp nutmeg
- 1 tsp horseradish powder
- 2 pork chops

Directions:
1. Preheat air fryer at 350ºF/175°C. Whisk egg and mustard in a bowl. In another bowl, combine Parmesan cheese, cumin powder, nutmeg, horseradish powder, bran cereal, and black pepper. Dip pork chops in the egg mixture, then dredge them in the cheese mixture. Place pork chops in the frying basket and Air Fry for 12 minutes, tossing once. Let rest onto a cutting board for 5 minutes. Serve.

Original Köttbullar

Servings: 4
Cooking Time: 30 Minutes
Ingredients:
- 1 lb ground beef
- 1 small onion, chopped
- 1 clove garlic, minced
- 1/3 cup bread crumbs
- 1 egg, beaten
- Salt and pepper to taste
- 1 cup beef broth
- 1/3 cup heavy cream
- 2 tbsp flour

Directions:
1. Preheat air fryer to 370°F/185°C. Combine beef, onion, garlic, crumbs, egg, salt and pepper in a bowl. Scoop 2 tbsp of mixture and form meatballs with hands. Place the meatballs in the greased frying basket. Bake for 14 minutes.
2. Meanwhile, stir-fry beef broth and heavy cream in a saucepan over medium heat for 2 minutes; stir in flour. Cover and simmer for 4 minutes or until the sauce thicken. Transfer meatballs to a serving dish and drizzle with sauce. Serve and enjoy!

Santorini Steak Bowls

Servings:2
Cooking Time: 15 Minutes
Ingredients:
- 5 pitted Kalamata olives, halved
- 1 cucumber, diced
- 2 tomatoes, diced
- 1 tbsp apple cider vinegar
- 2 tsp olive oil
- ¼ cup feta cheese crumbles
- ½ tsp Greek oregano
- ½ tsp dried dill
- ¼ tsp garlic powder

- ⅛ tsp ground nutmeg
- Salt and pepper to taste
- 1 (¾-lb) strip steak

Directions:
1. In a large bowl, combine cucumber, tomatoes, vinegar, olive oil, olives, and feta cheese. Let chill covered in the fridge until ready to use. Preheat air fryer to 400ºF/205°C. Combine all spices in a bowl, then coat strip steak with this mixture. Add steak in the lightly greased frying basket and Air Fry for 10 minutes or until you reach your desired doneness, flipping once. Let sit onto a cutting board for 5 minutes.Thinly slice against the grain and divide between 2 bowls. Top with the cucumber mixture. Serve.

Sloppy Joes

Servings: 4
Cooking Time: 17 Minutes
Ingredients:
- oil for misting or cooking spray
- 1 pound very lean ground beef
- 1 teaspoon onion powder
- ⅓ cup ketchup
- ¼ cup water
- ½ teaspoon celery seed
- 1 tablespoon lemon juice
- 1½ teaspoons brown sugar
- 1¼ teaspoons low-sodium Worcestershire sauce
- ½ teaspoon salt (optional)
- ½ teaspoon vinegar
- ⅛ teaspoon dry mustard
- hamburger or slider buns

Directions:
1. Spray air fryer basket with nonstick cooking spray or olive oil.
2. Break raw ground beef into small chunks and pile into basket.
3. Cook at 390°F/200°C for 5minutes. Stir to break apart and cook 3minutes. Stir and cook 4 minutes longer or until meat is well done.
4. Remove meat from air fryer, drain, and use a knife and fork to crumble into small pieces.
5. Give your air fryer basket a quick rinse to remove any bits of meat.
6. Place all the remaining ingredients except the buns in a 6 x 6-inch baking pan and mix together.
7. Add meat and stir well.
8. Cook at 330°F/165°C for 5minutes. Stir and cook for 2minutes.
9. Scoop onto buns.

Beef Al Carbon (street Taco Meat)

Servings: 6
Cooking Time: 8 Minutes
Ingredients:
- 1½ pounds sirloin steak, cut into ½-inch cubes
- ¾ cup lime juice
- ½ cup extra-virgin olive oil
- 1 teaspoon ground cumin
- 2 teaspoons garlic powder
- 1 teaspoon salt

Directions:
1. In a large bowl, toss together the steak, lime juice, olive oil, cumin, garlic powder, and salt. Allow the meat to marinate for 30 minutes. Drain off all the marinade and pat the meat dry with paper towels.
2. Preheat the air fryer to 400°F/205°C.
3. Place the meat in the air fryer basket and spray with cooking spray. Cook the meat for 5 minutes, toss the meat, and continue cooking another 3 minutes, until slightly crispy.

Beef Fajitas

Servings:2
Cooking Time: 15 Minutes
Ingredients:
- 8 oz sliced mushrooms
- ½ onion, cut into half-moons
- 1 tbsp olive oil
- Salt and pepper to taste
- 1 strip steak
- ½ tsp smoked paprika
- ½ tsp fajita seasoning
- 2 tbsp corn

Directions:
1. Preheat air fryer to 400°F/205°C. Combine the olive oil, onion, and salt in a bowl. Add the mushrooms and toss to coat. Spread in the frying basket. Sprinkle steak with salt, paprika, fajita seasoning and black pepper. Place steak on top of the mushroom mixture and Air Fry for 9 minutes, flipping steak once. Let rest onto a cutting board for 5 minutes before cutting in half. Divide steak, mushrooms, corn, and onions between 2 plates and serve.

Teriyaki Country-style Pork Ribs

Servings: 3
Cooking Time: 30 Minutes
Ingredients:
- 3 tablespoons Regular or low-sodium soy sauce or gluten-free tamari sauce
- 3 tablespoons Honey
- ¾ teaspoon Ground dried ginger
- ¾ teaspoon Garlic powder
- 3 8-ounce boneless country-style pork ribs
- Vegetable oil spray

Directions:
1. Preheat the air fryer to 350°F/175°C .
2. Mix the soy or tamari sauce, honey, ground ginger, and garlic powder in another bowl until uniform.
3. Smear about half of this teriyaki sauce over all sides of the country-style ribs. Reserve the remainder of the teriyaki sauce. Generously coat the meat with vegetable oil spray.
4. When the machine is at temperature, place the country-style ribs in the basket with as much air space between them as possible. Air-fry undisturbed for 15 minutes. Turn the country-style ribs (but keep the space between them) and brush them all over with the remaining teriyaki sauce. Continue air-frying undisturbed for 15 minutes, or until an instant-read meat thermometer inserted into the center of one rib registers at least 145°F/60°C.
5. Use kitchen tongs to transfer the country-style ribs to a wire rack. Cool for 5 minutes before serving.

Easy Tex-mex Chimichangas

Servings: 2
Cooking Time: 8 Minutes
Ingredients:
- ¼ pound Thinly sliced deli roast beef, chopped
- ½ cup (about 2 ounces) Shredded Cheddar cheese or shredded Tex-Mex cheese blend
- ¼ cup Jarred salsa verde or salsa rojo
- ½ teaspoon Ground cumin
- ½ teaspoon Dried oregano
- 2 Burrito-size (12-inch) flour tortilla(s), not corn tortillas (gluten-free, if a concern)
- ⅔ cup Canned refried beans
- Vegetable oil spray

Directions:
1. Preheat the air fryer to 375°F/190°C .
2. Stir the roast beef, cheese, salsa, cumin, and oregano in a bowl until well mixed.
3. Lay a tortilla on a clean, dry work surface. Spread ⅓ cup of the refried beans in the center lower third of the tortilla(s), leaving an inch on either side of the spread beans.
4. For one chimichanga, spread all of the roast beef mixture on top of the beans. For two, spread half of the roast beef mixture on each tortilla.
5. At either "end" of the filling mixture, fold the sides of the tortilla up and over the filling, partially covering it. Starting with the unfolded side of the tortilla just below the filling, roll the tortilla closed. Fold and roll the second filled tortilla, as necessary.
6. Coat the exterior of the tortilla(s) with vegetable oil spray. Set the chimichanga(s) seam side down in the basket, with at least ½ inch air space between them if you're working with two. Air-fry undisturbed for 8 minutes, or until the tortilla is lightly browned and crisp.
7. Use kitchen tongs to gently transfer the chimichanga(s) to a wire rack. Cool for at last 5 minutes or up to 20 minutes before serving.

Korean-style Lamb Shoulder Chops

Servings: 3
Cooking Time: 28 Minutes
Ingredients:
- ⅓ cup Regular or low-sodium soy sauce or gluten-free tamari sauce
- 1½ tablespoons Toasted sesame oil
- 1½ tablespoons Granulated white sugar
- 2 teaspoons Minced peeled fresh ginger
- 1 teaspoon Minced garlic
- ¼ teaspoon Red pepper flakes
- 3 6-ounce bone-in lamb shoulder chops, any excess fat trimmed
- ⅔ cup Tapioca flour
- Vegetable oil spray

Directions:
1. Put the soy or tamari sauce, sesame oil, sugar, ginger, garlic, and red pepper flakes in a large, heavy zip-closed plastic bag. Add the chops, seal, and rub the marinade evenly over them through the bag. Refrigerate for at least 2 hours or up to 6 hours, turning the bag at least once so the chops move around in the marinade.
2. Set the bag out on the counter as the air fryer heats. Preheat the air fryer to 375°F/190°C .
3. Pour the tapioca flour on a dinner plate or in a small pie plate. Remove a chop from the marinade and dredge it on both sides in the tapioca flour, coating it evenly and well. Coat both sides with vegetable oil spray, set it in the basket, and dredge and spray the remaining chop(s), setting them in the basket in a single layer with space between them. Discard the bag with the marinade.
4. Air-fry, turning once, for 25 minutes, or until the chops are well browned and tender when pierced with the point of a paring knife. If the machine is at 360°F/180°C, you may need to add up to 3 minutes to the cooking time.
5. Use kitchen tongs to transfer the chops to a wire rack. Cool for just a couple of minutes before serving.

Steakhouse Filets Mignons

Servings: 3
Cooking Time: 12-15 Minutes
Ingredients:
- ¾ ounce Dried porcini mushrooms
- ¼ teaspoon Granulated white sugar
- ¼ teaspoon Ground white pepper
- ¼ teaspoon Table salt
- 6 ¼-pound filets mignons or beef tenderloin steaks
- 6 Thin-cut bacon strips (gluten-free, if a concern)

Directions:
1. Preheat the air fryer to 400°F/205°C.
2. Grind the dried mushrooms in a clean spice grinder until powdery. Add the sugar, white pepper, and salt. Grind to blend.
3. Rub this mushroom mixture into both cut sides of each filet. Wrap the circumference of each filet with a strip of bacon. (It will loop around the beef about 1½ times.)
4. Set the filets mignons in the basket on their sides with the bacon seam side down. Do not let the filets touch; keep at least ¼ inch open between them. Air-fry undisturbed for 12 minutes for rare, or until an instant-read meat thermometer inserted into the center of a filet registers 125°F/50°C (not USDA-approved); 13 minutes for medium-rare, or until an instant-read meat thermometer inserted into the center of a filet registers 132°F/55°C (not USDA-approved); or 15 minutes for medium, or until an instant-read meat thermometer inserted into the center of a filet registers 145°F (USDA-approved).
5. Use kitchen tongs to transfer the filets to a wire rack, setting them cut side down. Cool for 5 minutes before serving.

Tender Steak With Salsa Verde

Servings:4
Cooking Time: 20 Minutes
Ingredients:
- 1 flank steak, halved
- 1 ½ cups salsa verde
- ½ tsp black pepper

Directions:
1. Toss steak and 1 cup of salsa verde in a bowl and refrigerate covered for 2 hours. Preheat air fryer to 400ºF/205°C.Add steaks to the lightly greased frying basket and Air Fry for 10-12 minutes or until you reach your desired doneness, flipping once. Let sit onto a cutting board for 5 minutes. Thinly slice against the grain and divide between 4 plates. Spoon over the remaining salsa verde and serve sprinkled with black pepper to serve.

Italian Sausage Rolls

Servings: 4
Cooking Time: 20 Minutes
Ingredients:
- 1 red bell pepper, cut into strips
- 4 Italian sausages
- 1 zucchini, cut into strips
- ½ onion, cut into strips
- 1 tsp dried oregano
- ½ tsp garlic powder
- 5 Italian rolls

Directions:
1. Preheat air fryer to 360°F/180°C. Place all sausages in the air fryer. Bake for 10 minutes. While the sausages are cooking, season the bell pepper, zucchini and onion with oregano and garlic powder. When the time is up, flip the sausages, then add the peppers and onions. Cook for another 5 minutes or until the vegetables are soft and the sausages are cooked through. Put the sausage on Italian rolls, then top with peppers and onions. Serve.

Sriracha Pork Strips With Rice

Servings: 4
Cooking Time: 30 Minutes + Chilling Time
Ingredients:
- ½ cup lemon juice
- 2 tbsp lemon marmalade
- 1 tbsp avocado oil
- 1 tbsp tamari
- 2 tsp sriracha
- 1 tsp yellow mustard
- 1 lb pork shoulder strips
- 4 cups cooked white rice
- ¼ cup chopped cilantro
- 1 tsp black pepper

Directions:
1. Whisk the lemon juice, lemon marmalade, avocado oil, tamari, sriracha, and mustard in a bowl. Reserve half of the marinade. Toss pork strips with half of the marinade and let marinate covered in the fridge for 30 minutes.
2. Preheat air fryer at 350ºF/175°C. Place pork strips in the frying basket and Air Fry for 17 minutes, tossing twice. Transfer them to a bowl and stir in the remaining marinade. Serve over cooked rice and scatter with cilantro and pepper.

Steakhouse Burgers With Red Onion Compote

Servings: 4
Cooking Time: 22 Minutes
Ingredients:
- 1½ pounds lean ground beef
- 2 cloves garlic, minced and divided
- 1 teaspoon Worcestershire sauce
- 1 teaspoon sea salt, divided
- ½ teaspoon black pepper
- 1 tablespoon extra-virgin olive oil
- 1 red onion, thinly sliced
- ¼ cup balsamic vinegar
- 1 teaspoon sugar
- 1 tablespoon tomato paste
- 2 tablespoons mayonnaise
- 2 tablespoons sour cream
- 4 brioche hamburger buns
- 1 cup arugula

Directions:
1. In a large bowl, mix together the ground beef, 1 of the minced garlic cloves, the Worcestershire sauce, ½ teaspoon of the salt, and the black pepper. Form the meat into 1-inch-thick patties. Make a dent in the center (this helps the center cook evenly). Let the meat sit for 15 minutes.
2. Meanwhile, in a small saucepan over medium heat, cook the olive oil and red onion for 4 minutes, stirring frequently to avoid burning. Add in the balsamic vinegar, sugar, and tomato paste, and cook for an additional 3 minutes, stirring frequently. Transfer the onion compote to a small bowl.
3. Preheat the air fryer to 350°F/175°C.
4. In another small bowl, mix together the remaining minced garlic, the mayonnaise, and the sour cream. Spread the mayo mixture on the insides of the brioche buns.
5. Cook the hamburgers for 6 minutes, flip the burgers, and cook an additional 2 to 6 minutes. Check the internal temperature to avoid under- or overcooking. Hamburgers

should be cooked to at least 160°F/70°C. After cooking, cover with foil and let the meat rest for 5 minutes.

6. Meanwhile, place the buns inside the air fryer and toast them for 3 minutes.

7. To assemble the burgers, place the hamburger on one side of the bun, top with onion compote and ¼ cup arugula, and then place the other half of the bun on top.

Barbecue-style London Broil

Servings: 5
Cooking Time: 17 Minutes
Ingredients:
- ¾ teaspoon Mild smoked paprika
- ¾ teaspoon Dried oregano
- ¾ teaspoon Table salt
- ¾ teaspoon Ground black pepper
- ¼ teaspoon Garlic powder
- ¼ teaspoon Onion powder
- 1½ pounds Beef London broil (in one piece)
- Olive oil spray

Directions:
1. Preheat the air fryer to 400°F/205°C.
2. Mix the smoked paprika, oregano, salt, pepper, garlic powder, and onion powder in a small bowl until uniform.
3. Pat and rub this mixture across all surfaces of the beef. Lightly coat the beef on all sides with olive oil spray.
4. When the machine is at temperature, lay the London broil flat in the basket and air-fry undisturbed for 8 minutes for the small batch, 10 minutes for the medium batch, or 12 minutes for the large batch for medium-rare, until an instant-read meat thermometer inserted into the center of the meat registers 130°F/55°C (not USDA-approved). Add 1, 2, or 3 minutes, respectively (based on the size of the cut) for medium, until an instant-read meat thermometer registers 135°F/55°C (not USDA-approved). Or add 3, 4, or 5 minutes respectively for medium, until an instant-read meat thermometer registers 145°F/60°C (USDA-approved).
5. Use kitchen tongs to transfer the London broil to a cutting board. Let the meat rest for 10 minutes. It needs a long time for the juices to be reincorporated into the meat's fibers. Carve it against the grain into very thin (less than ¼-inch-thick) slices to serve.

Horseradish Mustard Pork Chops

Servings:2
Cooking Time: 20 Minutes
Ingredients:
- ½ cup grated Pecorino cheese
- 1 egg white
- 1 tbsp horseradish mustard
- ¼ tsp black pepper
- 2 pork chops
- ¼ cup chopped cilantro

Directions:
1. Preheat air fryer to 350°F/175°C. Whisk egg white and horseradish mustard in a bowl. In another bowl, combine Pecorino cheese and black pepper. Dip pork chops in the mustard mixture, then dredge them in the Parmesan mixture. Place pork chops in the frying basket lightly greased with olive oil and Air Fry for 12-14 minutes until cooked through and tender, flipping twice. Transfer the chops to a cutting board and let sit for 5 minutes. Scatter with cilantro to serve.

Better-than-chinese-take-out Sesame Beef

Servings: 4

Cooking Time: 14 Minutes
Ingredients:
- 1¼ pounds Beef flank steak
- 2½ tablespoons Regular or low-sodium soy sauce or gluten-free tamari sauce
- 2 tablespoons Toasted sesame oil
- 2½ teaspoons Cornstarch
- 1 pound 2 ounces (about 4½ cups) Frozen mixed vegetables for stir-fry, thawed, seasoning packet discarded
- 3 tablespoons Unseasoned rice vinegar (see here)
- 3 tablespoons Thai sweet chili sauce
- 2 tablespoons Light brown sugar
- 2 tablespoons White sesame seeds
- 2 teaspoons Water
- Vegetable oil spray
- 1½ tablespoons Minced peeled fresh ginger
- 1 tablespoon Minced garlic

Directions:
1. Set the flank steak on a cutting board and run your clean fingers across it to figure out which way the meat's fibers are running. (Usually, they run the long way from end to end, or perhaps slightly at an angle lengthwise along the cut.) Cut the flank steak into three pieces parallel to the meat's grain. Then cut each of these pieces into ½-inch-wide strips against the grain.
2. Put the meat strips in a large bowl. For a small batch, add 2 teaspoons of the soy or tamari sauce, 2 teaspoons of the sesame oil, and ½ teaspoon of the cornstarch; for a medium batch, add 1 tablespoon of the soy or tamari sauce, 1 tablespoon of the sesame oil, and 1 teaspoon of the cornstarch; and for a large batch, add 1½ tablespoons of the soy or tamari sauce, 1½ tablespoons of the sesame oil, and 1½ teaspoons of the cornstarch. Toss well until the meat is thoroughly coated in the marinade. Set aside at room temperature.
3. Preheat the air fryer to 400°F/205°C.
4. When the machine is at temperature, place the beef strips in the basket in as close to one layer as possible. The strips will overlap or even cover each other. Air-fry for 10 minutes, tossing and rearranging the strips three times so that the covered parts get exposed, until browned and even a little crisp. Pour the strips into a clean bowl.
5. Spread the vegetables in the basket and air-fry undisturbed for 4 minutes, just until they are heated through and somewhat softened. Pour these into the bowl with the meat strips. Turn off the air fryer.
6. Whisk the rice vinegar, sweet chili sauce, brown sugar, sesame seeds, the remaining soy sauce, and the remaining sesame oil in a small bowl until well combined. For a small batch, whisk the remaining 1 teaspoon cornstarch with the water in a second small bowl to make a smooth slurry; for medium batch, whisk the remaining 1½ teaspoons cornstarch with the water in a second small bowl to make a smooth slurry; and for a large batch, whisk the remaining 2 teaspoons cornstarch with the water in a second small bowl to make a smooth slurry.
7. Generously coat the inside of a large wok with vegetable oil spray, then set the wok over high heat for a few minutes. Add the ginger and garlic; stir-fry for 10 seconds or so, just until fragrant. Add the meat and vegetables; stir-fry for 1 minute to heat through.
8. Add the rice vinegar mixture and continue stir-frying until the sauce is bubbling, less than 1 minute. Add the cornstarch slurry and stir-fry until the sauce has thickened, just a few seconds. Remove the wok from the heat and serve hot.

Italian Sausage Bake

Servings: 4
Cooking Time: 25 Minutes
Ingredients:
- 1 cup red bell pepper, strips
- ¾ lb Italian sausage, sliced
- ½ cup minced onions
- 3 tbsp brown sugar
- 1/3 cup ketchup
- 2 tbsp mustard
- 2 tbsp apple cider vinegar
- ½ cup chicken broth

Directions:
1. Preheat air fryer to 350°F/175°C. Combine the Italian sausage, bell pepper, and minced onion into a bowl. Stir well. Mix together brown sugar, ketchup, mustard, apple cider vinegar, and chicken broth in a small bowl. Pour over the sausage. Place the bowl in the air fryer, and Bake until the sausage is hot, the vegetables are tender, and the sauce is bubbling and thickened, 10-15 minutes. Serve and enjoy!

Rib Eye Cheesesteaks With Fried Onions

Servings: 2
Cooking Time: 20 Minutes
Ingredients:
- 1 (12-ounce) rib eye steak
- 2 tablespoons Worcestershire sauce
- salt and freshly ground black pepper
- ½ onion, sliced
- 2 tablespoons butter, melted
- 4 ounces sliced Cheddar or provolone cheese
- 2 long hoagie rolls, lightly toasted

Directions:
1. Place the steak in the freezer for 30 minutes to make it easier to slice. When it is well-chilled, thinly slice the steak against the grain and transfer it to a bowl. Pour the Worcestershire sauce over the steak and season it with salt and pepper. Allow the meat to come to room temperature.
2. Preheat the air fryer to 400°F/205°C.
3. Toss the sliced onion with the butter and transfer it to the air fryer basket. Air-fry at 400°F/205°C for 12 minutes, shaking the basket a few times during the cooking process. Place the steak on top of the onions and air-fry for another 6 minutes, stirring the meat and onions together halfway through the cooking time.
4. When the air fryer has finished cooking, divide the steak and onions in half in the air fryer basket, pushing each half to one side of the air fryer basket. Place the cheese on top of each half, push the drawer back into the turned off air fryer and let it sit for 2 minutes, until the cheese has melted.
5. Transfer each half of the cheesesteak mixture into a toasted roll with the cheese side up and dig in!

Pork Kabobs With Pineapple

Servings: 4
Cooking Time: 30 Minutes
Ingredients:
- 2 cans juice-packed pineapple chunks, juice reserved
- 1 green bell pepper, cut into ½-inch chunks
- 1 red bell pepper, cut into ½-inch chunks
- 1 lb pork tenderloin, cubed
- Salt and pepper to taste
- 1 tbsp honey
- ½ tsp ground ginger
- ½ tsp ground coriander
- 1 red chili, minced

Directions:
1. Preheat the air fryer to 375°F/190°C. Mix the coriander, chili, salt, and pepper in a bowl. Add the pork and toss to coat. Then, thread the pork pieces, pineapple chunks, and bell peppers onto skewers. Combine the pineapple juice, honey, and ginger and mix well. Use all the mixture as you brush it on the kebabs. Put the kebabs in the greased frying basket and Air Fry for 10-14 minutes or until cooked through. Serve and enjoy!

Pork Cutlets With Almond-lemon Crust

Servings: 3
Cooking Time: 14 Minutes
Ingredients:
- ¾ cup Almond flour
- ¾ cup Plain dried bread crumbs (gluten-free, if a concern)
- 1½ teaspoons Finely grated lemon zest
- 1¼ teaspoons Table salt
- ¾ teaspoon Garlic powder
- ¾ teaspoon Dried oregano
- 1 Large egg white(s)
- 2 tablespoons Water
- 3 6-ounce center-cut boneless pork loin chops (about ¾ inch thick)
- Olive oil spray

Directions:
1. Preheat the air fryer to 375°F/190°C .
2. Mix the almond flour, bread crumbs, lemon zest, salt, garlic powder, and dried oregano in a large bowl until well combined.
3. Whisk the egg white(s) and water in a shallow soup plate or small pie plate until uniform.
4. Dip a chop in the egg white mixture, turning it to coat all sides, even the ends. Let any excess egg white mixture slip back into the rest, then set it in the almond flour mixture. Turn it several times, pressing gently to coat it evenly. Generously coat the chop with olive oil spray, then set aside to dip and coat the remaining chop(s).
5. Set the chops in the basket with as much air space between them as possible. Air-fry undisturbed for 12 minutes, or until browned and crunchy. You may need to add 2 minutes to the cooking time if the machine is at 360°F/180°C.
6. Use kitchen tongs to transfer the chops to a wire rack. Cool for a few minutes before serving.

Pepper Steak

Servings: 4
Cooking Time: 30 Minutes
Ingredients:
- 2 tablespoons cornstarch
- 1 tablespoon sugar
- ¾ cup beef broth
- ¼ cup hoisin sauce
- 3 tablespoons soy sauce
- 1 teaspoon sesame oil
- ½ teaspoon freshly ground black pepper
- 1½ pounds boneless New York strip steaks, sliced into ½-inch strips
- 1 onion, sliced
- 3 small bell peppers, red, yellow and green, sliced

Directions:
1. Whisk the cornstarch and sugar together in a large bowl to break up any lumps in the cornstarch. Add the beef broth

and whisk until combined and smooth. Stir in the hoisin sauce, soy sauce, sesame oil and freshly ground black pepper. Add the beef, onion and peppers, and toss to coat. Marinate the beef and vegetables at room temperature for 30 minutes, stirring a few times to keep meat and vegetables coated.
2. Preheat the air fryer to 350°F/175°C.
3. Transfer the beef, onion, and peppers to the air fryer basket with tongs, reserving the marinade. Air-fry the beef and vegetables for 30 minutes, stirring well two or three times during the cooking process.
4. While the beef is air-frying, bring the reserved marinade to a simmer in a small saucepan over medium heat on the stovetop. Simmer for 5 minutes until the sauce thickens.
5. When the steak and vegetables have finished cooking, transfer them to a serving platter. Pour the hot sauce over the pepper steak and serve with white rice.

Traditional Italian Beef Meatballs

Servings:4
Cooking Time: 35 Minutes
Ingredients:
- 1/3 cup grated Parmesan
- 1 lb ground beef
- 1 egg, beaten
- 2 tbsp tomato paste
- ½ tsp Italian seasonings
- ¼ cup ricotta cheese
- 3 cloves garlic, minced
- ¼ cup grated yellow onion
- Salt and pepper to taste
- ¼ cup almond flour
- ¼ cup chopped basil
- 2 cups marinara sauce

Directions:
1. Preheat air fryer to 400ºF/205°C. In a large bowl, combine ground beef, egg, tomato paste, Italian seasoning, ricotta cheese, Parmesan cheese, garlic, onion, salt, pepper, flour, and basil. Form mixture into 4 meatballs. Add them to the greased frying basket and Air Fry for 20 minutes. Warm the marinara sauce in a skillet over medium heat for 3 minutes. Add in cooked meatballs and roll them around in sauce for 2 minutes. Serve with sauce over the top.

Pork & Beef Egg Rolls

Servings: 8
Cooking Time: 8 Minutes
Ingredients:
- ¼ pound very lean ground beef
- ¼ pound lean ground pork
- 1 tablespoon soy sauce
- 1 teaspoon olive oil
- ½ cup grated carrots
- 2 green onions, chopped
- 2 cups grated Napa cabbage
- ¼ cup chopped water chestnuts
- ¼ teaspoon salt
- ¼ teaspoon garlic powder
- ¼ teaspoon black pepper
- 1 egg
- 1 tablespoon water
- 8 egg roll wraps
- oil for misting or cooking spray

Directions:
1. In a large skillet, brown beef and pork with soy sauce. Remove cooked meat from skillet, drain, and set aside.
2. Pour off any excess grease from skillet. Add olive oil, carrots, and onions. Sauté until barely tender, about 1 minute.

3. Stir in cabbage, cover, and cook for 1 minute or just until cabbage slightly wilts. Remove from heat.
4. In a large bowl, combine the cooked meats and vegetables, water chestnuts, salt, garlic powder, and pepper. Stir well. If needed, add more salt to taste.
5. Beat together egg and water in a small bowl.
6. Fill egg roll wrappers, using about ¼ cup of filling for each wrap. Roll up and brush all over with egg wash to seal. Spray very lightly with olive oil or cooking spray.
7. Place 4 egg rolls in air fryer basket and cook at 390°F/200°C for 4minutes. Turn over and cook 4 more minutes, until golden brown and crispy.
8. Repeat to cook remaining egg rolls.

Broccoli & Mushroom Beef

Servings: 4
Cooking Time: 30 Minutes
Ingredients:
- 1 lb sirloin strip steak, cubed
- 1 cup sliced cremini mushrooms
- 2 tbsp potato starch
- ½ cup beef broth
- 1 tsp soy sauce
- 2 ½ cups broccoli florets
- 1 onion, chopped
- 1 tbsp grated fresh ginger
- 1 cup cooked quinoa

Directions:
1. Add potato starch, broth, and soy sauce to a bowl and mix, then add in the beef and coat thoroughly. Marinate for 5 minutes. Preheat air fryer to 400°F/205°C. Set aside the broth and move the beef to a bowl. Add broccoli, onion, mushrooms, and ginger and transfer the bowl to the air fryer. Bake for 12-15 minutes until the beef is golden brown and the veggies soft. Pour the reserved broth over the beef and cook for 2-3 more minutes until the sauce is bubbling. Serve warm over cooked quinoa.

Double Cheese & Beef Burgers

Servings: 4
Cooking Time: 30 Minutes
Ingredients:
- 4 toasted onion buns, split
- ¼ cup breadcrumbs
- 2 tbsp milk
- 1 tp smoked paprika
- 6 tbsp salsa
- 2 tsp cayenne pepper
- 2 tbsp grated Cotija cheese
- 1 ¼ lb ground beef
- 4 Colby Jack cheese slices
- ¼ cup sour cream

Directions:
1. Preheat the air fryer to 375°F/190°C. Combine the breadcrumbs, milk, paprika, 2 tbsp of salsa, cayenne, and Cotija cheese in a bowl and mix. Let stand for 5 minutes. Add the ground beef and mix with your hands. Form into 4 patties and lay them on wax paper. Place the patties into the greased frying basket and Air Fry for 11-14 minutes, flipping once during cooking until golden and crunchy on the outside. Put a slice of Colby jack on top of each and cook for another minute until the cheese melts. Combine the remaining salsa with sour cream. Spread the mix on the bun bottoms, lay the patties on top, and spoon the rest of the mix over. Add the top buns and serve.

Perfect Strip Steaks

Servings: 2
Cooking Time: 17 Minutes
Ingredients:
- 1½ tablespoons Olive oil
- 1½ tablespoons Minced garlic
- 2 teaspoons Ground black pepper
- 1 teaspoon Table salt
- 2 ¾-pound boneless beef strip steak(s)

Directions:
1. Preheat the air fryer to 375°F/190°C (or 380°F/195°C or 390°F/200°C, if one of these is the closest setting).
2. Mix the oil, garlic, pepper, and salt in a small bowl, then smear this mixture over both sides of the steak(s).
3. When the machine is at temperature, put the steak(s) in the basket with as much air space as possible between them for the larger batch. They should not overlap or even touch. That said, even just a ¼-inch between them will work. Air-fry for 12 minutes, turning once, until an instant-read meat thermometer inserted into the thickest part of a steak registers 127°F/50°C for rare (not USDA-approved). Or air-fry for 15 minutes, turning once, until an instant-read meat thermometer registers 145°F/60°C for medium (USDA-approved). If the machine is at 390°F/200°C, the steaks may cook 2 minutes more quickly than the stated timing.
4. Use kitchen tongs to transfer the steak(s) to a wire rack. Cool for 5 minutes before serving.

Crunchy Fried Pork Loin Chops

Servings: 3
Cooking Time: 12 Minutes
Ingredients:
- 1 cup All-purpose flour or tapioca flour
- 1 Large egg(s), well beaten
- 1½ cups Seasoned Italian-style dried bread crumbs (gluten-free, if a concern)
- 3 4- to 5-ounce boneless center-cut pork loin chops
- Vegetable oil spray

Directions:
1. Preheat the air fryer to 350°F/175°C .
2. Set up and fill three shallow soup plates or small pie plates on your counter: one for the flour, one for the beaten egg(s), and one for the bread crumbs.
3. Dredge a pork chop in the flour, coating both sides as well as around the edge. Gently shake off any excess, then dip the chop in the egg(s), again coating both sides and the edge. Let any excess egg slip back into the rest, then set the chop in the bread crumbs, turning it and pressing gently to coat well on both sides and the edge. Coat the pork chop all over with vegetable oil spray and set aside so you can dredge, coat, and spray the additional chop(s).
4. Set the chops in the basket with as much air space between them as possible. Air-fry undisturbed for 12 minutes, or until brown and crunchy and an instant-read meat thermometer inserted into the center of a chop registers 145°F/60°C.
5. Use kitchen tongs to transfer the chops to a wire rack. Cool for 5 minutes before serving.

Ground Beef Calzones

Servings: 6
Cooking Time: 30 Minutes
Ingredients:
- 1 refrigerated pizza dough
- 1 cup shredded mozzarella
- ½ cup chopped onion
- 2 garlic cloves, minced
- ¼ cup chopped mushrooms
- 1 lb ground beef
- 1 tbsp pizza seasoning
- Salt and pepper to taste
- 1 ½ cups marinara sauce
- 1 tsp flour

Directions:
1. Warm 1 tbsp of oil in a skillet over medium heat. Stir-fry onion, garlic and mushrooms for 2-3 minutes or until aromatic. Add beef, pizza seasoning, salt and pepper. Use a large spoon to break up the beef. Cook for 3 minutes or until brown. Stir in marinara sauce and set aside.
2. On a floured work surface, roll out pizza dough and cut into 6 equal-sized rectangles. On each rectangle, add ½ cup of beef and top with 1 tbsp of shredded cheese. Fold one side of the dough over the filling to the opposite side. Press the edges using the back of a fork to seal them. Preheat air fryer to 400°F/205°C. Place the first batch of calzones in the air fryer and spray with cooking oil. Bake for 10 minutes. Let cool slightly and serve warm.

Argentinian Steak Asado Salad

Servings: 2
Cooking Time: 35 Minutes
Ingredients:
- 1 jalapeño pepper, sliced thin
- ¼ cup shredded pepper Jack cheese
- 1 avocado, peeled and pitted
- ¼ cup diced tomatoes
- ½ diced shallot
- 2 tsp chopped cilantro
- 2 tsp lime juice
- ½ lb flank steak
- 1 garlic clove, minced
- 1 tsp ground cumin
- Salt and pepper to taste
- ¼ lime
- 3 cups mesclun mix
- ½ cup pico de gallo

Directions:
1. Mash the avocado in a small bowl. Add tomatoes, shallot, cilantro, lime juice, salt, and pepper. Set aside. Season the steak with garlic, salt, pepper, and cumin.
2. Preheat air fryer to 400°F/205°C. Put the steak into the greased frying basket. Bake 8-10 minutes, flipping once until your desired doneness. Remove and let rest. Squeeze the lime over the steak and cut into thin slices. For one serving, plate half of mesclun, 2 tbsp of cheese, and ¼ cup guacamole. Place half of the steak slices on top t, then add ¼ cup pico de gallo and jalapeño if desired.

Pepperoni Pockets

Servings: 4
Cooking Time: 8 Minutes
Ingredients:
- 4 bread slices, 1-inch thick
- olive oil for misting
- 24 slices pepperoni (about 2 ounces)
- 1 ounce roasted red peppers, drained and patted dry
- 1 ounce Pepper Jack cheese cut into 4 slices
- pizza sauce (optional)

Directions:
1. Spray both sides of bread slices with olive oil.

2. Stand slices upright and cut a deep slit in the top to create a pocket—almost to the bottom crust but not all the way through.
3. Stuff each bread pocket with 6 slices of pepperoni, a large strip of roasted red pepper, and a slice of cheese.
4. Place bread pockets in air fryer basket, standing up. Cook at 360°F/180°C for 8 minutes, until filling is heated through and bread is lightly browned. Serve while hot as is or with pizza sauce for dipping.

Pesto-rubbed Veal Chops

Servings: 2
Cooking Time: 12-15 Minutes
Ingredients:
*   ¼ cup Purchased pesto
*   2 10-ounce bone-in veal loin or rib chop(s)
*   ½ teaspoon Ground black pepper
Directions:
1. Preheat the air fryer to 400°F/205°C.
2. Rub the pesto onto both sides of the veal chop(s). Sprinkle one side of the chop(s) with the ground black pepper. Set aside at room temperature as the machine comes up to temperature.
3. Set the chop(s) in the basket. If you're cooking more than one chop, leave as much air space between them as possible. Air-fry undisturbed for 12 minutes for medium-rare, or until an instant-read meat thermometer inserted into the center of a chop (without touching bone) registers 135°F/55°C (not USDA-approved). Or air-fry undisturbed for 15 minutes for medium-well, or until an instant-read meat thermometer registers 145°F/60°C (USDA-approved).
4. Use kitchen tongs to transfer the chops to a cutting board or a wire rack. Cool for 5 minutes before serving.

Cheeseburger Sliders With Pickle Sauce

Servings: 4
Cooking Time: 20 Minutes
Ingredients:
*   4 iceberg lettuce leaves, each halved lengthwise
*   2 red onion slices, rings separated
*   ¼ cup shredded Swiss cheese
*   1 lb ground beef
*   1 tbsp Dijon mustard
*   Salt and pepper to taste
*   ¼ tsp shallot powder
*   2 tbsp mayonnaise
*   2 tsp ketchup
*   ½ tsp mustard powder
*   ½ tsp dill pickle juice
*   ⅛ tsp onion powder
*   ⅛ tsp garlic powder
*   ⅛ tsp sweet paprika
*   8 tomato slices
*   ½ cucumber, thinly sliced
Directions:
1. In a large bowl, use your hands to mix beef, Swiss cheese, mustard, salt, shallot, and black pepper. Do not overmix. Form 8 patties ½-inch thick. Mix together mayonnaise, ketchup, mustard powder, pickle juice, onion and garlic powder, and paprika in a medium bowl. Stir until smooth.
2. Preheat air fryer to 400°F/205°C. Place the sliders in the greased frying basket and Air Fry for about 8-10 minutes, flipping once until preferred doneness. Serve on top of lettuce

halves with a slice of tomato, a slider, onion, a smear of special sauce, and cucumber.

Crispy Pork Medallions With Radicchio And Endive Salad

Servings: 4
Cooking Time: 7 Minutes
Ingredients:
*   1 (8-ounce) pork tenderloin
*   salt and freshly ground black pepper
*   ¼ cup flour
*   2 eggs, lightly beaten
*   ¾ cup cracker meal
*   1 teaspoon paprika
*   1 teaspoon dry mustard
*   1 teaspoon garlic powder
*   1 teaspoon dried thyme
*   1 teaspoon salt
*   vegetable or canola oil, in spray bottle
*   Vinaigrette
*   ¼ cup white balsamic vinegar
*   2 tablespoons agave syrup (or honey or maple syrup)
*   1 tablespoon Dijon mustard
*   juice of ½ lemon
*   2 tablespoons chopped chervil or flat-leaf parsley
*   salt and freshly ground black pepper
*   ½ cup extra-virgin olive oil
*   Radicchio and Endive Salad
*   1 heart romaine lettuce, torn into large pieces
*   ½ head radicchio, coarsely chopped
*   2 heads endive, sliced
*   ½ cup cherry tomatoes, halved
*   3 ounces fresh mozzarella, diced
*   salt and freshly ground black pepper
Directions:
1. Slice the pork tenderloin into 1-inch slices. Using a meat pounder, pound the pork slices into thin ½-inch medallions. Generously season the pork with salt and freshly ground black pepper on both sides.
2. Set up a dredging station using three shallow dishes. Place the flour in one dish and the beaten eggs in a second dish. Combine the cracker meal, paprika, dry mustard, garlic powder, thyme and salt in a third dish.
3. Preheat the air fryer to 400°F/205°C.
4. Dredge the pork medallions in flour first and then into the beaten egg. Let the excess egg drip off and coat both sides of the medallions with the cracker meal crumb mixture. Spray both sides of the coated medallions with vegetable or canola oil.
5. Air-fry the medallions in two batches at 400°F/205°C for 5 minutes. Once you have air-fried all the medallions, flip them all over and return the first batch of medallions back into the air fryer on top of the second batch. Air-fry at 400°F/205°C for an additional 2 minutes.
6. While the medallions are cooking, make the salad and dressing. Whisk the white balsamic vinegar, agave syrup, Dijon mustard, lemon juice, chervil, salt and pepper together in a small bowl. Whisk in the olive oil slowly until combined and thickened.
7. Combine the romaine lettuce, radicchio, endive, cherry tomatoes, and mozzarella cheese in a large salad bowl. Drizzle the dressing over the vegetables and toss to combine. Season with salt and freshly ground black pepper.
8. Serve the pork medallions warm on or beside the salad.

Wasabi-coated Pork Loin Chops

Servings: 3
Cooking Time: 14 Minutes
Ingredients:
- 1½ cups Wasabi peas
- ¼ cup Plain panko bread crumbs
- 1 Large egg white(s)
- 2 tablespoons Water
- 3 5- to 6-ounce boneless center-cut pork loin chops (about ½ inch thick)

Directions:
1. Preheat the air fryer to 375°F/190°C .
2. Put the wasabi peas in a food processor. Cover and process until finely ground, about like panko bread crumbs. Add the bread crumbs and pulse a few times to blend.
3. Set up and fill two shallow soup plates or small pie plates on your counter: one for the egg white(s), whisked with the water until uniform; and one for the wasabi pea mixture.
4. Dip a pork chop in the egg white mixture, coating the chop on both sides as well as around the edge. Allow any excess egg white mixture to slip back into the rest, then set the chop in the wasabi pea mixture. Press gently and turn it several times to coat evenly on both sides and around the edge. Set aside, then dip and coat the remaining chop(s).
5. Set the chops in the basket with as much air space between them as possible. Air-fry, turning once at the 6-minute mark, for 12 minutes, or until the chops are crisp and browned and an instant-read meat thermometer inserted into the center of a chop registers 145°F/60°C. If the machine is at 360°F, you may need to add 2 minutes to the cooking time.
6. Use kitchen tongs to transfer the chops to a wire rack. Cool for a couple of minutes before serving.

Egg Stuffed Pork Meatballs

Servings: 2
Cooking Time: 40 Minutes
Ingredients:
- 3 soft boiled eggs, peeled
- 8 oz ground pork
- 2 tsp dried tarragon
- ½ tsp hot paprika
- 2 tsp garlic powder
- Salt and pepper to taste

Directions:
1. Preheat air fryer to 350°F/175°C. Combine the pork, tarragon, hot paprika, garlic powder, salt, and pepper in a bowl and stir until all spices are evenly spread throughout the meat. Divide the meat mixture into three equal portions in the mixing bowl, and shape each into balls.
2. Flatten one of the meatballs on top to make a wide, flat meat circle. Place an egg in the middle. Use your hands to mold the mixture up and around to enclose the egg. Repeat with the remaining eggs. Place the stuffed balls in the air fryer. Air Fry for 18-20 minutes, shaking the basket once until the meat is crispy and golden brown. Serve.

Chipotle Pork Meatballs

Servings:4
Cooking Time: 35 Minutes
Ingredients:
- 1 lb ground pork
- 1 egg
- ¼ cup chipotle sauce
- ¼ cup grated celery
- ¼ cup chopped parsley
- ¼ cup chopped cilantro
- ¼ cup flour
- ¼ tsp salt

Directions:
1. Preheat air fryer to 350ºF/175°C. In a large bowl, combine the ground pork, egg, chipotle sauce, celery, parsley, cilantro, flour, and salt. Form mixture into 16 meatballs. Place the meatballs in the lightly greased frying basket and Air Fry for 8-10 minutes, flipping once. Serve immediately!

Flank Steak With Chimichurri Sauce

Servings: 4
Cooking Time: 25 Minutes + Chilling Time
Ingredients:
- For Marinade
- 2/3 cup olive oil
- 1 tbsp Dijon mustard
- 1 orange, juiced and zested
- 1 lime, juiced and zested
- 1/3 cup tamari sauce
- 2 tbsp red wine vinegar
- 4 cloves garlic, minced
- 1 flank steak
- For Chimichurri Sauce
- 2 red jalapeños, minced
- 1 cup Italian parsley leaves
- ¼ cup cilantro leaves
- ¼ cup oregano leaves
- ¼ cup olive oil
- ½ onion, diced
- 4 cloves garlic, minced
- 2 tbsp lime juice
- 2 tsp lime zest
- 2 tbsp red wine vinegar
- ½ tsp ground cumin
- ½ tsp salt

Directions:
1. Whisk all the marinade ingredients in a large bowl. Toss in flank steak and let marinate covered for at least 1 hour. In a food processor, blend parsley, cilantro, oregano, red jalapeños, olive oil, onion, garlic, lime juice, lime zest, vinegar, cumin, and salt until you reach your desired consistency. Let chill in the fridge until ready to use.
2. Preheat air fryer at 325ºF/160°C. Place flank steak in the greased frying basket and Bake for 18-20 minutes until rare, turning once. Let rest onto a cutting board for 5 minutes before slicing thinly against the grain. Serve with chimichurri sauce on the side.

Kentucky-style Pork Tenderloin

Servings:2
Cooking Time: 30 Minutes
Ingredients:
- 1 lb pork tenderloin, halved crosswise
- 1 tbsp smoked paprika
- 2 tsp ground cumin
- 1 tsp garlic powder
- 1 tsp shallot powder
- ¼ tsp chili pepper
- Salt and pepper to taste
- 1 tsp Italian seasoning
- 2 tbsp butter, melted
- 1 tsp Worcestershire sauce

Directions:

1. Preheat air fryer to 350ºF/175°C. In a shallow bowl, combine all spices. Set aside. In another bowl, whisk butter and Worcestershire sauce and brush over pork tenderloin. Sprinkle with the seasoning mix. Place pork in the lightly greased frying basket and Air Fry for 16 minutes, flipping once. Let sit onto a cutting board for 5 minutes before slicing. Serve immediately.

Indian Fry Bread Tacos

Servings: 4
Cooking Time: 20 Minutes
Ingredients:
- 1 cup all-purpose flour
- 1½ teaspoons salt, divided
- 1½ teaspoons baking powder
- ¼ cup milk
- ¼ cup warm water
- ½ pound lean ground beef
- One 14.5-ounce can pinto beans, drained and rinsed
- 1 tablespoon taco seasoning
- ½ cup shredded cheddar cheese
- 2 cups shredded lettuce
- ¼ cup black olives, chopped
- 1 Roma tomato, diced
- 1 avocado, diced
- 1 lime

Directions:
1. In a large bowl, whisk together the flour, 1 teaspoon of the salt, and baking powder. Make a well in the center and add in the milk and water. Form a ball and gently knead the dough four times. Cover the bowl with a damp towel, and set aside.
2. Preheat the air fryer to 380°F/195°C.
3. In a medium bowl, mix together the ground beef, beans, and taco seasoning. Crumble the meat mixture into the air fryer basket and cook for 5 minutes; toss the meat and cook an additional 2 to 3 minutes, or until cooked fully. Place the cooked meat in a bowl for taco assembly; season with the remaining ½ teaspoon salt as desired.
4. On a floured surface, place the dough. Cut the dough into 4 equal parts. Using a rolling pin, roll out each piece of dough to 5 inches in diameter. Spray the dough with cooking spray and place in the air fryer basket, working in batches as needed. Cook for 3 minutes, flip over, spray with cooking spray, and cook for an additional 1 to 3 minutes, until golden and puffy.
5. To assemble, place the fry breads on a serving platter. Equally divide the meat and bean mixture on top of the fry bread. Divide the cheese, lettuce, olives, tomatoes, and avocado among the four tacos. Squeeze lime over the top prior to serving.

Kielbasa Chunks With Pineapple & Peppers

Servings: 2
Cooking Time: 10 Minutes
Ingredients:
- ¾ pound kielbasa sausage
- 1 cup bell pepper chunks (any color)
- 1 8-ounce can pineapple chunks in juice, drained
- 1 tablespoon barbeque seasoning
- 1 tablespoon soy sauce
- cooking spray

Directions:
1. Cut sausage into ½-inch slices.
2. In a medium bowl, toss all ingredients together.

3. Spray air fryer basket with nonstick cooking spray.
4. Pour sausage mixture into the basket.
5. Cook at 390°F/200°C for approximately 5minutes. Shake basket and cook an additional 5minutes.

Tandoori Lamb Samosas

Servings: 2
Cooking Time: 20 Minutes
Ingredients:
- 6 oz ground lamb, sautéed
- ¼ cup spinach, torn
- ½ onion, minced
- 1 tsp tandoori masala
- ½ tsp ginger-garlic paste
- ½ tsp red chili powder
- ½ tsp turmeric powder
- Salt and pepper to taste
- 3 puff dough sheets

Directions:
1. Preheat air fryer to 350°F/175°C. Put the ground lamb, tandoori masala, ginger garlic paste, red chili powder, turmeric powder, salt, and pepper in a bowl and stir to combine. Add in the spinach and onion and stir until the ingredients are evenly blended. Divide the mixture into three equal segments.
2. Lay the pastry dough sheets out on a lightly floured surface. Fill each sheet of dough with one of the three portions of lamb mix, then fold the pastry over into a triangle, sealing the edges with a bit of water. Transfer the samosas to the greased frying basket and Air Fry for 12 minutes, flipping once until the samosas are crispy and flaky. Remove and leave to cool for 5 minutes. Serve.

Easy Carnitas

Servings: 3
Cooking Time: 25 Minutes
Ingredients:
- 1½ pounds Boneless country-style pork ribs, cut into 2-inch pieces
- ¼ cup Orange juice
- 2 tablespoons Brine from a jar of pickles, any type, even pickled jalapeño rings (gluten-free, if a concern)
- 2 teaspoons Minced garlic
- 2 teaspoons Minced fresh oregano leaves
- ¾ teaspoon Ground cumin
- ¾ teaspoon Table salt
- ¾ teaspoon Ground black pepper

Directions:
1. Mix the country-style pork rib pieces, orange juice, pickle brine, garlic, oregano, cumin, salt, and pepper in a large bowl. Cover and refrigerate for at least 2 hours or up to 10 hours, stirring the mixture occasionally.
2. Preheat the air fryer to 400°F/205°C. Set the rib pieces in their bowl on the counter as the machine heats.
3. Use kitchen tongs to transfer the rib pieces to the basket, arranging them in one layer. Some may touch. Air-fry for 25 minutes, turning and rearranging the pieces at the 10- and 20-minute marks to make sure all surfaces have been exposed to the air currents, until browned and sizzling.
4. Use clean kitchen tongs to transfer the rib pieces to a wire rack. Cool for a couple of minutes before serving.

Rosemary Lamb Chops

Servings: 4
Cooking Time: 6 Minutes
Ingredients:
- 8 lamb chops
- 1 tablespoon extra-virgin olive oil
- 1 teaspoon dried rosemary, crushed
- 2 cloves garlic, minced
- 1 teaspoon sea salt
- ¼ teaspoon black pepper

Directions:
1. In a large bowl, mix together the lamb chops, olive oil, rosemary, garlic, salt, and pepper. Let sit at room temperature for 10 minutes.
2. Meanwhile, preheat the air fryer to 380°F/195°C.
3. Cook the lamb chops for 3 minutes, flip them over, and cook for another 3 minutes.

Stuffed Pork Chops

Servings: 4
Cooking Time: 12 Minutes
Ingredients:
- 4 boneless pork chops
- ½ teaspoon salt
- ½ teaspoon black pepper
- ¼ teaspoon paprika
- 1 cup frozen spinach, defrosted and squeezed dry
- 2 cloves garlic, minced
- 2 ounces cream cheese
- ¼ cup grated Parmesan cheese
- 1 tablespoon extra-virgin olive oil

Directions:
1. Pat the pork chops with a paper towel. Make a slit in the side of each pork chop to create a pouch.
2. Season the pork chops with the salt, pepper, and paprika.
3. In a small bowl, mix together the spinach, garlic, cream cheese, and Parmesan cheese.
4. Divide the mixture into fourths and stuff the pork chop pouches. Secure the pouches with toothpicks.
5. Preheat the air fryer to 400°F/205°C.
6. Place the stuffed pork chops in the air fryer basket and spray liberally with cooking spray. Cook for 6 minutes, flip and coat with more cooking spray, and cook another 6 minutes. Check to make sure the meat is cooked to an internal temperature of 145°F/60°C. Cook the pork chops in batches, as needed.

Aromatic Pork Tenderloin

Servings: 6
Cooking Time: 65 Minutes
Ingredients:
- 1 pork tenderloin
- 2 tbsp olive oil
- 2 garlic cloves, minced
- 1 tsp dried sage
- 1 tsp dried marjoram
- 1 tsp dried thyme
- 1 tsp paprika
- Salt and pepper to taste

Directions:
1. Preheat air fryer to 360°F/180°C. Drizzle oil over the tenderloin, then rub garlic, sage, marjoram, thyme, paprika, salt and pepper all over. Place the tenderloin in the greased frying basket and Bake for 45 minutes. Flip the pork and cook for another 15 minutes. Check the temperature for doneness. Let the cooked tenderloin rest for 10 minutes before slicing. Serve and enjoy!

Exotic Pork Skewers

Servings: 4
Cooking Time: 30 Minutes
Ingredients:
- 1/3 cup apricot jam
- 2 tbsp lemon juice
- 2 tsp olive oil
- ½ tsp dried tarragon
- 1 lb pork tenderloin, cubed
- 4 pitted cherries, halved
- 4 pitted apricots, halved

Directions:
1. Preheat air fryer to 380°F/195°C. Toss the jam, lemon juice, olive oil, and tarragon in a big bowl and mix well. Place the pork in the bowl, then stir well to coat. Allow marinating for 10 minutes. Poke 4 metal skewers through the pork, cherries, and apricots, alternating ingredients. Use a cooking brush to rub the marinade on the skewers, then place them in the air fryer. Toss the rest of the marinade. Air Fry the kebabs for 4-6 minutes on each side until the pork is cooked through and the fruit is soft. Serve!

Lamb Burger With Feta And Olives

Servings: 3
Cooking Time: 16 Minutes
Ingredients:
- 2 teaspoons olive oil
- 1/3 onion, finely chopped
- 1 clove garlic, minced
- 1 pound ground lamb
- 2 tablespoons fresh parsley, finely chopped
- 1½ teaspoons fresh oregano, finely chopped
- ½ cup black olives, finely chopped
- 1/3 cup crumbled feta cheese
- ½ teaspoon salt
- freshly ground black pepper
- 4 thick pita breads
- toppings and condiments

Directions:
1. Preheat a medium skillet over medium-high heat on the stovetop. Add the olive oil and cook the onion until tender, but not browned – about 4 to 5 minutes. Add the garlic and cook for another minute. Transfer the onion and garlic to a mixing bowl and add the ground lamb, parsley, oregano, olives, feta cheese, salt and pepper. Gently mix the ingredients together.
2. Divide the mixture into 3 or 4 equal portions and then form the hamburgers, being careful not to over-handle the meat. One good way to do this is to throw the meat back and forth between your hands like a baseball, packing the meat each time you catch it. Flatten the balls into patties, making an indentation in the center of each patty. Flatten the sides of the patties as well to make it easier to fit them into the air fryer basket.
3. Preheat the air fryer to 370°F/185°C.
4. If you don't have room for all four burgers, air-fry two or three burgers at a time for 8 minutes at 370°F. Flip the burgers over and air-fry for another 8 minutes. If you cooked your burgers in batches, return the first batch of burgers to the air fryer for the last two minutes of cooking to re-heat. This should give you a medium-well burger. If you'd prefer a medium-rare burger, shorten the cooking time to about 13

minutes. Remove the burgers to a resting plate and let the burgers rest for a few minutes before dressing and serving.

5. While the burgers are resting, toast the pita breads in the air fryer for 2 minutes. Tuck the burgers into the toasted pita breads, or wrap the pitas around the burgers and serve with a tzatziki sauce or some mayonnaise.

Mongolian Beef

Servings: 4
Cooking Time: 15 Minutes
Ingredients:
- 1½ pounds flank steak, thinly sliced
- on the bias into ¼-inch strips
- Marinade
- 2 tablespoons soy sauce*
- 1 clove garlic, smashed
- big pinch crushed red pepper flakes
- Sauce
- 1 tablespoon vegetable oil
- 2 cloves garlic, minced
- 1 tablespoon finely grated fresh ginger
- 3 dried red chili peppers
- ¾ cup soy sauce*
- ¾ cup chicken stock
- 5 to 6 tablespoons brown sugar (depending on how sweet you want the sauce)
- ½ cup cornstarch, divided
- 1 bunch scallions, sliced into 2-inch pieces

Directions:
1. Marinate the beef in the soy sauce, garlic and red pepper flakes for one hour.
2. In the meantime, make the sauce. Preheat a small saucepan over medium heat on the stovetop. Add the oil, garlic, ginger and dried chili peppers and sauté for just a minute or two. Add the soy sauce, chicken stock and brown sugar and continue to simmer for a few minutes. Dissolve 3 tablespoons of cornstarch in 3 tablespoons of water and stir this into the saucepan. Stir the sauce over medium heat until it thickens. Set this aside.
3. Preheat the air fryer to 400°F/205°C.
4. Remove the beef from the marinade and transfer it to a zipper sealable plastic bag with the remaining cornstarch. Shake it around to completely coat the beef and transfer the coated strips of beef to a baking sheet or plate, shaking off any excess cornstarch. Spray the strips with vegetable oil on all sides and transfer them to the air fryer basket.
5. Air-fry at 400°F/205°C for 15 minutes, shaking the basket to toss and rotate the beef strips throughout the cooking process. Add the scallions for the last 4 minutes of the cooking. Transfer the hot beef strips and scallions to a bowl and toss with the sauce (warmed on the stovetop if necessary), coating all the beef strips with the sauce. Serve warm over white rice.

Minted Lamb Chops

Servings: 4
Cooking Time: 20 Minutes
Ingredients:
- 8 lamb chops
- 2 tsp olive oil
- 1 ½ tsp chopped mint leaves
- 1 tsp ground coriander
- 1 lemon, zested
- ½ tsp baharat seasoning
- 1 garlic clove, minced
- Salt and pepper to taste

Directions:

1. Preheat air fryer to 390°F/200°C. Coat the lamb chops with olive oil. Set aside. Mix mint, coriander, baharat, zest, garlic, salt and pepper in a bowl. Rub the seasoning onto both sides of the chops. Place the chops in the greased frying basket and Air Fry for 10 minutes. Flip the lamb chops and cook for another 5 minutes. Let the lamb chops rest for a few minutes. Serve right away.

Chile Con Carne Galette

Servings: 4
Cooking Time: 30 Minutes
Ingredients:
- 1 can chili beans in chili sauce
- ½ cup canned fire-roasted diced tomatoes, drained
- ½ cup grated Mexican cheese blend
- 2 tsp olive oil
- ½ lb ground beef
- ½ cup dark beer
- ½ onion, diced
- 1 carrot, peeled and diced
- 1 celery stalk, diced
- ½ tsp ground cumin
- ½ tsp chili powder
- ¼ tsp salt
- 1 cup corn chips
- 3 tbsp beef broth
- 2 tsp corn masa

Directions:
1. Warm the olive oil in a skillet over -high heat for 30 seconds. Add in ground beef, onion, carrot, and celery and cook for 5 minutes until the beef is no longer pink. Drain the fat. Mix 3 tbsp beef broth and 2 tsp corn mass until smooth and then toss it in beans, chili sauce, dark beer, tomatoes, cumin, chili powder, and salt. Cook until thickened. Turn the heat off.
2. Preheat air fryer at 350ºF/175°C. Spoon beef mixture into a cake pan, then top with corn chips, followed by cheese blend. Place cake pan in the frying basket and Bake for 6 minutes. Let rest for 10 minutes before serving.

Tasty Filet Mignon

Servings:2
Cooking Time: 30 Minutes
Ingredients:
- 2 filet mignon steaks
- ¼ tsp garlic powder
- Salt and pepper to taste
- 1 tbsp butter, melted

Directions:
1. Preheat air fryer to 370ºF/185°C. Sprinkle the steaks with salt, garlic and pepper on both sides. Place them in the greased frying basket and Air Fry for 12 minutes to yield a medium-rare steak, turning twice. Transfer steaks to a cutting board, brush them with butter and let rest 5 minutes before serving.

Sausage-cheese Calzone

Servings: 8
Cooking Time: 8 Minutes
Ingredients:
- Crust
- 2 cups white wheat flour, plus more for kneading and rolling
- 1 package (¼ ounce) RapidRise yeast
- 1 teaspoon salt
- ½ teaspoon dried basil
- 1 cup warm water (115°F to 125°F)
- 2 teaspoons olive oil

- Filling
- ¼ pound Italian sausage
- ½ cup ricotta cheese
- 4 ounces mozzarella cheese, shredded
- ¼ cup grated Parmesan cheese
- oil for misting or cooking spray
- marinara sauce for serving

Directions:
1. Crumble Italian sausage into air fryer baking pan and cook at 390°F/200°C for 5 minutes. Stir, breaking apart, and cook for 3 to 4 minutes, until well done. Remove and set aside on paper towels to drain.
2. To make dough, combine flour, yeast, salt, and basil. Add warm water and oil and stir until a soft dough forms. Turn out onto lightly floured board and knead for 3 or 4 minutes. Let dough rest for 10 minutes.
3. To make filling, combine the three cheeses in a medium bowl and mix well. Stir in the cooked sausage.
4. Cut dough into 8 pieces.
5. Working with 4 pieces of the dough, press each into a circle about 5 inches in diameter. Top each dough circle with 2 heaping tablespoons of filling. Fold over to create a half-moon shape and press edges firmly together. Be sure that edges are firmly sealed to prevent leakage. Spray both sides with oil or cooking spray.
6. Place 4 calzones in air fryer basket and cook at 360°F/180°C for 5 minutes. Mist with oil and cook for 3 minutes, until crust is done and nicely browned.
7. While the first batch is cooking, press out the remaining dough, fill, and shape into calzones.
8. Spray both sides with oil and cook for 5 minutes. If needed, mist with oil and continue cooking for 3 minutes longer. This second batch will cook a little faster than the first because your air fryer is already hot.
9. Serve with marinara sauce on the side for dipping.

Pork Taco Gorditas

Servings: 4
Cooking Time: 21 Minutes
Ingredients:
- 1 pound lean ground pork
- 2 tablespoons chili powder
- 2 tablespoons ground cumin
- 1 teaspoon dried oregano
- 2 teaspoons paprika
- 1 teaspoon garlic powder
- ½ cup water
- 1 (15-ounce) can pinto beans, drained and rinsed
- ½ cup taco sauce
- salt and freshly ground black pepper
- 2 cups grated Cheddar cheese
- 5 (12-inch) flour tortillas
- 4 (8-inch) crispy corn tortilla shells
- 4 cups shredded lettuce
- 1 tomato, diced
- ⅓ cup sliced black olives
- sour cream, for serving
- tomato salsa, for serving

Directions:
1. Preheat the air fryer to 400°F/205°C.
2. Place the ground pork in the air fryer basket and air-fry at 400°F/205°C for 10 minutes, stirring a few times during the cooking process to gently break up the meat. Combine the chili powder, cumin, oregano, paprika, garlic powder and water in a small bowl. Stir the spice mixture into the browned pork. Stir in the beans and taco sauce and air-fry for an additional minute. Transfer the pork mixture to a bowl. Season to taste with salt and freshly ground black pepper.

3. Sprinkle ½ cup of the shredded cheese in the center of four of the flour tortillas, making sure to leave a 2-inch border around the edge free of cheese and filling. Divide the pork mixture among the four tortillas, placing it on top of the cheese. Place a crunchy corn tortilla on top of the pork and top with shredded lettuce, diced tomatoes, and black olives. Cut the remaining flour tortilla into 4 quarters. These quarters of tortilla will serve as the bottom of the gordita. Place one quarter tortilla on top of each gordita and fold the edges of the bottom flour tortilla up over the sides, enclosing the filling. While holding the seams down, brush the bottom of the gordita with olive oil and place the seam side down on the countertop while you finish the remaining three gorditas.
4. Preheat the air fryer to 380°F/195°C.
5. Air-fry one gordita at a time. Transfer the gordita carefully to the air fryer basket, seam side down. Brush or spray the top tortilla with oil and air-fry for 5 minutes. Carefully turn the gordita over and air-fry for an additional 5 minutes, until both sides are browned. When finished air frying all four gorditas, layer them back into the air fryer for an additional minute to make sure they are all warm before serving with sour cream and salsa.

Taco Pie With Meatballs

Servings: 4
Cooking Time: 40 Minutes + Cooling Time
Ingredients:
- 1 cup shredded quesadilla cheese
- 1 cup shredded Colby cheese
- 10 cooked meatballs, halved
- 1 cup salsa
- 1 cup canned refried beans
- 2 tsp chipotle powder
- ½ tsp ground cumin
- 4 corn tortillas

Directions:
1. Preheat the air fryer to 375°F/190°C. Combine the meatball halves, salsa, refried beans, chipotle powder, and cumin in a bowl. In a baking pan, add a tortilla and top with one-quarter of the meatball mixture. Sprinkle one-quarter of the cheeses on top and repeat the layers three more times, ending with cheese. Put the pan in the fryer. Bake for 15-20 minutes until the pie is bubbling and the cheese has melted. Let cool on a wire rack for 10 minutes. Run a knife around the edges of the pan and remove the sides of the pan, then cut into wedges to serve.

Coffee-rubbed Pork Tenderloin

Servings: 4
Cooking Time: 30 Minutes
Ingredients:
- 1 tbsp packed brown sugar
- 2 tsp espresso powder
- 1 tsp bell pepper powder
- ½ tsp dried parsley
- 1 tbsp honey
- ½ tbsp lemon juice
- 2 tsp olive oil
- 1 pound pork tenderloin

Directions:
1. Preheat air fryer to 400°F/205°C. Toss the brown sugar, espresso powder, bell pepper powder, and parsley in a bowl and mix together. Add the honey, lemon juice, and olive oil, then stir well. Smear the pork with the mix, then allow to marinate for 10 minutes before putting it in the air fryer. Roast for 9-11 minutes until the pork is cooked through. Slice before serving.

Tuscan Chimichangas

Servings: 2
Cooking Time: 8 Minutes
Ingredients:

- ¼ pound Thinly sliced deli ham, chopped
- 1 cup Drained and rinsed canned white beans
- ½ cup (about 2 ounces) Shredded semi-firm mozzarella
- ¼ cup Chopped sun-dried tomatoes
- ¼ cup Bottled Italian salad dressing, vinaigrette type
- 2 Burrito-size (12-inch) flour tortilla(s)
- Olive oil spray

Directions:

1. Preheat the air fryer to 375°F/190°C .
2. Mix the ham, beans, cheese, tomatoes, and salad dressing in a bowl.
3. Lay a tortilla on a clean, dry work surface. Put all of the ham mixture in a narrow oval in the middle of the tortilla, if making one burrito; or half of this mixture, if making two. Fold the parts of the tortilla that are closest to the ends of the filling oval up and over the filling, then roll the tortilla tightly closed, but don't press down hard. Generously coat the tortilla with olive oil spray. Make a second filled tortilla, if necessary.
4. Set the filled tortilla(s) seam side down in the basket, with at least ½ inch between them, if making two. Air-fry undisturbed for 8 minutes, or until crisp and lightly browned.
5. Use kitchen tongs and a nonstick-safe spatula to transfer the chimichanga(s) to a wire rack. Cool for 5 minutes before serving.

Balsamic Beef & Veggie Skewers

Servings: 4
Cooking Time: 25 Minutes
Ingredients:

- 2 tbsp balsamic vinegar
- 2 tsp olive oil
- ½ tsp dried oregano
- Salt and pepper to taste
- ¾ lb round steak, cubed
- 1 red bell pepper, sliced
- 1 yellow bell pepper, sliced
- 1 cup cherry tomatoes

Directions:

1. Preheat air fryer to 390°F/200°C. Put the balsamic vinegar, olive oil, oregano, salt, and black pepper in a bowl and stir. Toss the steak in and allow to marinate for 10 minutes. Poke 8 metal skewers through the beef, bell peppers, and cherry tomatoes, alternating ingredients as you go. Place the skewers in the air fryer and Air Fry for 5-7 minutes, turning once until the beef is golden and cooked through and the veggies are tender. Serve and enjoy!

Friendly Bbq Baby Back Ribs

Servings: 4
Cooking Time: 35 Minutes
Ingredients:

- 1 rack baby back ribs, halved
- 1 tsp onion powder
- 1 tsp garlic powder
- 1 tsp brown sugar
- 1 tsp dried oregano
- 1 tsp ancho chili powder
- 1 tsp mustard powder
- Salt and pepper to taste
- ½ cup barbecue sauce

Directions:

1. Mix the onion powder, garlic powder, brown sugar, oregano, salt, mustard, ancho chili and pepper in a small bowl. Rub the seasoning all over the meat of the ribs. Cover the ribs in plastic wrap or foil. Sit for 30 minutes.
2. Preheat air fryer to 360°F/180°C. Place all of the ribs in the air fryer. Bake for 15 minutes, then use tongs to flip the ribs. Cook for another 15 minutes. Transfer to a serving dish and drizzle with barbecue sauce. Serve and enjoy!

Tex-mex Beef Carnitas

Servings: 4
Cooking Time: 30 Minutes
Ingredients:

- 1 ¼ lb flank steak, cut into strips
- 1 ½ cups grated Colby cheese
- Salt and pepper to taste
- 2 tbsp lime juice
- 4 garlic cloves, minced
- 2 tsp chipotle powder
- 1 red bell pepper, sliced
- 1 yellow bell pepper, sliced
- 1 tbsp chili oil
- ½ cup salsa
- 8 corn tortillas

Directions:

1. Preheat the air fryer to 400°F/205°C. Lay the strips in a bowl and sprinkle with salt, pepper, lime juice, garlic, and chipotle powder. Toss well and let marinate. In the frying basket, combine the bell peppers and chili oil and toss.
2. Air Fry for 6 minutes or until crispy but tender. Drain the steak and discard the liquid. Lay the steak in the basket on top of the peppers and fry for 7-9 minutes more until browned. Divide the strips among tortillas and top with pepper strips, salsa, and cheese. Fold and serve.

Cal-mex Chimichangas

Servings: 4
Cooking Time: 30 Minutes
Ingredients:

- 1 can diced tomatoes with chiles
- 1 cup shredded cheddar
- ½ cup chopped onions
- 2 garlic cloves, minced
- 1 lb ground beef
- 2 tbsp taco seasoning
- Salt and pepper to taste
- 4 flour tortillas
- ½ cup Pico de Gallo

Directions:

1. Warm the olive oil in a skillet over medium heat and stir-fry the onion and garlic for 3 minutes or until fragrant. Add ground beef, taco seasoning, salt and pepper. Stir and break up the beef with a spoon. Cook for 3-4 minutes or until it is browned. Stir in diced tomatoes with chiles. Scoop ½ cup of beef onto each tortilla. Form chimichangas by folding the sides of the tortilla into the middle, then roll up from the bottom. Use a toothpick to secure the chimichanga.
2. Preheat air fryer to 400°F/205°C. Lightly spray the chimichangas with cooking oil. Place the first batch in the fryer and Bake for 8 minutes. Transfer to a serving dish and top with shredded cheese and pico de gallo.

Vietnamese Beef Lettuce Wraps

Servings: 4
Cooking Time: 12 Minutes
Ingredients:
- ⅓ cup low-sodium soy sauce*
- 2 teaspoons fish sauce*
- 2 teaspoons brown sugar
- 1 tablespoon chili paste
- juice of 1 lime
- 2 cloves garlic, minced
- 2 teaspoons fresh ginger, minced
- 1 pound beef sirloin
- Sauce
- ⅓ cup low-sodium soy sauce*
- juice of 2 limes
- 1 tablespoon mirin wine
- 2 teaspoons chili paste
- Serving
- 1 head butter lettuce
- ½ cup julienned carrots
- ½ cup julienned cucumber
- ½ cup sliced radishes, sliced into half moons
- 2 cups cooked rice noodles
- ⅓ cup chopped peanuts

Directions:
1. Combine the soy sauce, fish sauce, brown sugar, chili paste, lime juice, garlic and ginger in a bowl. Slice the beef into thin slices, then cut those slices in half. Add the beef to the marinade and marinate for 1 to 3 hours in the refrigerator. When you are ready to cook, remove the steak from the refrigerator and let it sit at room temperature for 30 minutes.
2. Preheat the air fryer to 400°F/205°C.
3. Transfer the beef and marinade to the air fryer basket. Air-fry at 400°F/205°C for 12 minutes, shaking the basket a few times during the cooking process.
4. While the beef is cooking, prepare a wrap-building station. Combine the soy sauce, lime juice, mirin wine and chili paste in a bowl and transfer to a little pouring vessel. Separate the lettuce leaves from the head of lettuce and put them in a serving bowl. Place the carrots, cucumber, radish, rice noodles and chopped peanuts all in separate serving bowls.
5. When the beef has finished cooking, transfer it to another serving bowl and invite your guests to build their wraps. To build the wraps, place some beef in a lettuce leaf and top with carrots, cucumbers, some rice noodles and chopped peanuts. Drizzle a little sauce over top, fold the lettuce around the ingredients and enjoy!

Suwon Pork Meatballs

Servings: 4
Cooking Time: 30 Minutes
Ingredients:
- 1 lb ground pork
- 1 egg
- 1 tsp cumin
- 1 tbsp gochujang
- 1 tsp tamari
- ¼ tsp ground ginger
- ¼ cup bread crumbs
- 1 scallion, sliced
- 4 tbsp plum jam
- 1 tsp toasted sesame seeds

Directions:

1. Preheat air fryer at 350ºF/175°C. In a bowl, combine all ingredients, except scallion greens, sesame seeds and plum jam. Form mixture into meatballs. Place meatballs in the greased frying basket and Air Fry for 8 minutes, flipping once. Garnish with scallion greens, plum jam and toasted sesame seeds to serve.

Zesty London Broil

Servings: 4
Cooking Time: 28 Minutes
Ingredients:
- ⅔ cup ketchup
- ¼ cup honey
- ¼ cup olive oil
- 2 tablespoons apple cider vinegar
- 2 tablespoons Worcestershire sauce
- 2 tablespoons minced onion
- ½ teaspoon paprika
- 1 teaspoon salt
- 1 teaspoon freshly ground black pepper
- 2 pounds London broil, top round or flank steak (about 1-inch thick)

Directions:
1. Combine the ketchup, honey, olive oil, apple cider vinegar, Worcestershire sauce, minced onion, paprika, salt and pepper in a small bowl and whisk together.
2. Generously pierce both sides of the meat with a fork or meat tenderizer and place it in a shallow dish. Pour the marinade mixture over the steak, making sure all sides of the meat get coated with the marinade. Cover and refrigerate overnight.
3. Preheat the air fryer to 400°F/205°C.
4. Transfer the London broil to the air fryer basket and air-fry for 28 minutes, depending on how rare or well done you like your steak. Flip the steak over halfway through the cooking time.
5. Remove the London broil from the air fryer and let it rest for five minutes on a cutting board. To serve, thinly slice the meat against the grain and transfer to a serving platter.

Lamb Chops In Currant Sauce

Servings: 4
Cooking Time: 30 Minutes
Ingredients:
- ½ cup chicken broth
- 2 tbsp red currant jelly
- 2 tbsp Dijon mustard
- 1 tbsp lemon juice
- ½ tsp dried thyme
- ½ tsp dried mint
- 8 lamb chops
- Salt and pepper to taste

Directions:
1. Preheat the air fryer to 375°F/190°C. Combine the broth, jelly, mustard, lemon juice, mint, and thyme and mix with a whisk until smooth. Sprinkle the chops with salt and pepper and brush with some of the broth mixture.
2. Set 4 chops in the frying basket in a single layer, then add a raised rack and lay the rest of the chops on top. Bake for 15-20 minutes. Then, lay them in a cake pan and add the chicken broth mix. Put in the fryer and Bake for 3-5 more minutes or until the sauce is bubbling and the chops are tender.

Peppered Steak Bites

Servings: 4
Cooking Time: 14 Minutes
Ingredients:
- 1 pound sirloin steak, cut into 1-inch cubes
- ½ teaspoon coarse sea salt
- 1 teaspoon coarse black pepper
- 2 teaspoons Worcestershire sauce
- ½ teaspoon garlic powder
- ¼ teaspoon red pepper flakes
- ¼ cup chopped parsley

Directions:
1. Preheat the air fryer to 390°F/200°C.
2. In a large bowl, place the steak cubes and toss with the salt, pepper, Worcestershire sauce, garlic powder, and red pepper flakes.
3. Pour the steak into the air fryer basket and cook for 10 to 14 minutes, depending on how well done you prefer your bites. Starting at the 8-minute mark, toss the steak bites every 2 minutes to check for doneness.
4. When the steak is cooked, remove it from the basket to a serving bowl and top with the chopped parsley. Allow the steak to rest for 5 minutes before serving.

Traditional Moo Shu Pork Lettuce Wraps

Servings: 4
Cooking Time: 40 Minutes
Ingredients:
- ½ cup sliced shiitake mushrooms
- 1 lb boneless pork loin, cubed
- 3 tbsp cornstarch
- 2 tbsp rice vinegar
- 3 tbsp hoisin sauce
- 1 tsp oyster sauce
- 3 tsp sesame oil
- 1 tsp sesame seeds
- ¼ tsp ground ginger
- 1 egg
- 2 tbsp flour
- 1 bag coleslaw mix
- 1 cup chopped baby spinach
- 3 green onions, sliced
- 8 iceberg lettuce leaves

Directions:
1. Preheat air fryer at 350ºF/175°C. Make a slurry by whisking 1 tbsp of cornstarch and 1 tbsp of water in a bowl. Set aside. Warm a saucepan over heat, add in rice vinegar, hoisin sauce, oyster sauce, 1 tsp of sesame oil, and ginger, and cook for 3 minutes, stirring often. Add in cornstarch slurry and cook for 1 minute. Set aside and let the mixture thicken. Beat the egg, flour, and the remaining cornstarch in a bowl. Set aside.
2. Dredge pork cubes in the egg mixture. Shake off any excess. Place them in the greased frying basket and Air Fry for 8 minutes, shaking once. Warm the remaining sesame oil in a skillet over medium heat. Add in coleslaw mix, baby spinach, green onions, and mushrooms and cook for 5 minutes until the coleslaw wilts. Turn the heat off. Add in cooked pork, pour in oyster sauce mixture, and toss until coated. Divide mixture between lettuce leaves, sprinkle with sesame seed, roll them up, and serve.

Garlic And Oregano Lamb Chops

Servings: 4
Cooking Time: 17 Minutes
Ingredients:
- 1½ tablespoons Olive oil
- 1 tablespoon Minced garlic
- 1 teaspoon Dried oregano
- 1 teaspoon Finely minced orange zest
- ¾ teaspoon Fennel seeds
- ¾ teaspoon Table salt
- ¾ teaspoon Ground black pepper
- 6 4-ounce, 1-inch-thick lamb loin chops

Directions:
1. Mix the olive oil, garlic, oregano, orange zest, fennel seeds, salt, and pepper in a large bowl. Add the chops and toss well to coat. Set aside as the air fryer heats, tossing one more time.
2. Preheat the air fryer to 400°F/205°C.
3. Set the chops bone side down in the basket (that is, so they stand up on their bony edge) with as much air space between them as possible. Air-fry undisturbed for 14 minutes for medium-rare, or until an instant-read meat thermometer inserted into the thickest part of a chop (without touching bone) registers 132°F/55°C (not USDA-approved). Or air-fry undisturbed for 17 minutes for well done, or until an instant-read meat thermometer registers 145°F/60°C (USDA-approved).
4. Use kitchen tongs to transfer the chops to a wire rack. Cool for 5 minutes before serving.

Beef & Barley Stuffed Bell Peppers

Servings: 4
Cooking Time: 30 Minutes
Ingredients:
- 1 cup pulled cooked roast beef
- 4 bell peppers, tops removed
- 1 onion, chopped
- ½ cup grated carrot
- 2 tsp olive oil
- 2 tomatoes, chopped
- 1 cup cooked barley
- 1 tsp dried marjoram

Directions:
1. Preheat air fryer to 400°F/205°C. Cut the tops of the bell peppers, then remove the stems. Put the onion, carrots, and olive oil in a baking pan and cook for 2-4 minutes. The veggies should be crispy but soft. Put the veggies in a bowl, toss in the tomatoes, barley, roast beef, and marjoram, and mix to combine. Spoon the veggie mix into the cleaned bell peppers and put them in the frying basket. Bake for 12-16 minutes or until the peppers are tender. Serve warm.

Basil Cheese & Ham Stromboli

Servings: 6
Cooking Time: 30 Minutes
Ingredients:
- 1 can refrigerated pizza dough
- ½ cup shredded mozzarella
- ½ red bell pepper, sliced
- 2 tsp all-purpose flour
- 6 Havarti cheese slices
- 12 deli ham slices
- ½ tsp dried basil
- 1 tsp garlic powder
- ½ tsp oregano
- Black pepper to taste

Directions:

1. Preheat air fryer to 400°F/205°C. Flour a flat work surface and roll out the pizza dough. Use a knife to cut into 6 equal-sized rectangles. On each rectangle, add 1 slice of Havarti, 1 tbsp of mozzarella, 2 slices of ham, and some red pepper slices. Season with basil, garlic, oregano, and black pepper. Fold one side of the dough over the filling to the opposite side. Press the edges with the back of a fork to seal them.Place one batch of stromboli in the fryer and lightly spray with cooking oil. Air Fry for 10 minutes. Serve and enjoy!

Wasabi Pork Medallions

Servings: 4
Cooking Time: 20 Minutes + Marinate Time
Ingredients:
- 1 lb pork medallions
- 1 cup soy sauce
- 1 tbsp mirin
- ½ cup olive oil
- 3 cloves garlic, crushed
- 1 tsp fresh grated ginger
- 1 tsp wasabi paste
- 1 tbsp brown sugar

Directions:
1. Place all ingredients, except for the pork, in a resealable bag and shake to combine. Add the pork medallions to the bag, shake again, and place in the fridge to marinate for 2 hours. Preheat air fryer to 360°F/180°C. Remove pork medallions from the marinade and place them in the frying basket in rows. Air Fry for 14-16 minutes or until the medallions are cooked through and juicy. Serve.

City "chicken"

Servings: 3
Cooking Time: 10 Minutes
Ingredients:
- 1 pound Pork tenderloin, cut into 2-inch cubes
- ½ cup All-purpose flour or tapioca flour
- 1 Large egg(s)
- 1 teaspoon Dried poultry seasoning blend
- 1¼ cups Plain panko bread crumbs (gluten-free, if a concern)
- Vegetable oil spray

Directions:
1. Preheat the air fryer to 350°F/175°C .
2. Thread 3 or 4 pieces of pork on a 4-inch bamboo skewer. You'll need 2 or 3 skewers for a small batch, 3 or 4 for a medium, and up to 6 for a large batch.
3. Set up and fill three shallow soup plates or small pie plates on your counter: one for the flour; one for the egg(s), beaten with the poultry seasoning until foamy; and one for the bread crumbs.
4. Dip and roll one skewer into the flour, coating all sides of the meat. Gently shake off any excess flour, then dip and roll the skewer in the egg mixture. Let any excess egg mixture slip back into the rest, then set the skewer in the bread crumbs and roll it around, pressing gently, until the exterior surfaces of the meat are evenly coated. Generously coat the meat on the skewer with vegetable oil spray. Set aside and continue dredging, dipping, coating, and spraying the remaining skewers.
5. Set the skewers in the basket in one layer and air-fry undisturbed for 10 minutes, or until brown and crunchy.
6. Use kitchen tongs to transfer the skewers to a wire rack. Cool for a minute or two before serving.

Provençal Grilled Rib-eye

Servings: 4
Cooking Time: 25 Minutes
Ingredients:
- 4 ribeye steaks
- 1 tbsp herbs de Provence
- Salt and pepper to taste

Directions:
1. Preheat air fryer to 360°F/180°C. Season the steaks with herbs, salt and pepper. Place them in the greased frying basket and cook for 8-12 minutes, flipping once. Use a thermometer to check for doneness and adjust time as needed. Let the steak rest for a few minutes and serve.

Oktoberfest Bratwursts

Servings:4
Cooking Time: 35 Minutes
Ingredients:
- ½ onion, cut into half-moons
- 1 lb pork bratwurst links
- 2 cups beef broth
- 1 cup beer
- 2 cups drained sauerkraut
- 2 tbsp German mustard

Directions:
1. Pierce each bratwurst with a fork twice. Place them along with beef broth, beer, 1 cup of water, and onion in a saucepan over high heat and bring to a boil. Lower the heat and simmer for 15 minutes. Drain.
2. Preheat air fryer to 400°F/205°C. Place bratwursts and onion in the frying basket and Air Fry for 3 minutes. Flip bratwursts, add the sauerkraut and cook for 3 more minutes. Serve warm with mustard on the side.

Pizza Tortilla Rolls

Servings: 4
Cooking Time: 8 Minutes
Ingredients:
- 1 teaspoon butter
- ½ medium onion, slivered
- ½ red or green bell pepper, julienned
- 4 ounces fresh white mushrooms, chopped
- 8 flour tortillas (6- or 7-inch size)
- ½ cup pizza sauce
- 8 thin slices deli ham
- 24 pepperoni slices (about 1½ ounces)
- 1 cup shredded mozzarella cheese (about 4 ounces)
- oil for misting or cooking spray

Directions:
1. Place butter, onions, bell pepper, and mushrooms in air fryer baking pan. Cook at 390°F/200°C for 3minutes. Stir and cook 4 minutes longer until just crisp and tender. Remove pan and set aside.
2. To assemble rolls, spread about 2 teaspoons of pizza sauce on one half of each tortilla. Top with a slice of ham and 3 slices of pepperoni. Divide sautéed vegetables among tortillas and top with cheese.
3. Roll up tortillas, secure with toothpicks if needed, and spray with oil.
4. Place 4 rolls in air fryer basket and cook for 4minutes. Turn and cook 4 minutes, until heated through and lightly browned.
5. Repeat step 4 to cook remaining pizza rolls.

Chorizo & Veggie Bake

Servings: 4
Cooking Time: 40 Minutes
Ingredients:
- 1 cup halved Brussels sprouts
- 1 lb baby potatoes, halved
- 1 cup baby carrots
- 1 onion, sliced
- 2 garlic cloves, sliced
- 2 tbsp olive oil
- Salt and pepper to taste
- 1 lb chorizo sausages, sliced
- 2 tbsp Dijon mustard

Directions:
1. Preheat the air fryer to 370°F/185°C. Put the potatoes, Brussels sprouts, baby carrots, garlic, and onion in the frying basket and drizzle with olive oil. Sprinkle with salt and pepper; toss to coat. Bake for 15 minutes or until the veggies are crisp but tender, shaking once during cooking. Add the chorizo sausages to the fryer and cook for 8-12 minutes, shaking once until the sausages are hot and the veggies tender. Drizzle with the mustard to serve.

Indonesian Pork Satay

Servings: 4
Cooking Time: 30 Minutes
Ingredients:
- 1 lb pork tenderloin, cubed
- ¼ cup minced onion
- 2 garlic cloves, minced
- 1 jalapeño pepper, minced
- 2 tbsp lime juice
- 2 tbsp coconut milk
- ½ tbsp ground coriander
- ½ tsp ground cumin
- 2 tbsp peanut butter
- 2 tsp curry powder

Directions:
1. Combine the pork, onion, garlic, jalapeño, lime juice, coconut milk, peanut butter, ground coriander, cumin, and curry powder in a bowl. Stir well and allow to marinate for 10 minutes.
2. Preheat air fryer to 380°F/195°C. Use a holey spoon and take the pork out of the marinade and set the marinade aside. Poke 8 bamboo skewers through the meat, then place the skewers in the air fryer. Use a cooking brush to rub the marinade on each skewer, then Grill for 10-14 minutes, adding more marinade if necessary. The pork should be golden and cooked through when finished. Serve warm.

Kielbasa Sausage With Pierogies And Caramelized Onions

Servings: 3
Cooking Time: 30 Minutes
Ingredients:
- 1 Vidalia or sweet onion, sliced
- olive oil
- salt and freshly ground black pepper
- 2 tablespoons butter, cut into small cubes
- 1 teaspoon sugar
- 1 pound light Polish kielbasa sausage, cut into 2-inch chunks
- 1 (13-ounce) package frozen mini pierogies
- 2 teaspoons vegetable or olive oil
- chopped scallions

Directions:
1. Preheat the air fryer to 400°F/205°C.
2. Toss the sliced onions with a little olive oil, salt and pepper and transfer them to the air fryer basket. Dot the onions with pieces of butter and air-fry at 400°F/205°C for 2 minutes. Then sprinkle the sugar over the onions and stir. Pour any melted butter from the bottom of the air fryer drawer over the onions (do this over the sink – some of the butter will spill through the basket). Continue to air-fry for another 13 minutes, stirring or shaking the basket every few minutes to cook the onions evenly.
3. Add the kielbasa chunks to the onions and toss. Air-fry for another 5 minutes, shaking the basket halfway through the cooking time. Transfer the kielbasa and onions to a bowl and cover with aluminum foil to keep warm.
4. Toss the frozen pierogies with the vegetable or olive oil and transfer them to the air fryer basket. Air-fry at 400°F/205°C for 8 minutes, shaking the basket twice during the cooking time.
5. When the pierogies have finished cooking, return the kielbasa and onions to the air fryer and gently toss with the pierogies. Air-fry for 2 more minutes and then transfer everything to a serving platter. Garnish with the chopped scallions and serve hot with the spicy sour cream sauce below.
6. Kielbasa Sausage with Pierogies and Caramelized Onions

Pork Cutlets With Aloha Salsa

Servings: 4
Cooking Time: 9 Minutes
Ingredients:
- Aloha Salsa
- 1 cup fresh pineapple, chopped in small pieces
- ¼ cup red onion, finely chopped
- ¼ cup green or red bell pepper, chopped
- ½ teaspoon ground cinnamon
- 1 teaspoon low-sodium soy sauce
- ⅛ teaspoon crushed red pepper
- ⅛ teaspoon ground black pepper
- 2 eggs
- 2 tablespoons milk
- ¼ cup flour
- ¼ cup panko breadcrumbs
- 4 teaspoons sesame seeds
- 1 pound boneless, thin pork cutlets (⅜- to ½-inch thick)
- lemon pepper and salt
- ¼ cup cornstarch
- oil for misting or cooking spray

Directions:
1. In a medium bowl, stir together all ingredients for salsa. Cover and refrigerate while cooking pork.
2. Preheat air fryer to 390°F/200°C.
3. Beat together eggs and milk in shallow dish.
4. In another shallow dish, mix together the flour, panko, and sesame seeds.
5. Sprinkle pork cutlets with lemon pepper and salt to taste. Most lemon pepper seasoning contains salt, so go easy adding extra.
6. Dip pork cutlets in cornstarch, egg mixture, and then panko coating. Spray both sides with oil or cooking spray.
7. Cook cutlets for 3minutes. Turn cutlets over, spraying both sides, and continue cooking for 6 minutes or until well done.
8. Serve fried cutlets with salsa on the side.

Pork Tenderloin With Apples & Celery

Servings: 4
Cooking Time: 30 Minutes
Ingredients:
- 1 lb pork tenderloin, cut into 4 pieces
- 2 Granny Smith apples, sliced
- 1 tbsp butter, melted
- 2 tsp olive oil
- 3 celery stalks, sliced
- 1 onion, sliced
- 2 tsp dried thyme
- 1/3 cup apple juice

Directions:
1. Preheat air fryer to 400°F/205°C. Brush olive oil and butter all over the pork, then toss the pork, apples, celery, onion, thyme, and apple juice in a bowl and mix well. Put the bowl in the air fryer and Roast for 15-19 minutes until the pork is cooked through and the apples and veggies are soft, stirring once during cooking. Serve warm.

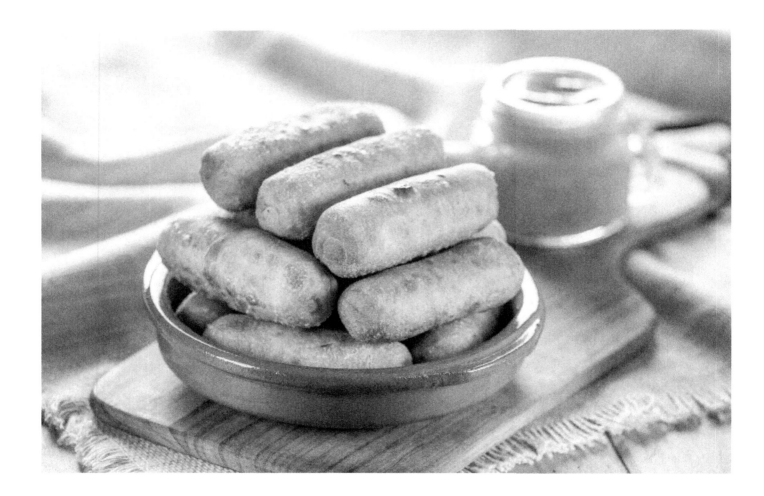

Vegetable Side Dishes Recipes

Five-spice Roasted Sweet Potatoes

Servings: 4
Cooking Time: 12 Minutes
Ingredients:
- ½ teaspoon ground cinnamon
- ¼ teaspoon ground cumin
- ¼ teaspoon paprika
- 1 teaspoon chile powder
- ⅛ teaspoon turmeric
- ½ teaspoon salt (optional)
- freshly ground black pepper
- 2 large sweet potatoes, peeled and cut into ¾-inch cubes (about 3 cups)
- 1 tablespoon olive oil

Directions:
1. In a large bowl, mix together cinnamon, cumin, paprika, chile powder, turmeric, salt, and pepper to taste.
2. Add potatoes and stir well.
3. Drizzle the seasoned potatoes with the olive oil and stir until evenly coated.
4. Place seasoned potatoes in the air fryer baking pan or an ovenproof dish that fits inside your air fryer basket.
5. Cook for 6minutes at 390°F/200°C, stop, and stir well.
6. Cook for an additional 6minutes.

Crispy Herbed Potatoes

Servings: 6
Cooking Time: 20 Minutes
Ingredients:
- 3 medium baking potatoes, washed and cubed
- ½ teaspoon dried thyme
- 1 teaspoon minced dried rosemary
- ½ teaspoon garlic powder
- 1 teaspoon sea salt
- ½ teaspoon black pepper
- 2 tablespoons extra-virgin olive oil
- ¼ cup chopped parsley

Directions:
1. Preheat the air fryer to 390°F/200°C.
2. Pat the potatoes dry. In a large bowl, mix together the cubed potatoes, thyme, rosemary, garlic powder, sea salt, and pepper. Drizzle and toss with olive oil.
3. Pour the herbed potatoes into the air fryer basket. Cook for 20 minutes, stirring every 5 minutes.
4. Toss the cooked potatoes with chopped parsley and serve immediately.
5. VARY IT! Potatoes are versatile — add any spice or seasoning mixture you prefer and create your own favorite side dish.

Perfect Broccoli

Servings: 4
Cooking Time: 12 Minutes
Ingredients:
- 5 cups (about 1 pound 10 ounces) 1- to 1½-inch fresh broccoli florets (not frozen)
- Olive oil spray
- ¾ teaspoon Table salt

Directions:
1. Preheat the air fryer to 375°F/190°C .
2. Put the broccoli florets in a big bowl, coat them generously with olive oil spray, then toss to coat all surfaces, even down into the crannies, spraying them in a couple of times more. Sprinkle the salt on top and toss again.
3. When the machine is at temperature, pour the florets into the basket. Air-fry for 10 minutes, tossing and rearranging the pieces twice so that all the covered or touching bits are eventually exposed to the air currents, until lightly browned but still crunchy. (If the machine is at 360°F/180°C, you may have to add 2 minutes to the cooking time.)
4. Pour the florets into a serving bowl. Cool for a minute or two, then serve hot.

Buttery Radish Wedges

Servings:2
Cooking Time: 20 Minutes
Ingredients:
- 2 tbsp butter, melted
- 2 cloves garlic, minced
- ¼ tsp salt
- 20 radishes, quartered
- 2 tbsp feta cheese crumbles
- 1 tbsp chopped parsley

Directions:
1. Preheat air fryer to 370ºF/185°C. Mix the butter, garlic, and salt in a bowl. Stir in radishes. Place the radish wedges in the frying basket and Roast for 10 minutes, shaking once. Transfer to a large serving dish and stir in feta cheese. Scatter with parsley and serve.

Brussels Sprouts

Serving: 3
Cooking Time: 5 Minutes
Ingredients:
- 1 10-ounce package frozen brussels sprouts, thawed and halved
- 2 teaspoons olive oil
- salt and pepper

Directions:
1. Toss the brussels sprouts and olive oil together.
2. Place them in the air fryer basket and season to taste with salt and pepper.
3. Cook at 360°F/180°C for approximately 5minutes, until the edges begin to brown.

Classic Stuffed Shells

Servings: 4
Cooking Time: 35 Minutes
Ingredients:
- 1 cup chopped spinach, cooked
- 1 cup shredded mozzarella
- 4 cooked jumbo shells
- 1 tsp dry oregano
- 1 cup ricotta cheese
- 1 egg, beaten
- 1 cup marinara sauce
- 1 tbsp basil leaves

Directions:
1. Preheat air fryer to 360°F/180°C. Place the beaten egg, oregano, ricotta, mozzarella, and chopped spinach in a bowl and mix until all the ingredients are combined. Fill the mixture into the cooked pasta shells. Spread half of the marinara sauce on a baking pan, then place the stuffed shells over the sauce. Spoon the remaining marinara sauce over the shells. Bake in the air fryer for 25 minutes or until the stuffed shells are wonderfully cooked, crispy on the outside with the spinach and cheeses inside gooey and delicious. Sprinkle with basil leaves and serve warm.

Chili-oiled Brussels Sprouts

Servings: 4
Cooking Time: 30 Minutes
Ingredients:
- 1 cup Brussels sprouts, quartered
- 1 tsp olive oil
- 1 tsp chili oil
- Salt and pepper to taste

Directions:
1. Preheat air fryer to 350°F/175°C. Coat the Brussels sprouts with olive oil, chili oil, salt, and black pepper in a bowl. Transfer to the frying basket. Bake for 20 minutes, shaking the basket several times throughout cooking until the sprouts are crispy, browned on the outside, and juicy inside. Serve and enjoy!

Breaded Artichoke Hearts

Servings: 2
Cooking Time: 25 Minutes
Ingredients:
- 1 can artichoke hearts in water, drained
- 1 egg
- ¼ cup bread crumbs
- ¼ tsp salt
- ¼ tsp hot paprika
- ½ lemon
- ¼ cup garlic aioli

Directions:
1. Preheat air fryer to 380°F/195°C. Whisk together the egg and 1 tbsp of water in a bowl until frothy. Mix together the bread crumbs, salt, and hot paprika in a separate bowl. Dip the artichoke hearts into the egg mixture, then coat in the bread crumb mixture. Put the artichoke hearts in a single layer in the frying basket. Air Fry for 15 minutes.
2. Remove the artichokes from the air fryer, and squeeze fresh lemon juice over the top. Serve with garlic aioli.

Grilled Lime Scallions

Servings:6
Cooking Time: 15 Minutes
Ingredients:
- 2 bunches of scallions
- 1 tbsp olive oil
- 2 tsp lime juice
- Salt and pepper to taste
- ¼ tsp Italian seasoning
- 2 tsp lime zest

Directions:
1. Preheat air fryer to 370ºF/185°C. Trim the scallions and cut them in half lengthwise. Place them in a bowl and add olive oil and lime juice. Toss to coat. Place the mix in the frying basket and Air Fry for 7 minutes, tossing once. Transfer to a serving dish and stir in salt, pepper, Italian seasoning and lime zest. Serve immediately.

Honey-mustard Asparagus Puffs

Servings: 4
Cooking Time: 35 Minutes
Ingredients:
- 8 asparagus spears
- ½ sheet puff pastry
- 2 tbsp honey mustard
- 1 egg, lightly beaten

Directions:
1. Preheat the air fryer to 375°F/190°C. Spread the pastry with honey mustard and cut it into 8 strips. Wrap the pastry, honey mustard–side in, around the asparagus. Put a rack in the frying basket and lay the asparagus spears on the rack. Brush all over pastries with beaten egg and Air Fry for 12-17 minutes or until the pastry is golden. Serve.

Jerk Rubbed Corn On The Cob

Servings: 4
Cooking Time: 6 Minutes
Ingredients:
- 1 teaspoon ground allspice
- 1 teaspoon dried thyme
- ½ teaspoon ground ginger
- ½ teaspoon ground cinnamon
- ¼ teaspoon ground nutmeg
- ⅛ teaspoon ground cayenne pepper
- 1 teaspoon salt
- 2 tablespoons butter, melted
- 4 ears of corn, husked

Directions:
1. Preheat the air fryer to 380°F/195°C.
2. Combine all the spices in a bowl. Brush the corn with the melted butter and then sprinkle the spices generously on all sides of each ear of corn.
3. Transfer the ears of corn to the air fryer basket. It's ok if they are crisscrossed on top of each other. Air-fry at 380°F/195°C for 6 minutes, rotating the ears as they cook.
4. Brush more butter on at the end and sprinkle with any remaining spice mixture.

Home Fries

Servings: 4
Cooking Time: 20 Minutes
Ingredients:
- 3 pounds potatoes, cut into 1-inch cubes
- ½ teaspoon oil
- salt and pepper

Directions:
1. In a large bowl, mix the potatoes and oil thoroughly.
2. Cook at 390°F/200°C for 10minutes and shake the basket to redistribute potatoes.
3. Cook for an additional 10 minutes, until brown and crisp.
4. Season with salt and pepper to taste.

Tasty Brussels Sprouts With Guanciale

Servings: 4
Cooking Time: 50 Minutes
Ingredients:
- 3 guanciale slices, halved
- 1 lb Brussels sprouts, halved
- 2 tbsp olive oil
- ¼ tsp salt
- ¼ tsp dried thyme

Directions:

1. Preheat air fryer to 350°F/175°C. Air Fry Lay the guanciale in the air fryer, until crispy, 10 minutes. Remove and drain on a paper towel. Give the guanciale a rough chop and Set aside. Coat Brussels sprouts with olive oil in a large bowl. Add salt and thyme, then toss. Place the sprouts in the frying basket. Air Fry for about 12-15 minutes, shake the basket once until the sprouts are golden and tender. Top with guanciale and serve.

Glazed Carrots

Servings: 4
Cooking Time: 10 Minutes
Ingredients:
- 2 teaspoons honey
- 1 teaspoon orange juice
- ½ teaspoon grated orange rind
- ⅛ teaspoon ginger
- 1 pound baby carrots
- 2 teaspoons olive oil
- ¼ teaspoon salt

Directions:
1. Combine honey, orange juice, grated rind, and ginger in a small bowl and set aside.
2. Toss the carrots, oil, and salt together to coat well and pour them into the air fryer basket.
3. Cook at 390°F/200°C for 5minutes. Shake basket to stir a little and cook for 4 minutes more, until carrots are barely tender.
4. Pour carrots into air fryer baking pan.
5. Stir the honey mixture to combine well, pour glaze over carrots, and stir to coat.
6. Cook at 360°F/180°C for 1 minute or just until heated through.

Blistered Shishito Peppers

Servings:2
Cooking Time: 15 Minutes
Ingredients:
- 20 shishito peppers
- 1 tsp sesame oil
- ½ tsp soy sauce
- ½ tsp grated ginger
- Salt to taste
- 1 tsp sesame seeds

Directions:
1. Preheat air fryer to 375ºF/190°C. Coat the peppers with sesame oil and salt in a bowl. Transfer them to the frying basket and Air Fry for 8 minutes or until blistered and softened, shaking the basket to turn the peppers. Drizzle with soy sauce and sprinkle with ginger and sesame seeds to serve.

Mexican-style Frittata

Servings: 4
Cooking Time: 35 Minutes
Ingredients:
- ½ cup shredded Cotija cheese
- ½ cup cooked black beans
- 1 cooked potato, sliced
- 3 eggs, beaten
- Salt and pepper to taste

Directions:
1. Preheat air fryer to 350°F/175°C. Mix the eggs, beans, half of Cotija cheese, salt, and pepper in a bowl. Pour the mixture into a greased baking dish. Top with potato slices. Place the baking dish in the frying basket and Air Fry for 10 minutes. Slide the basket out and sprinkle the remaining Cotija cheese over the dish. Cook for 10 more minutes or until golden and bubbling. Slice into wedges to serve.

Southwestern Sweet Potato Wedges

Servings: 4
Cooking Time: 30 Minutes
Ingredients:
- 2 sweet potatoes, peeled and cut into ½-inch wedges
- 2 tsp olive oil
- 2 tbsp cornstarch
- 1 tsp garlic powder
- ¼ tsp ground allspice
- ¼ tsp paprika
- ⅛ tsp cayenne pepper

Directions:
1. Preheat air fryer to 400°F/205°C. Place the sweet potatoes in a bowl. Add some olive oil and toss to coat, then transfer to the frying basket. Roast for 8 minutes. Sprinkle the potatoes with cornstarch, garlic powder, allspice, paprika, and cayenne, then toss. Put the potatoes back into the fryer and Roast for 12-17 more minutes. Shake the basket a couple of times while cooking. The potatoes should be golden and crispy. Serve warm.

Mediterranean Roasted Vegetables

Servings: 4
Cooking Time: 30 Minutes
Ingredients:
- 1 red bell pepper, cut into chunks
- 1 cup sliced mushrooms
- 1 cup green beans, diced
- 1 zucchini, sliced
- 1/3 cup diced red onion
- 3 garlic cloves, sliced
- 2 tbsp olive oil
- 1 tsp rosemary
- ½ tsp flaked sea salt

Directions:
1. Preheat air fryer to 350°F/175°C. Add the bell pepper, mushrooms, green beans, red onion, zucchini, rosemary, and garlic to a bowl and mix, then spritz with olive oil. Stir until well-coated. Put the veggies in the frying basket and Air Fry for 14-18 minutes. The veggies should be soft and crispy. Serve sprinkled with flaked sea salt.

Broccoli Au Gratin

Servings: 2
Cooking Time: 25 Minutes
Ingredients:
- 2 cups broccoli florets, chopped
- 6 tbsp grated Gruyère cheese
- 1 tbsp grated Pecorino cheese
- ½ tbsp olive oil
- 1 tbsp flour
- 1/3 cup milk
- ½ tsp ground coriander
- Salt and black pepper
- 2 tbsp panko bread crumbs

Directions:
1. Whisk the olive oil, flour, milk, coriander, salt, and pepper in a bowl. Incorporate broccoli, Gruyere cheese, panko bread crumbs, and Pecorino cheese until well combined. Pour in a greased baking dish.
2. Preheat air fryer to 330°F/165°C. Put the baking dish into the frying basket. Bake until the broccoli is crisp-tender and the top is golden, or about 12-15 minutes. Serve warm.

Okra

Servings: 4
Cooking Time: 12 Minutes
Ingredients:
- 7–8 ounces fresh okra
- 1 egg
- 1 cup milk
- 1 cup breadcrumbs
- ½ teaspoon salt
- oil for misting or cooking spray

Directions:
1. Remove stem ends from okra and cut in ½-inch slices.
2. In a medium bowl, beat together egg and milk. Add okra slices and stir to coat.
3. In a sealable plastic bag or container with lid, mix together the breadcrumbs and salt.
4. Remove okra from egg mixture, letting excess drip off, and transfer into bag with breadcrumbs.
5. Shake okra in crumbs to coat well.
6. Place all of the coated okra into the air fryer basket and mist with oil or cooking spray. Okra doesn't need to cook in a single layer, nor is it necessary to spray all sides at this point. A good spritz on top will do.
7. Cook at 390°F/200°C for 5minutes. Shake basket to redistribute and give it another spritz as you shake.
8. Cook 5 more minutes. Shake and spray again. Cook for 2 minutes longer or until golden brown and crispy.

Hasselback Garlic-and-butter Potatoes

Servings: 3
Cooking Time: 48 Minutes
Ingredients:
- 3 8-ounce russet potatoes
- 6 Brown button or Baby Bella mushrooms, very thinly sliced
- Olive oil spray
- 3 tablespoons Butter, melted and cooled
- 1 tablespoon Minced garlic
- ¾ teaspoon Table salt
- 3 tablespoons (about ½ ounce) Finely grated Parmesan cheese

Directions:
1. Preheat the air fryer to 350°F/175°C .
2. Cut slits down the length of each potato, about three-quarters down into the potato and spaced about ¼ inch apart. Wedge a thin mushroom slice in each slit. Generously coat the potatoes on all sides with olive oil spray.
3. When the machine is at temperature, set the potatoes mushroom side up in the basket with as much air space between them as possible. Air-fry undisturbed for 45 minutes, or tender when pricked with a fork.
4. Increase the machine's temperature to 400°F/205°C. Use kitchen tongs, and perhaps a flatware fork for balance, to gently transfer the potatoes to a cutting board. Brush each evenly with butter, then sprinkle the minced garlic and salt over them. Sprinkle the cheese evenly over the potatoes.
5. Use those same tongs to gently transfer the potatoes cheese side up to the basket in one layer with some space for air flow between them. Air-fry undisturbed for 3 minutes, or until the cheese has melted and begun to brown.
6. Use those same tongs to gently transfer the potatoes back to the wire rack. Cool for 5 minutes before serving.

Crunchy Roasted Potatoes

Servings: 5
Cooking Time: 25 Minutes
Ingredients:
- 2 pounds Small (1- to 1½-inch-diameter) red, white, or purple potatoes
- 2 tablespoons Olive oil
- 2 teaspoons Table salt
- ¾ teaspoon Garlic powder
- ½ teaspoon Ground black pepper

Directions:
1. Preheat the air fryer to 400°F/205°C.
2. Toss the potatoes, oil, salt, garlic powder, and pepper in a large bowl until the spuds are evenly and thoroughly coated.
3. When the machine is at temperature, pour the potatoes into the basket, spreading them into an even layer (although they may be stacked on top of each other). Air-fry for 25 minutes, tossing twice, until the potatoes are tender but crunchy.
4. Pour the contents of the basket into a serving bowl. Cool for 5 minutes before serving.

Chicken Salad With Sunny Citrus Dressing

Servings: 4
Cooking Time: 8 Minutes
Ingredients:
- Sunny Citrus Dressing
- 1 cup first cold-pressed extra virgin olive oil
- ⅓ cup red wine vinegar
- 2 tablespoons all natural orange marmalade
- 1 teaspoon dry mustard
- 1 teaspoon ground black pepper
- California Chicken
- 4 large chicken tenders
- 1 teaspoon olive oil
- juice of 1 small orange or clementine
- salt and pepper
- ½ teaspoon rosemary
- Salad
- 8 cups romaine or leaf lettuce, chopped or torn into bite-size pieces
- 2 clementines or small oranges, peeled and sectioned
- ½ cup dried cranberries
- 4 tablespoons sliced almonds

Directions:
1. In a 2-cup jar or container with lid, combine all dressing ingredients and shake until well blended. Refrigerate for at least 30minutes for flavors to blend.
2. Brush chicken tenders lightly with oil.
3. Drizzle orange juice over chicken.
4. Sprinkle with salt and pepper to taste.
5. Crush the rosemary and sprinkle over chicken.
6. Cook at 390°F/200°C for 3minutes, turn over, and cook for an additional 5 minutes or until chicken is tender and juices run clear.
7. When ready to serve, toss lettuce with 2 tablespoons of dressing to coat.
8. Divide lettuce among 4 plates or bowls. Arrange chicken and clementines on top and sprinkle cranberries and almonds. Pass extra dressing at the table.

Roasted Brussels Sprouts

Servings: 4
Cooking Time: 25 Minutes
Ingredients:
- ½ cup balsamic vinegar
- 2 tablespoons honey
- 1 pound Brussels sprouts, halved lengthwise
- 2 slices bacon, chopped
- ½ teaspoon garlic powder
- 1 teaspoon salt
- 1 tablespoon extra-virgin olive oil
- ¼ cup grated Parmesan cheese

Directions:
1. Preheat the air fryer to 370°F/185°C.
2. In a small saucepan, heat the vinegar and honey for 8 to 10 minutes over medium-low heat, or until the balsamic vinegar reduces by half to create a thick balsamic glazing sauce.
3. While the balsamic glaze is reducing, in a large bowl, toss together the Brussels sprouts, bacon, garlic powder, salt, and olive oil. Pour the mixture into the air fryer basket and cook for 10 minutes; check for doneness. Cook another 2 to 5 minutes or until slightly crispy and tender.
4. Pour the balsamic glaze into a serving bowl and add the cooked Brussels sprouts to the dish, stirring to coat. Top with grated Parmesan cheese and serve.

Brussels Sprout And Ham Salad

Servings: 3
Cooking Time: 12 Minutes
Ingredients:
- 1 pound 2-inch-in-length Brussels sprouts, quartered through the stem
- 6 ounces Smoked ham steak, any rind removed, diced (gluten-free, if a concern)
- ¼ teaspoon Caraway seeds
- Vegetable oil spray
- ¼ cup Brine from a jar of pickles (gluten-free, if a concern)
- ¾ teaspoon Ground black pepper

Directions:
1. Preheat the air fryer to 375°F/190°C .
2. Toss the Brussels sprout quarters, ham, and caraway seeds in a bowl until well combined. Generously coat the top of the mixture with vegetable oil spray, toss again, spray again, and repeat a couple of times until the vegetables and ham are glistening.
3. When the machine is at temperature, scrape the contents of the bowl into the basket, spreading it into as close to one layer as you can. Air-fry for 12 minutes, tossing and rearranging the pieces at least twice so that any covered or touching parts are eventually exposed to the air currents, until the Brussels sprouts are tender and a little brown at the edges.
4. Dump the contents of the basket into a serving bowl. Scrape any caraway seeds from the bottom of the basket or the tray under the basket attachment into the bowl as well. Add the pickle brine and pepper. Toss well to coat. Serve warm.

Air-fried Potato Salad

Servings: 4
Cooking Time: 15 Minutes
Ingredients:
- 1⅓ pounds Yellow potatoes, such as Yukon Golds, cut into ½-inch chunks
- 1 large Sweet white onion(s), such as Vidalia, chopped into ½-inch pieces
- 1 tablespoon plus 2 teaspoons Olive oil
- ¾ cup Thinly sliced celery
- 6 tablespoons Regular or low-fat mayonnaise (gluten-free, if a concern)
- 2½ tablespoons Apple cider vinegar
- 1½ teaspoons Dijon mustard (gluten-free, if a concern)
- ¾ teaspoon Table salt
- ¼ teaspoon Ground black pepper

Directions:
1. Preheat the air fryer to 400°F/205°C.
2. Toss the potatoes, onion(s), and oil in a large bowl until the vegetables are glistening with oil.
3. When the machine is at temperature, transfer the vegetables to the basket, spreading them out into as even a layer as you can. Air-fry for 15 minutes, tossing and rearranging the vegetables every 3 minutes so that all surfaces get exposed to the air currents, until the vegetables are tender and even browned at the edges.
4. Pour the contents of the basket into a serving bowl. Cool for at least 5 minutes or up to 30 minutes. Add the celery, mayonnaise, vinegar, mustard, salt, and pepper. Stir well to coat. The potato salad can be made in advance; cover and refrigerate for up to 4 days.

Acorn Squash Halves With Maple Butter Glaze

Servings: 2
Cooking Time: 33 Minutes
Ingredients:
- 1 medium (1 to 1¼ pounds) Acorn squash
- Vegetable oil spray
- ¼ teaspoon Table salt
- 1½ tablespoons Butter, melted
- 1½ tablespoons Maple syrup

Directions:
1. Preheat the air fryer to 325°F/160°C (or 330°F/165°C, if that's the closest setting).
2. Cut a squash in half through the stem end. Use a flatware spoon (preferably, a serrated grapefruit spoon) to scrape out and discard the seeds and membranes in each half. Use a paring knife to make a crisscross pattern of cuts about ½ inch apart and ¼ inch deep across the "meat" of the squash. If working with a second squash, repeat this step for that one.
3. Generously coat the cut side of the squash halves with vegetable oil spray. Sprinkle the halves with the salt. Set them in the basket cut side up with at least ¼ inch between them. Air-fry undisturbed for 30 minutes.
4. Increase the machine's temperature to 400°F. Mix the melted butter and syrup in a small bowl until uniform. Brush this mixture over the cut sides of the squash(es), letting it pool in the center. Air-fry undisturbed for 3 minutes, or until the glaze is bubbling.
5. Use a nonstick-safe spatula and kitchen tongs to transfer the squash halves cut side up to a wire rack. Cool for 5 to 10 minutes before serving.

Truffle Vegetable Croquettes

Servings: 4
Cooking Time: 40 Minutes
Ingredients:
- 2 cooked potatoes, mashed
- 1 cooked carrot, mashed
- 1 tbsp onion, minced
- 2 eggs, beaten

- 2 tbsp melted butter
- 1 tbsp truffle oil
- ½ tbsp flour
- Salt and pepper to taste

Directions:

1. Preheat air fryer to 350°F/175°C. Sift the flour, salt, and pepper in a bowl and stir to combine. Add the potatoes, carrot, onion, butter, and truffle oil to a separate bowl and mix well. Shape the potato mixture into small bite-sized patties. Dip the potato patties into the beaten eggs, coating thoroughly, then roll in the flour mixture to cover all sides. Arrange the croquettes in the greased frying basket and Air Fry for 14-16 minutes. Halfway through cooking, shake the basket. The croquettes should be crispy and golden. Serve hot and enjoy!

Almond Green Beans

Servings: 4
Cooking Time: 20 Minutes
Ingredients:

- 2 cups green beans, trimmed
- ¼ cup slivered almonds
- 2 tbsp butter, melted
- Salt and pepper to taste
- 2 tsp lemon juice
- Lemon zest and slices

Directions:

1. Preheat air fryer at 375ºF/190°C. Add almonds to the frying basket and Air Fry for 2 minutes, tossing once. Set aside in a small bowl. Combine the remaining ingredients, except 1 tbsp of butter, in a bowl.
2. Place green beans in the frying basket and Air Fry for 10 minutes, tossing once. Then, transfer them to a large serving dish. Scatter with the melted butter, lemon juice and roasted almonds and toss. Serve immediately garnished with lemon zest and lemon slices.

Roasted Brussels Sprouts With Bacon

Cooking Time: 20 Minutes
Servings: 4
Ingredients:

- 4 slices thick-cut bacon, chopped (about ¼ pound)
- 1 pound Brussels sprouts, halved (or quartered if large)
- freshly ground black pepper

Directions:

1. Preheat the air fryer to 380°F/195°C.
2. Air-fry the bacon for 5 minutes, shaking the basket once or twice during the cooking time.
3. Add the Brussels sprouts to the basket and drizzle a little bacon fat from the bottom of the air fryer drawer into the basket. Toss the sprouts to coat with the bacon fat. Air-fry for an additional 15 minutes, or until the Brussels sprouts are tender to a knifepoint.
4. Season with freshly ground black pepper.

Rosemary Roasted Potatoes With Lemon

Cooking Time: 12 Minutes
Servings: 4
Ingredients:

- 1 pound small red-skinned potatoes, halved or cut into bite-sized chunks
- 1 tablespoon olive oil
- 1 teaspoon finely chopped fresh rosemary
- ¼ teaspoon salt
- freshly ground black pepper

- 1 tablespoon lemon zest

Directions:

1. Preheat the air fryer to 400°F/205°C.
2. Toss the potatoes with the olive oil, rosemary, salt and freshly ground black pepper.
3. Air-fry for 12 minutes (depending on the size of the chunks), tossing the potatoes a few times throughout the cooking process.
4. As soon as the potatoes are tender to a knifepoint, toss them with the lemon zest and more salt if desired.

Beet Fries

Servings: 3
Cooking Time: 22 Minutes
Ingredients:

- 3 6-ounce red beets
- Vegetable oil spray
- To taste Coarse sea salt or kosher salt

Directions:

1. Preheat the air fryer to 375°F/190°C .
2. Remove the stems from the beets and peel them with a knife or vegetable peeler. Slice them into ½-inch-thick circles. Lay these flat on a cutting board and slice them into ½-inch-thick sticks. Generously coat the sticks on all sides with vegetable oil spray.
3. When the machine is at temperature, drop them into the basket, shake the basket to even the sticks out into as close to one layer as possible, and air-fry for 20 minutes, tossing and rearranging the beet matchsticks every 5 minutes, or until brown and even crisp at the ends. If the machine is at 360°F, you may need to add 2 minutes to the cooking time.
4. Pour the fries into a big bowl, add the salt, toss well, and serve warm.

Horseradish Potato Mash

Servings: 4
Cooking Time: 50 Minutes
Ingredients:

- 1 lb baby potatoes
- 1 tbsp horseradish sauce
- ½ cup vegetable broth
- ½ tsp sea salt
- 3 tbsp butter
- 2 garlic cloves, minced
- 2 tsp chili powder

Directions:

1. Preheat the air fryer to 400°F/205°C. Combine the potatoes, broth, and salt in a cake pan, then cover with foil and put it in the frying basket. Bake for 20 minutes, stirring once until they are almost tender. Drain and place them on a baking sheet. With the bottom of a glass, smash the potatoes, but don't break them apart. Put a small saucepan on the stove and mix butter, garlic, chili powder, and horseradish sauce. Melt the butter over low heat, then brush over the potatoes. Put as many as will fit in the basket in a single layer, butter-side down. Brush the tops with more of the butter mix, and Bake for 12-17 minutes, turning once until they're crisp. Keep the cooked potatoes warm in the oven at 250°F while air frying the rest of the potatoes.

Dauphinoise (potatoes Au Gratin)

Servings: 4
Cooking Time: 30 Minutes
Ingredients:

- ½ cup grated cheddar cheese
- 3 peeled potatoes, sliced
- ½ cup milk

- ½ cup heavy cream
- Salt and pepper to taste
- 1 tsp ground nutmeg

Directions:
1. Preheat air fryer to 350°F/175°C. Place the milk, heavy cream, salt, pepper, and nutmeg in a bowl and mix well. Dip in the potato slices and arrange on a baking dish. Spoon the remaining mixture over the potatoes. Scatter the grated cheddar cheese on top. Place the baking dish in the air fryer and Bake for 20 minutes. Serve warm and enjoy!

Lemony Fried Fennel Slices

Servings:2
Cooking Time: 15 Minutes
Ingredients:
- 1 tbsp minced fennel fronds
- 1 fennel bulb
- 2 tsp olive oil
- ¼ tsp salt
- 2 lemon wedges
- 1 tsp fennel seeds

Directions:
1. Preheat air fryer to 350ºF/175°C. Remove the fronds from the fennel bulb and reserve them. Cut the fennel into thin slices. Rub fennel chips with olive oil on both sides and sprinkle with salt and fennel seeds. Place fennel slices in the frying basket and Bake for 8 minutes. Squeeze lemon on top and scatter with chopped fronds. Serve.

Savory Brussels Sprouts

Servings: 4
Cooking Time: 15 Minutes
Ingredients:
- 1 lb Brussels sprouts, quartered
- 2 tbsp balsamic vinegar
- 1 tbsp olive oil
- 1 tbsp honey
- Salt and pepper to taste
- 1 ½ tbsp lime juice
- Parsley for sprinkling

Directions:
1. Preheat air fryer at 350ºF/175°C. Combine all ingredients in a bowl. Transfer them to the frying basket. Air Fry for 10 minutes, tossing once. Top with lime juice and parsley.

Roast Sweet Potatoes With Parmesan

Servings: 4
Cooking Time: 30 Minutes
Ingredients:
- 2 peeled sweet potatoes, sliced
- ¼ cup grated Parmesan
- 1 tsp olive oil
- 1 tbsp balsamic vinegar
- 1 tsp dried rosemary

Directions:
1. Preheat air fryer to 400°F/205°C. Place the sweet potatoes and some olive oil in a bowl and shake to coat. Spritz with balsamic vinegar and rosemary, then shake again. Put the potatoes in the frying basket and Roast for 18-25 minutes, shaking at least once until the potatoes are soft. Sprinkle with Parmesan cheese and serve warm.

Sage Hasselback Potatoes

Servings: 4

Cooking Time: 45 Minutes
Ingredients:
- 1 lb fingerling potatoes
- 1 tbsp olive oil
- 1 tbsp butter
- 1tsp dried sage
- Salt and pepper to taste

Directions:
1. Preheat the air fryer to 400°F/205°C. Rinse the potatoes dry, then set them on a work surface and put two chopsticks lengthwise on either side of each so you won't cut all the way through. Make vertical, crosswise cuts in the potato, about ⅛ inch apart. Repeat with the remaining potatoes. Combine the olive oil and butter in a bowl and microwave for 30 seconds or until melted. Stir in the sage, salt, and pepper. Put the potatoes in a large bowl and drizzle with the olive oil mixture. Toss to coat, then put the potatoes in the fryer and Air Fry for 22-27 minutes, rearranging them after 10-12 minutes. Cook until the potatoes are tender. Serve hot and enjoy!

Smooth & Silky Cauliflower Purée

Servings:4
Cooking Time: 25 Minutes
Ingredients:
- 1 head cauliflower, cut into florets
- 1 rutabaga, diced
- 4 tbsp butter, divided
- Salt and pepper to taste
- 3 cloves garlic, peeled
- 2 oz cream cheese, softened
- ½ cup milk
- 1 tsp dried thyme

Directions:
1. Preheat air fryer to 350ºF/175°C. Combine cauliflower, rutabaga, 2 tbsp of butter, and salt to taste in a bowl. Add veggie mixture to the frying basket and Air Fry for 10 minutes, tossing once. Put in garlic and Air Fry for 5 more minutes. Let them cool a bit, then transfer them to a blender. Blend them along with 2 tbsp of butter, salt, black pepper, cream cheese, thyme and milk until smooth. Serve immediately.

Perfect French Fries

Servings: 3
Cooking Time: 37 Minutes
Ingredients:
- 1 pound Large russet potato(es)
- Vegetable oil or olive oil spray
- ½ teaspoon Table salt

Directions:
1. Cut each potato lengthwise into ¼-inch-thick slices. Cut each of these lengthwise into ¼-inch-thick matchsticks.
2. Set the potato matchsticks in a big bowl of cool water and soak for 5 minutes. Drain in a colander set in the sink, then spread the matchsticks out on paper towels and dry them very well.
3. Preheat the air fryer to 225°F/105°C (or 230°F/110°C, if that's the closest setting).
4. When the machine is at temperature, arrange the matchsticks in an even layer (if overlapping but not compact) in the basket. Air-fry for 20 minutes, tossing and rearranging the fries twice.
5. Pour the contents of the basket into a big bowl. Increase the air fryer's temperature to 325°F/160°C (or 330°F/165°C, if that's the closest setting).
6. Generously coat the fries with vegetable or olive oil spray. Toss well, then coat them again to make sure they're

covered on all sides, tossing (and maybe spraying) a couple of times to make sure.

7.   When the machine is at temperature, pour the fries into the basket and air-fry for 12 minutes, tossing and rearranging the fries at least twice.

8.   Increase the machine's temperature to 375°F/190°C (or 380°F/195°C or 390°F/200°C, if one of these is the closest setting). Air-fry for 5 minutes more (from the moment you raise the temperature), tossing and rearranging the fries at least twice to keep them from burning and to make sure they all get an even measure of the heat, until brown and crisp.

9.   Pour the contents of the basket into a serving bowl. Toss the fries with the salt and serve hot.

Mouth-watering Provençal Mushrooms

Servings: 4
Cooking Time: 35 Minutes
Ingredients:
- 2 lb mushrooms, quartered
- 2-3 tbsp olive oil
- ½ tsp garlic powder
- 2 tsp herbs de Provence
- 2 tbsp dry white wine

Directions:
1.   Preheat air fryer to 320°F/160°C. Beat together the olive oil, garlic powder, herbs de Provence, and white wine in a bowl. Add the mushrooms and toss gently to coat. Spoon the mixture onto the frying basket and Bake for 16-18 minutes, stirring twice. Serve hot and enjoy!

Garlicky Bell Pepper Mix

Servings: 4
Cooking Time: 30 Minutes
Ingredients:
- 2 tbsp vegetable oil
- ½ tsp dried cilantro
- 1 red bell pepper
- 1 yellow bell pepper
- 1 orange bell pepper
- 1 green bell pepper
- Salt and pepper to taste
- 1 head garlic

Directions:
1.   Preheat air fryer to 330°F/165°C. Slice the peppers into 1-inch strips. Transfer them to a large bowl along with 1 tbsp of vegetable oil. Toss to coat. Season with cilantro, salt, and pepper. Cut the top of a garlic head and place it cut-side up on an oiled square of aluminium foil. Drizzle with vegetable oil and wrap completely in the foil.

2.   Roast the wrapped garlic in the air fryer for 15 minutes. Next, add the pepper strips and roast until the peppers are tender and the garlic is soft, 6-8 minutes. Transfer the peppers to a serving dish. Remove the garlic and unwrap the foil carefully. Once cooled, squeeze the cloves out of the garlic head and mix into the peppers' dish. Serve.

Citrusy Brussels Sprouts

Servings: 4
Cooking Time: 15 Minutes
Ingredients:
- 1 lb Brussels sprouts, quartered
- 1 clementine, cut into rings
- 2 garlic cloves, minced
- 1 tbsp olive oil
- 1 tbsp butter, melted
- ½ tsp salt

Directions:
1.   Preheat air fryer to 360°F/180°C. Add the quartered Brussels sprouts with the garlic, olive oil, butter and salt in a bowl and toss until well coated. Pour the Brussels sprouts into the air fryer, top with the clementine slices, and Roast for 10 minutes. Remove from the air fryer and set the clementines aside. Toss the Brussels sprouts and serve.

Spicy Bean Stuffed Potatoes

Servings: 4
Cooking Time: 60 Minutes
Ingredients:
- 1 lb russet potatoes, scrubbed and perforated with a fork
- 1 can diced green chilies, including juice
- 1/3 cup grated Mexican cheese blend
- 1 green bell pepper, diced
- 1 yellow bell pepper, diced
- ¼ cup torn iceberg lettuce
- 2 tsp olive oil
- 2 tbsp sour cream
- ½ tsp chili powder
- 2-3 jalapeños, sliced
- 1 red bell pepper, chopped
- Salt and pepper to taste
- 1/3 cup canned black beans
- 4 grape tomatoes, sliced
- ¼ cup chopped parsley

Directions:
1.   Preheat air fryer at 400°F/205°C. Brush olive oil over potatoes. Place them in the frying basket and Bake for 45 minutes, turning at 30 minutes mark. Let cool on a cutting board for 10 minutes until cool enough to handle. Slice each potato lengthwise and scoop out all but a ¼" layer of potato to form 4 boats.

2.   Mash potato flesh, sour cream, green chilies, cheese, chili powder, jalapeños, green, yellow, and red peppers, salt, and pepper in a bowl until smooth. Fold in black beans. Divide between potato skin boats. Place potato boats in the frying basket and Bake for 2 minutes. Remove them to a serving plate. Top each boat with lettuce, tomatoes, and parsley. Sprinkle tops with salt and serve.

Cheesy Potato Pot

Servings: 4
Cooking Time: 13 Minutes
Ingredients:
- 3 cups cubed red potatoes (unpeeled, cut into ½-inch cubes)
- ½ teaspoon garlic powder
- salt and pepper
- 1 tablespoon oil
- chopped chives for garnish (optional)
- Sauce
- 2 tablespoons milk
- 1 tablespoon butter
- 2 ounces sharp Cheddar cheese, grated
- 1 tablespoon sour cream

Directions:
1.   Place potato cubes in large bowl and sprinkle with garlic, salt, and pepper. Add oil and stir to coat well.

2.   Cook at 390°F/200°C for 13 minutes or until potatoes are tender. Stir every 4 or 5minutes during cooking time.

3.   While potatoes are cooking, combine milk and butter in a small saucepan. Warm over medium-low heat to melt butter. Add cheese and stir until it melts. The melted cheese will

remain separated from the milk mixture. Remove from heat until potatoes are done.

4. When ready to serve, add sour cream to cheese mixture and stir over medium-low heat just until warmed. Place cooked potatoes in serving bowl. Pour sauce over potatoes and stir to combine.

5. Garnish with chives if desired.

Homemade Potato Puffs

Servings: 4
Cooking Time: 15 Minutes
Ingredients:
- 1¾ cups Water
- 4 tablespoons (¼ cup/½ stick) Butter
- 2 cups plus 2 tablespoons Instant mashed potato flakes
- 1½ teaspoons Table salt
- ¾ teaspoon Ground black pepper
- ¼ teaspoon Mild paprika
- ¼ teaspoon Dried thyme
- 1¼ cups Seasoned Italian-style dried bread crumbs (gluten-free, if a concern)
- Olive oil spray

Directions:
1. Heat the water with the butter in a medium saucepan set over medium-low heat just until the butter melts. Do not bring to a boil.
2. Remove the saucepan from the heat and stir in the potato flakes, salt, pepper, paprika, and thyme until smooth. Set aside to cool for 5 minutes.
3. Preheat the air fryer to 400°F/205°C. Spread the bread crumbs on a dinner plate.
4. Scrape up 2 tablespoons of the potato flake mixture and form it into a small, oblong puff, like a little cylinder about 1½ inches long. Gently roll the puff in the bread crumbs until coated on all sides. Set it aside and continue making more, about 12 for the small batch, 18 for the medium batch, or 24 for the large.
5. Coat the potato cylinders with olive oil spray on all sides, then arrange them in the basket in one layer with some air space between them. Air-fry undisturbed for 15 minutes, or until crisp and brown.
6. Gently dump the contents of the basket onto a wire rack. Cool for 5 minutes before serving.

Latkes

Servings: 12
Cooking Time: 13 Minutes
Ingredients:
- 1 russet potato
- ¼ onion
- 2 eggs, lightly beaten
- ⅓ cup flour*
- ½ teaspoon baking powder
- 1 teaspoon salt
- freshly ground black pepper
- canola or vegetable oil, in a spray bottle
- chopped chives, for garnish
- apple sauce
- sour cream

Directions:
1. Shred the potato and onion with a coarse box grater or a food processor with the shredding blade. Place the shredded vegetables into a colander or mesh strainer and squeeze or press down firmly to remove the excess water.
2. Transfer the onion and potato to a large bowl and add the eggs, flour, baking powder, salt and black pepper. Mix to combine and then shape the mixture into patties, about ¼-cup of mixture each. Brush or spray both sides of the latkes with oil.
3. Preheat the air fryer to 400°F/205°C.
4. Air-fry the latkes in batches. Transfer one layer of the latkes to the air fryer basket and air-fry at 400°F/205°C for 12 to 13 minutes, flipping them over halfway through the cooking time. Transfer the finished latkes to a platter and cover with aluminum foil, or place them in a warm oven to keep warm.
5. Garnish the latkes with chopped chives and serve with sour cream and applesauce.

Zucchini Boats With Ham And Cheese

Servings: 4
Cooking Time: 12 Minutes
Ingredients:
- 2 6-inch-long zucchini
- 2 ounces Thinly sliced deli ham, any rind removed, meat roughly chopped
- 4 Dry-packed sun-dried tomatoes, chopped
- ⅓ cup Purchased pesto
- ¼ cup Packaged mini croutons
- ¼ cup (about 1 ounce) Shredded semi-firm mozzarella cheese

Directions:
1. Preheat the air fryer to 375°F/190°C .
2. Split the zucchini in half lengthwise and use a flatware spoon or a serrated grapefruit spoon to scoop out the insides of the halves, leaving at least a ¼-inch border all around the zucchini half. (You can save the scooped out insides to add to soups and stews—or even freeze it for a much later use.)
3. Mix the ham, sun-dried tomatoes, pesto, croutons, and half the cheese in a bowl until well combined. Pack this mixture into the zucchini "shells." Top them with the remaining cheese.
4. Set them stuffing side up in the basket without touching (even a fraction of an inch between them is enough room). Air-fry undisturbed for 12 minutes, or until softened and browned, with the cheese melted on top.
5. Use a nonstick-safe spatula to transfer the zucchini boats stuffing side up on a wire rack. Cool for 5 or 10 minutes before serving.

Bacon-wrapped Asparagus

Servings: 4
Cooking Time: 10 Minutes
Ingredients:
- 1 tablespoon extra-virgin olive oil
- ½ teaspoon sea salt
- ¼ cup grated Parmesan cheese
- 1 pound asparagus, ends trimmed
- 8 slices bacon

Directions:
1. Preheat the air fryer to 380°F/195°C.
2. In large bowl, mix together the olive oil, sea salt, and Parmesan cheese. Toss the asparagus in the olive oil mixture.
3. Evenly divide the asparagus into 8 bundles. Wrap 1 piece of bacon around each bundle, not overlapping the bacon but spreading it across the bundle.
4. Place the asparagus bundles into the air fryer basket, not touching. Work in batches as needed.
5. Cook for 8 minutes; check for doneness, and cook another 2 minutes.

French Fries

Servings: 4
Cooking Time: 25 Minutes
Ingredients:
- 2 cups fresh potatoes
- 2 teaspoons oil
- ½ teaspoon salt

Directions:
1. Cut potatoes into ½-inch-wide slices, then lay slices flat and cut into ½-inch sticks.
2. Rinse potato sticks and blot dry with a clean towel.
3. In a bowl or sealable plastic bag, mix the potatoes, oil, and salt together.
4. Pour into air fryer basket.
5. Cook at 390°F/200°C for 10minutes. Shake basket to redistribute fries and continue cooking for approximately 15minutes, until fries are golden brown.

Simple Green Bake

Servings: 4
Cooking Time: 15 Minutes
Ingredients:
- 1 cup asparagus, chopped
- 2 cups broccoli florets
- 1 tbsp olive oil
- 1 tbsp lemon juice
- 1 cup green peas
- 2 tbsp honey mustard
- Salt and pepper to taste

Directions:
1. Preheat air fryer to 330°F/165°C. Add asparagus and broccoli to the frying basket. Drizzle with olive oil and lemon juice and toss. Bake for 6 minutes. Remove the basket and add peas. Steam for another 3 minutes or until the vegetables are hot and tender. Pour the vegetables into a serving dish. Drizzle with honey mustard and season with salt and pepper. Toss and serve warm.

Lovely Mac`n´cheese

Servings: 4
Cooking Time: 40 Minutes
Ingredients:
- 2 cups grated American cheese
- 4 cups elbow macaroni
- 3 egg, beaten
- ½ cup sour cream
- 4 tbsp butter
- ½ tsp mustard powder
- ½ tsp salt
- 1 cup milk

Directions:
1. Preheat air fryer to 350°F/175°C. Bring a pot of salted water to a boil and cook the macaroni following the packet instructions. Drain and place in a bowl.
2. Add 1 ½ cups of cheese and butter to the hot macaroni and stir to melt. Mix the beaten eggs, milk, sour cream, mustard powder, and salt in a bowl and add the mixture to the macaroni; mix gently. Spoon the macaroni mixture into a greased baking dish and transfer the dish to the air fryer. Bake for 15 minutes. Slide the dish out and sprinkle with the remaining American cheese. Cook for 5-8 more minutes until the top is bubbling and golden. Serve.

Cheese-rice Stuffed Bell Peppers

Servings: 4
Cooking Time: 30 Minutes
Ingredients:
- 2 red bell peppers, halved and seeds and stem removed
- 1 cup cooked brown rice
- 2 tomatoes, diced
- 1 garlic clove, minced
- Salt and pepper to taste
- 4 oz goat cheese
- 3 tbsp basil, chopped
- 3 tbsp oregano, chopped
- 1 tbsp parsley, chopped
- ¼ cup grated Parmesan

Directions:
1. Preheat air fryer to 360°F/180°C. Place the brown rice, tomatoes, garlic, salt, and pepper in a bowl and stir. Divide the rice filling evenly among the bell pepper halves. Combine the goat cheese, basil, parsley and oregano in a small bowl. Sprinkle each bell pepper with the herbed cheese. Arrange the bell peppers on the air fryer and Bake for 20 minutes. Serve topped with grated Parmesan and parsley.

Fried Pearl Onions With Balsamic Vinegar And Basil

Servings: 2
Cooking Time: 10 Minutes
Ingredients:
- 1 pound fresh pearl onions
- 1 tablespoon olive oil
- salt and freshly ground black pepper
- 1 teaspoon high quality aged balsamic vinegar
- 1 tablespoon chopped fresh basil leaves (or mint)

Directions:
1. Preheat the air fryer to 400°F/205°C.
2. Decide whether you want to peel the onions before or after they cook. Peeling them ahead of time is a little more laborious. Peeling after they cook is easier, but a little messier since the onions are hot and you may discard more of the onion than you'd like to. If you opt to peel them first, trim the tiny root of the onions off and pinch off any loose papery skins. (It's ok if there are some skins left on the onions.) Toss the pearl onions with the olive oil, salt and freshly ground black pepper.
3. Air-fry for 10 minutes, shaking the basket a couple of times during the cooking process. (If your pearl onions are very large, you may need to add a couple of minutes to this cooking time.)
4. Let the onions cool slightly and then slip off any remaining skins.
5. Toss the onions with the balsamic vinegar and basil and serve.

Parmesan Garlic Fries

Servings: 4
Cooking Time: 20 Minutes
Ingredients:
- 2 medium Yukon gold potatoes, washed
- 1 tablespoon extra-virgin olive oil
- 1 garlic clove, minced
- 2 tablespoons finely grated parmesan cheese
- ¼ teaspoon black pepper
- ¼ teaspoon salt
- 1 tablespoon freshly chopped parsley

Directions:
1. Preheat the air fryer to 400°F/205°C.
2. Slice the potatoes into long strips about ¼-inch thick. In a large bowl, toss the potatoes with the olive oil, garlic, cheese, pepper, and salt.
3. Place the fries into the air fryer basket and cook for 4 minutes; shake the basket and cook another 4 minutes.
4. Remove and serve warm.

Mushrooms

Servings: 4
Cooking Time: 12 Minutes
Ingredients:
- 8 ounces whole white button mushrooms
- ½ teaspoon salt
- ⅛ teaspoon pepper
- ¼ teaspoon garlic powder
- ¼ teaspoon onion powder
- 5 tablespoons potato starch
- 1 egg, beaten
- ¾ cup panko breadcrumbs
- oil for misting or cooking spray

Directions:
1. Place mushrooms in a large bowl. Add the salt, pepper, garlic and onion powders, and stir well to distribute seasonings.
2. Add potato starch to mushrooms and toss in bowl until well coated.
3. Dip mushrooms in beaten egg, roll in panko crumbs, and mist with oil or cooking spray.
4. Place mushrooms in air fryer basket. You can cook them all at once, and it's okay if a few are stacked.
5. Cook at 390°F/200°C for 5minutes. Shake basket, then continue cooking for 7 more minutes, until golden brown and crispy.

Roasted Bell Peppers With Garlic & Dill

Servings: 4
Cooking Time: 30 Minutes
Ingredients:
- 4 bell peppers, seeded and cut into fourths
- 1 tsp olive oil
- 4 garlic cloves, minced
- ½ tsp dried dill

Directions:
1. Preheat air fryer to 350°F/175°C. Add the peppers to the frying basket, spritz with olive oil, shake, and Roast for 15 minutes. Season with garlic and dill, then cook for an additional 3-5 minutes. The veggies should be soft. Serve.

Cinnamon Roasted Pumpkin

Servings: 2
Cooking Time: 25 Minutes
Ingredients:
- 1 lb pumpkin, halved crosswise and seeded
- 1 tsp coconut oil
- 1 tsp sugar
- ½ tsp ground nutmeg
- 1 tsp ground cinnamon

Directions:
1. Prepare the pumpkin by rubbing coconut oil on the cut sides. In a small bowl, combine sugar, nutmeg and cinnamon. Sprinkle over the pumpkin. Preheat air fryer to 325°F/160°C. Put the pumpkin in the greased frying basket, cut sides up. Bake until the squash is soft in the center, 15 minutes. Test with a knife to ensure softness. Serve.

Balsamic Beet Chips

Servings: 4
Cooking Time: 40 Minutes
Ingredients:
- ½ tsp balsamic vinegar
- 4 beets, peeled and sliced
- 1 garlic clove, minced
- 2 tbsp chopped mint
- Salt and pepper to taste
- 3 tbsp olive oil

Directions:
1. Preheat air fryer to 380°F/195°C. Coat all ingredients in a bowl, except balsamic vinegar. Pour the beet mixture into the frying basket and Roast for 25-30 minutes, stirring once. Serve, drizzled with vinegar and enjoy!

Roasted Peppers With Balsamic Vinegar And Basil

Servings: 6
Cooking Time: 12 Minutes
Ingredients:
- 4 Small or medium red or yellow bell peppers
- 3 tablespoons Olive oil
- 1 tablespoon Balsamic vinegar
- Up to 6 Fresh basil leaves, torn up

Directions:
1. Preheat the air fryer to 400°F/205°C.
2. When the machine is at temperature, put the peppers in the basket with at least ¼ inch between them. Air-fry undisturbed for 12 minutes, until blistered, even blackened in places.
3. Use kitchen tongs to transfer the peppers to a medium bowl. Cover the bowl with plastic wrap. Set aside at room temperature for 30 minutes.
4. Uncover the bowl and use kitchen tongs to transfer the peppers to a cutting board or work surface. Peel off the filmy exterior skin. If there are blackened bits under it, these can stay on the peppers. Cut off and remove the stem ends. Split open the peppers and discard any seeds and their spongy membranes. Slice the peppers into ½-inch- to 1-inch-wide strips.
5. Put these in a clean bowl and gently toss them with the oil, vinegar, and basil. Serve at once. Or cover and store at room temperature for up to 4 hours or in the refrigerator for up to 5 days.

Caraway Seed Pretzel Sticks

Servings: 4
Cooking Time: 30 Minutes
Ingredients:
- ½ pizza dough
- 1 tsp baking soda
- 2 tbsp caraway seeds

Directions:
1. Preheat air fryer to 400°F/205°C. Roll out the dough, on parchment paper, into a rectangle, then cut it into 8 strips.Whisk the baking soda and 1 cup of hot water until well dissolved in a bowl. Submerge each strip, shake off any excess, and stretch another 1 to 2 inches. Scatter with caraway seeds and let rise for 10 minutes in the frying basket. Grease with cooking spray and Air Fry for 8 minutes until golden brown, turning once. Serve.

Creole Potato Wedges

Servings: 4
Cooking Time: 10 Minutes
Ingredients:
- 1 pound medium Yukon gold potatoes
- ½ teaspoon cayenne pepper
- ½ teaspoon thyme
- ½ teaspoon garlic powder
- ½ teaspoon salt

- ½ teaspoon smoked paprika
- 1 cup dry breadcrumbs
- oil for misting or cooking spray

Directions:
1. Wash potatoes, cut into thick wedges, and drop wedges into a bowl of water to prevent browning.
2. Mix together the cayenne pepper, thyme, garlic powder, salt, paprika, and breadcrumbs and spread on a sheet of wax paper.
3. Remove potatoes from water and, without drying them, roll in the breadcrumb mixture.
4. Spray air fryer basket with oil or cooking spray and pile potato wedges into basket. It's okay if they form more than a single layer.
5. Cook at 390°F/200°C for 8minutes. Shake basket, then continue cooking for 2 minutes longer, until coating is crisp and potato centers are soft. Total cooking time will vary, depending on thickness of potato wedges.

Sesame Carrots And Sugar Snap Peas

Cooking Time: 16 Minutes
Servings: 4
Ingredients:
- 1 pound carrots, peeled sliced on the bias (½-inch slices)
- 1 teaspoon olive oil
- salt and freshly ground black pepper
- ⅓ cup honey
- 1 tablespoon sesame oil
- 1 tablespoon soy sauce
- ½ teaspoon minced fresh ginger
- 4 ounces sugar snap peas (about 1 cup)
- 1½ teaspoons sesame seeds

Directions:
1. Preheat the air fryer to 360°F/180°C.
2. Toss the carrots with the olive oil, season with salt and pepper and air-fry for 10 minutes, shaking the basket once or twice during the cooking process.
3. Combine the honey, sesame oil, soy sauce and minced ginger in a large bowl. Add the sugar snap peas and the air-fried carrots to the honey mixture, toss to coat and return everything to the air fryer basket.
4. Turn up the temperature to 400°F/205°C and air-fry for an additional 6 minutes, shaking the basket once during the cooking process.
5. Transfer the carrots and sugar snap peas to a serving bowl. Pour the sauce from the bottom of the cooker over the vegetables and sprinkle sesame seeds over top. Serve immediately.

Asiago Broccoli

Servings: 4
Cooking Time: 14 Minutes
Ingredients:
- 1 head broccoli, cut into florets
- 1 tablespoon extra-virgin olive oil
- 1 teaspoon minced garlic
- ¼ teaspoon ground black pepper
- ¼ teaspoon salt
- ¼ cup asiago cheese

Directions:
1. Preheat the air fryer to 360°F/180°C.
2. In a medium bowl, toss the broccoli florets with the olive oil, garlic, pepper, and salt. Lightly spray the air fryer basket with olive oil spray.
3. Place the broccoli florets into the basket and cook for 7 minutes. Shake the basket and sprinkle the broccoli with cheese. Cook another 7 minutes.

4. Remove from the basket and serve warm.

Southern Okra Chips

Servings: 2
Cooking Time: 20 Minutes
Ingredients:
- 2 eggs
- ¼ cup whole milk
- ¼ cup bread crumbs
- ¼ cup cornmeal
- 1 tbsp Cajun seasoning
- Salt and pepper to taste
- ⅛ tsp chili pepper
- ½ lb okra, sliced
- 1 tbsp butter, melted

Directions:
1. Preheat air fryer at 400°F/205°C. Beat the eggs and milk in a bowl. In another bowl, combine the remaining ingredients, except okra and butter. Dip okra chips in the egg mixture, then dredge them in the breadcrumbs mixture. Place okra chips in the greased frying basket and Roast for 7 minutes, shake once and brush with melted butter. Serve right away.

Roasted Garlic And Thyme Tomatoes

Servings: 2
Cooking Time: 15 Minutes
Ingredients:
- 4 Roma tomatoes
- 1 tablespoon olive oil
- salt and freshly ground black pepper
- 1 clove garlic, minced
- ½ teaspoon dried thyme

Directions:
1. Preheat the air fryer to 390°F/200°C.
2. Cut the tomatoes in half and scoop out the seeds and any pithy parts with your fingers. Place the tomatoes in a bowl and toss with the olive oil, salt, pepper, garlic and thyme.
3. Transfer the tomatoes to the air fryer, cut side up. Air-fry for 15 minutes. The edges should just start to brown. Let the tomatoes cool to an edible temperature for a few minutes and then use in pastas, on top of crostini, or as an accompaniment to any poultry, meat or fish.

Pork Tenderloin Salad

Servings: 4
Cooking Time: 25 Minutes
Ingredients:
- Pork Tenderloin
- ½ teaspoon smoked paprika
- ¼ teaspoon salt
- ¼ teaspoon garlic powder
- ½ teaspoon onion powder
- ⅛ teaspoon ginger
- 1 teaspoon extra-light olive oil
- ¾ pound pork tenderloin
- Dressing
- 3 tablespoons extra-light olive oil
- 2 tablespoons red wine vinegar
- 2 tablespoons Dijon mustard
- 1 tablespoon honey
- Salad
- ¼ sweet red bell pepper
- 1 large Granny Smith apple
- 8 cups shredded Napa cabbage

Directions:
1. Mix the tenderloin seasonings together with oil and rub all over surface of meat.

2. Place pork tenderloin in the air fryer basket and cook at 390°F/200°C for 25minutes, until meat registers 130°F on a meat thermometer.
3. Allow meat to rest while preparing salad and dressing.
4. In a jar, shake all dressing ingredients together until well mixed.
5. Cut the bell pepper into slivers, then core, quarter, and slice the apple crosswise.
6. In a large bowl, toss together the cabbage, bell pepper, apple, and dressing.
7. Divide salad mixture among 4 plates.
8. Slice pork tenderloin into ½-inch slices and divide among the 4 salads.
9. Serve with sweet potato or other vegetable chips.

Panzanella Salad With Crispy Croutons

Servings: 4
Cooking Time: 3 Minutes
Ingredients:
- ½ French baguette, sliced in half lengthwise
- 2 large cloves garlic
- 2 large ripe tomatoes, divided
- 2 small Persian cucumbers, quartered and diced
- ¼ cup Kalamata olives
- 1 tablespoon chopped, fresh oregano or 1 teaspoon dried oregano
- ¼ cup chopped fresh basil
- ¼ cup chopped fresh parsley
- ½ cup sliced red onion
- 2 tablespoons red wine vinegar
- ¼ cup extra-virgin olive oil
- Salt and pepper, to taste

Directions:
1. Preheat the air fryer to 380°F/195°C.
2. Place the baguette into the air fryer and toast for 3 to 5 minutes or until lightly golden brown.
3. Remove the bread from air fryer and immediately rub 1 raw garlic clove firmly onto the inside portion of each piece of bread, scraping the garlic onto the bread.
4. Slice 1 of the tomatoes in half and rub the cut edge of one half of the tomato onto the toasted bread. Season the rubbed bread with sea salt to taste.
5. Cut the bread into cubes and place in a large bowl. Cube the remaining 1½ tomatoes and add to the bowl. Add the cucumbers, olives, oregano, basil, parsley, and onion; stir to mix. Drizzle the red wine vinegar into the bowl, and stir. Drizzle the olive oil over the top, stir, and adjust the seasonings with salt and pepper.
6. Serve immediately or allow to sit at room temperature up to 1 hour before serving.

Turkish Mutabal (eggplant Dip)

Servings: 2
Cooking Time: 40 Minutes
Ingredients:
- 1 medium eggplant
- 2 tbsp tahini
- 2 tbsp lemon juice
- 1 tsp garlic powder
- ¼ tsp sumac
- 1 tsp chopped parsley

Directions:
1. Preheat air fryer to 400°F/205°C. Place the eggplant in a pan and Roast for 30 minutes, turning once. Let cool for 5-10 minutes. Scoop out the flesh and place it in a bowl. Squeeze any excess water; discard the water. Mix the flesh, tahini, lemon juice, garlic, and sumac until well combined. Scatter with parsley and serve.

Charred Radicchio Salad

Servings: 4
Cooking Time: 5 Minutes
Ingredients:
- 2 Small 5- to 6-ounce radicchio head(s)
- 3 tablespoons Olive oil
- ½ teaspoon Table salt
- 2 tablespoons Balsamic vinegar
- Up to ¼ teaspoon Red pepper flakes

Directions:
1. Preheat the air fryer to 375°F/190°C .
2. Cut the radicchio head(s) into quarters through the stem end. Brush the oil over the heads, particularly getting it between the leaves along the cut sides. Sprinkle the radicchio quarters with the salt.
3. When the machine is at temperature, set the quarters cut sides up in the basket with as much air space between them as possible. They should not touch. Air-fry undisturbed for 5 minutes, watching carefully because they burn quickly, until blackened in bits and soft.
4. Use a nonstick-safe spatula to transfer the quarters to a cutting board. Cool for a minute or two, then cut out the thick stems inside the heads. Discard these tough bits and chop the remaining heads into bite-size bits. Scrape them into a bowl. Add the vinegar and red pepper flakes. Toss well and serve warm.

Buttery Stuffed Tomatoes

Servings: 6
Cooking Time: 15 Minutes
Ingredients:
- 3 8-ounce round tomatoes
- ½ cup plus 1 tablespoon Plain panko bread crumbs (gluten-free, if a concern)
- 3 tablespoons (about ½ ounce) Finely grated Parmesan cheese
- 3 tablespoons Butter, melted and cooled
- 4 teaspoons Stemmed and chopped fresh parsley leaves
- 1 teaspoon Minced garlic
- ¼ teaspoon Table salt
- Up to ¼ teaspoon Red pepper flakes
- Olive oil spray

Directions:
1. Preheat the air fryer to 375°F/190°C .
2. Cut the tomatoes in half through their "equators" (that is, not through the stem ends). One at a time, gently squeeze the tomato halves over a trash can, using a clean finger to gently force out the seeds and most of the juice inside, working carefully so that the tomato doesn't lose its round shape or get crushed.
3. Stir the bread crumbs, cheese, butter, parsley, garlic, salt, and red pepper flakes in a bowl until the bread crumbs are moistened and the parsley is uniform throughout the mixture. Pile this mixture into the spaces left in the tomato halves. Press gently to compact the filling. Coat the tops of the tomatoes with olive oil spray.
4. Place the tomatoes cut side up in the basket. They may touch each other. Air-fry for 15 minutes, or until the filling is lightly browned and crunchy.
5. Use nonstick-safe spatula and kitchen tongs for balance to gently transfer the stuffed tomatoes to a platter or a cutting board. Cool for a couple of minutes before serving.

Crispy Cauliflower Puffs

Servings: 12
Cooking Time: 9 Minutes
Ingredients:
- 1½ cups Riced cauliflower
- 1 cup (about 4 ounces) Shredded Monterey Jack cheese
- ¾ cup Seasoned Italian-style panko bread crumbs (gluten-free, if a concern)
- 2 tablespoons plus 1 teaspoon All-purpose flour or potato starch
- 2 tablespoons plus 1 teaspoon Vegetable oil
- 1 plus 1 large yolk Large egg(s)
- ¾ teaspoon Table salt
- Vegetable oil spray

Directions:
1. Preheat the air fryer to 375°F/190°C .
2. Stir the riced cauliflower, cheese, bread crumbs, flour or potato starch, oil, egg(s) and egg yolk (if necessary), and salt in a large bowl to make a thick batter.
3. Using 2 tablespoons of the batter, form a compact ball between your clean, dry palms. Set it aside and continue forming more balls: 7 more for a small batch, 11 more for a medium batch, or 15 more for a large batch.
4. Generously coat the balls on all sides with vegetable oil spray. Set them in the basket with as much air space between them as possible. Air-fry undisturbed for 7 minutes, or until golden brown and crisp. If the machine is at 360°F/180°C, you may need to add 2 minutes to the cooking time.
5. Gently pour the contents of the basket onto a wire rack. Cool the puffs for 5 minutes before serving.

Buttered Brussels Sprouts

Servings: 4
Cooking Time: 30 Minutes
Ingredients:
- ¼ cup grated Parmesan
- 2 tbsp butter, melted
- 1 lb Brussels sprouts
- Salt and pepper to taste

Directions:
1. Preheat air fryer to 330°F/165°C. Trim the bottoms of the sprouts and remove any discolored leaves. Place the sprouts in a medium bowl along with butter, salt and pepper. Toss to coat, then place them in the frying basket. Roast for 20 minutes, shaking the basket twice. When done, the sprouts should be crisp with golden-brown color. Plate the sprouts in a serving dish and toss with Parmesan cheese.

Steamboat Shrimp Salad

Servings: 4
Cooking Time: 4 Minutes
Ingredients:
- Steamboat Dressing
- ½ cup mayonnaise
- ½ cup plain yogurt
- 2 teaspoons freshly squeezed lemon juice (no substitutes)
- 2 teaspoons grated lemon rind
- 1 teaspoon dill weed, slightly crushed
- ½ teaspoon hot sauce
- Steamed Shrimp
- 24 small, raw shrimp, peeled and deveined
- 1 teaspoon lemon juice
- ¼ teaspoon Old Bay Seasoning
- Salad
- 8 cups romaine or Bibb lettuce, chopped or torn

- ¼ cup red onion, cut in thin slivers
- 12 black olives, sliced
- 12 cherry or grape tomatoes, halved
- 1 medium avocado, sliced or cut into large chunks

Directions:
1. Combine all dressing ingredients and mix well. Refrigerate while preparing shrimp and salad.
2. Sprinkle raw shrimp with lemon juice and Old Bay Seasoning. Use more Old Bay if you like your shrimp bold and spicy.
3. Pour 4 tablespoons of water in bottom of air fryer.
4. Place shrimp in air fryer basket in single layer.
5. Cook at 390°F/200°C for 4 minutes. Remove shrimp from basket and place in refrigerator to cool.
6. Combine all salad ingredients and mix gently. Divide among 4 salad plates or bowls.
7. Top each salad with 6 shrimp and serve with dressing.

Buttered Garlic Broccolini

Servings: 2
Cooking Time: 20 Minutes
Ingredients:
- 1 bunch broccolini
- 2 tbsp butter, cubed
- ¼ tsp salt
- 2 minced cloves garlic
- 2 tsp lemon juice

Directions:
1. Preheat air fryer at 350ºF/175°C. Place salted water in a saucepan over high heat and bring it to a boil. Then, add in broccolini and boil for 3 minutes. Drain it and transfer it into a bowl. Mix in butter, garlic, and salt. Place the broccolini in the frying basket and Air Fry for 6 minutes. Serve immediately garnished with lemon juice.

Succulent Roasted Peppers

Servings:2
Cooking Time: 35 Minutes
Ingredients:
- 2 red bell peppers
- 2 tbsp olive oil
- Salt to taste
- 1 tsp dill, chopped

Directions:
1. Preheat air fryer to 400ºF/205°C. Remove the tops and bottoms of the peppers. Cut along rib sections and discard the seeds. Combine the bell peppers and olive oil in a bowl. Place bell peppers in the frying basket. Roast for 24 minutes, flipping once. Transfer the roasted peppers to a small bowl and cover for 15 minutes. Then, peel and discard the skins. Sprinkle with salt and dill and serve.

Rosemary Potato Salad

Servings: 4
Cooking Time: 30 Minutes
Ingredients:
- 3 tbsp olive oil
- 2 lb red potatoes, halved
- Salt and pepper to taste
- 1 red bell pepper, chopped
- 2 green onions, chopped
- 1/3 cup lemon juice
- 3 tbsp Dijon mustard
- 1 tbsp rosemary, chopped

Directions:

1. Preheat air fryer to 350°F/175°C. Add potatoes to the frying basket and drizzle with 1 tablespoon olive oil. Season with salt and pepper. Roast the potatoes for 25 minutes, shaking twice. Potatoes will be tender and lightly golden.
2. While the potatoes are roasting, add peppers and green onions in a bowl. In a separate bowl, whisk olive oil, lemon juice, and mustard. When the potatoes are done, transfer them to a large bowl. Pour the mustard dressing over and toss to coat. Serve sprinkled with rosemary.

Lemony Green Bean Sautée

Servings: 6
Cooking Time: 15 Minutes
Ingredients:
- 1 tbsp cilantro, chopped
- 1 lb green beans, trimmed
- ½ red onion, sliced
- 2 tbsp olive oil
- Salt and pepper to taste
- 1 tbsp grapefruit juice
- 6 lemon wedges

Directions:
1. Preheat air fryer to 360°F/180°C. Coat the green beans, red onion, olive oil, salt, pepper, cilantro and grapefruit juice in a bowl. Pour the mixture into the air fryer and Bake for 5 minutes. Stir well and cook for 5 minutes more. Serve with lemon wedges. Enjoy!

Salt And Pepper Baked Potatoes

Cooking Time: 40 Minutes
Servings: 4
Ingredients:

- 1 to 2 tablespoons olive oil
- 4 medium russet potatoes (about 9 to 10 ounces each)
- salt and coarsely ground black pepper
- butter, sour cream, chopped fresh chives, scallions or bacon bits (optional)

Directions:
1. Preheat the air fryer to 400°F/205°C.
2. Rub the olive oil all over the potatoes and season them generously with salt and coarsely ground black pepper. Pierce all sides of the potatoes several times with the tines of a fork.
3. Air-fry for 40 minutes, turning the potatoes over halfway through the cooking time.
4. Serve the potatoes, split open with butter, sour cream, fresh chives, scallions or bacon bits.

Sage & Thyme Potatoes

Servings: 4
Cooking Time: 30 Minutes
Ingredients:
- 2 red potatoes, peeled and cubed
- ¼ cup olive oil
- 1 tsp dried sage
- ½ tsp dried thyme
- ½ tsp salt
- 2 tbsp grated Parmesan

Directions:
1. Preheat air fryer to 360°F/180°C. Coat the red potatoes with olive oil, sage, thyme and salt in a bowl. Pour the potatoes into the air frying basket and Roast for 10 minutes. Stir the potatoes and sprinkle the Parmesan over the top. Continue roasting for 8 more minutes. Serve hot.

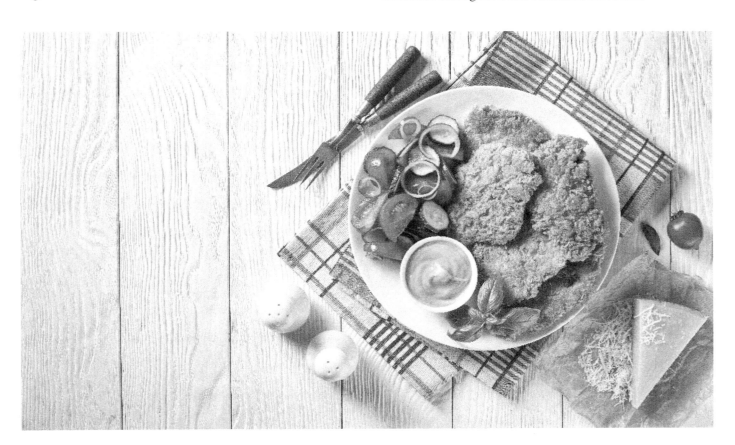

Desserts And Sweets

Peach Cobbler

Servings: 4
Cooking Time: 12 Minutes
Ingredients:
- 16 ounces frozen peaches, thawed, with juice (do not drain)
- 6 tablespoons sugar
- 1 tablespoon cornstarch
- 1 tablespoon water
- Crust
- ½ cup flour
- ¼ teaspoon salt
- 3 tablespoons butter
- 1½ tablespoons cold water
- ¼ teaspoon sugar

Directions:
1. Place peaches, including juice, and sugar in air fryer baking pan. Stir to mix well.
2. In a small cup, dissolve cornstarch in the water. Stir into peaches.
3. In a medium bowl, combine the flour and salt. Cut in butter using knives or a pastry blender. Stir in the cold water to make a stiff dough.
4. On a floured board or wax paper, pat dough into a square or circle slightly smaller than your air fryer baking pan. Cut diagonally into 4 pieces.
5. Place dough pieces on top of peaches, leaving a tiny bit of space between the edges. Sprinkle very lightly with sugar, no more than about ¼ teaspoon.
6. Cook at 360°F/180°C for 12 minutes, until fruit bubbles and crust browns.

Nutella® Torte

Servings: 6
Cooking Time: 55 Minutes
Ingredients:
- ¼ cup unsalted butter, softened
- ½ cup sugar
- 2 eggs
- 1 teaspoon vanilla
- 1¼ cups Nutella® (or other chocolate hazelnut spread), divided
- ¼ cup flour
- 1 teaspoon baking powder
- ¼ teaspoon salt
- dark chocolate fudge topping
- coarsely chopped toasted hazelnuts

Directions:
1. Cream the butter and sugar together with an electric hand mixer until light and fluffy. Add the eggs, vanilla, and ¾ cup of the Nutella® and mix until combined. Combine the flour, baking powder and salt together, and add these dry ingredients to the butter mixture, beating for 1 minute.
2. Preheat the air fryer to 350°F/175°C.
3. Grease a 7-inch cake pan with butter and then line the bottom of the pan with a circle of parchment paper. Grease the parchment paper circle as well. Pour the batter into the prepared cake pan and wrap the pan completely with aluminum foil. Lower the pan into the air fryer basket with an aluminum sling (fold a piece of aluminum foil into a strip about 2-inches wide by 24-inches long). Fold the ends of the aluminum foil over the top of the dish before returning the basket to the air fryer. Air-fry for 30 minutes. Remove the foil and air-fry for another 25 minutes.
4. Remove the cake from air fryer and let it cool for 10 minutes. Invert the cake onto a plate, remove the parchment paper and invert the cake back onto a serving platter. While the cake is still warm, spread the remaining ½ cup of Nutella® over the top of the cake. Melt the dark chocolate fudge in the microwave for about 10 seconds so it melts enough to be pourable. Drizzle the sauce on top of the cake in a zigzag motion. Turn the cake 90 degrees and drizzle more sauce in zigzags perpendicular to the first zigzags. Garnish the edges of the torte with the toasted hazelnuts and serve.

Dark Chocolate Peanut Butter S'mores

Servings: 4
Cooking Time: 6 Minutes
Ingredients:
- 4 graham cracker sheets
- 4 marshmallows
- 4 teaspoons chunky peanut butter
- 4 ounces dark chocolate
- ½ teaspoon ground cinnamon

Directions:
1. Preheat the air fryer to 390°F/200°C. Break the graham crackers in half so you have 8 pieces.
2. Place 4 pieces of graham cracker on the bottom of the air fryer. Top each with one of the marshmallows and bake for 6 or 7 minutes, or until the marshmallows have a golden brown center.
3. While cooking, slather each of the remaining graham crackers with 1 teaspoon peanut butter.
4. When baking completes, carefully remove each of the graham crackers, add 1 ounce of dark chocolate on top of the marshmallow, and lightly sprinkle with cinnamon. Top with the remaining peanut butter graham cracker to make the sandwich. Serve immediately.

Puff Pastry Apples

Servings: 4
Cooking Time: 10 Minutes
Ingredients:
- 3 Rome or Gala apples, peeled
- 2 tablespoons sugar
- 1 teaspoon all-purpose flour
- 1 teaspoon ground cinnamon
- ⅛ teaspoon ground ginger
- pinch ground nutmeg
- 1 sheet puff pastry
- 1 tablespoon butter, cut into 4 pieces
- 1 egg, beaten
- vegetable oil
- vanilla ice cream (optional)
- caramel sauce (optional)

Directions:

1. Remove the core from the apple by cutting the four sides off the apple around the core. Slice the pieces of apple into thin half-moons, about ¼-inch thick. Combine the sugar, flour, cinnamon, ginger, and nutmeg in a large bowl. Add the apples to the bowl and gently toss until the apples are evenly coated with the spice mixture. Set aside.
2. Cut the puff pastry sheet into a 12-inch by 12-inch square. Then quarter the sheet into four 6-inch squares. Save any remaining pastry for decorating the apples at the end.
3. Divide the spiced apples between the four puff pastry squares, stacking the apples in the center of each square and placing them flat on top of each other in a circle. Top the apples with a piece of the butter.
4. Brush the four edges of the pastry with the egg wash. Bring the four corners of the pastry together, wrapping them around the apple slices and pinching them together at the top in the style of a "beggars purse" appetizer. Fold the ends of the pastry corners down onto the apple making them look like leaves. Brush the entire apple with the egg wash.
5. Using the leftover dough, make leaves to decorate the apples. Cut out 8 leaf shapes, about 1½-inches long, "drawing" the leaf veins on the pastry leaves with a paring knife. Place 2 leaves on the top of each apple, tucking the ends of the leaves under the pastry in the center of the apples. Brush the top of the leaves with additional egg wash. Sprinkle the entire apple with some granulated sugar.
6. Preheat the air fryer to 350°F/175°C.
7. Spray or brush the inside of the air fryer basket with oil. Place the apples in the basket and air-fry for 6 minutes. Carefully turn the apples over – it's easiest to remove one apple, then flip the others over and finally return the last apple to the air fryer. Air-fry for an additional 4 minutes.
8. Serve the puff pastry apples warm with vanilla ice cream and drizzle with some caramel sauce.

Roasted Pears

Servings: 4
Cooking Time: 10 Minutes
Ingredients:
- 2 Ripe pears, preferably Anjou, stemmed, peeled, halved lengthwise, and cored
- 2 tablespoons Butter, melted
- 2 teaspoons Granulated white sugar
- Grated nutmeg
- ¼ cup Honey
- ½ cup (about 1½ ounces) Shaved Parmesan cheese

Directions:
1. Preheat the air fryer to 400°F/205°C.
2. Brush each pear half with about 1½ teaspoons of the melted butter, then sprinkle their cut sides with ½ teaspoon sugar. Grate a pinch of nutmeg over each pear.
3. When the machine is at temperature, set the pear halves cut side up in the basket with as much air space between them as possible. Air-fry undisturbed for 10 minutes, or until hot and softened.
4. Use a nonstick-safe spatula, and perhaps a flatware tablespoon for balance, to transfer the pear halves to a serving platter or plates. Cool for a minute or two, then drizzle each pear half with 1 tablespoon of the honey. Lay about 2 tablespoons of shaved Parmesan over each half just before serving.

Coconut Rice Cake

Servings: 8
Cooking Time: 30 Minutes
Ingredients:
- 1 cup all-natural coconut water

- 1 cup unsweetened coconut milk
- 1 teaspoon almond extract
- ¼ teaspoon salt
- 4 tablespoons honey
- cooking spray
- ¾ cup raw jasmine rice
- 2 cups sliced or cubed fruit

Directions:
1. In a medium bowl, mix together the coconut water, coconut milk, almond extract, salt, and honey.
2. Spray air fryer baking pan with cooking spray and add the rice.
3. Pour liquid mixture over rice.
4. Cook at 360°F/180°C for 15minutes. Stir and cook for 15 minutes longer or until rice grains are tender.
5. Allow cake to cool slightly. Run a dull knife around edge of cake, inside the pan. Turn the cake out onto a platter and garnish with fruit.

Chocolate Bars

Servings: 4
Cooking Time: 30 Minutes
Ingredients:
- 2 tbsp chocolate toffee chips
- ¼ cup chopped pecans
- 2 tbsp raisins
- 1 tbsp dried blueberries
- 2 tbsp maple syrup
- ¼ cup light brown sugar
- 1/3 cup peanut butter
- 2 tbsp chocolate chips
- 2 tbsp butter, melted
- ½ tsp vanilla extract
- Salt to taste

Directions:
1. Preheat air fryer at 350ºF/175°C. In a bowl, combine the pecans, maple syrup, sugar, peanut butter, toffee chips, raisins, dried blueberries, chocolate chips, butter, vanilla extract, and salt. Press mixture into a lightly greased cake pan and cover it with aluminum foil. Place cake pan in the frying basket and Bake for 15 minutes. Remove the foil and cook for 5 more minutes. Let cool completely for 15 minutes. Turn over on a place and cut into 6 bars. Enjoy!

Baked Apple

Servings: 6
Cooking Time: 20 Minutes
Ingredients:
- 3 small Honey Crisp or other baking apples
- 3 tablespoons maple syrup
- 3 tablespoons chopped pecans
- 1 tablespoon firm butter, cut into 6 pieces

Directions:
1. Put ½ cup water in the drawer of the air fryer.
2. Wash apples well and dry them.
3. Split apples in half. Remove core and a little of the flesh to make a cavity for the pecans.
4. Place apple halves in air fryer basket, cut side up.
5. Spoon 1½ teaspoons pecans into each cavity.
6. Spoon ½ tablespoon maple syrup over pecans in each apple.
7. Top each apple with ½ teaspoon butter.
8. Cook at 360°F/180°C for 20 minutes, until apples are tender.

Carrot Cake With Cream Cheese Icing

Servings: 6
Cooking Time: 55 Minutes
Ingredients:
- 1¼ cups all-purpose flour
- 1 teaspoon baking powder
- ½ teaspoon baking soda
- 1 teaspoon ground cinnamon
- ¼ teaspoon ground nutmeg
- ¼ teaspoon salt
- 2 cups grated carrot (about 3 to 4 medium carrots or 2 large)
- ¾ cup granulated sugar
- ¼ cup brown sugar
- 2 eggs
- ¾ cup canola or vegetable oil
- For the icing:
- 8 ounces cream cheese, softened at room , Temperature: 8 tablespoons butter (4 ounces or 1 stick), softened at room , Temperature: 1 cup powdered sugar
- 1 teaspoon pure vanilla extract

Directions:
1. Grease a 7-inch cake pan.
2. Combine the flour, baking powder, baking soda, cinnamon, nutmeg and salt in a bowl. Add the grated carrots and toss well. In a separate bowl, beat the sugars and eggs together until light and frothy. Drizzle in the oil, beating constantly. Fold the egg mixture into the dry ingredients until everything is just combined and you no longer see any traces of flour. Pour the batter into the cake pan and wrap the pan completely in greased aluminum foil.
3. Preheat the air fryer to 350°F/175°C.
4. Lower the cake pan into the air fryer basket using a sling made of aluminum foil (fold a piece of aluminum foil into a strip about 2-inches wide by 24-inches long). Fold the ends of the aluminum foil into the air fryer, letting them rest on top of the cake. Air-fry for 40 minutes. Remove the aluminum foil cover and air-fry for an additional 15 minutes or until a skewer inserted into the center of the cake comes out clean and the top is nicely browned.
5. While the cake is cooking, beat the cream cheese, butter, powdered sugar and vanilla extract together using a hand mixer, stand mixer or food processor (or a lot of elbow grease!).
6. Remove the cake pan from the air fryer and let the cake cool in the cake pan for 10 minutes or so. Then remove the cake from the pan and let it continue to cool completely. Frost the cake with the cream cheese icing and serve.

Hasselback Apple Crisp

Servings: 4
Cooking Time: 20 Minutes
Ingredients:
- 2 large Gala apples, peeled, cored and cut in half
- ¼ cup butter, melted
- ½ teaspoon ground cinnamon
- 2 tablespoons sugar
- Topping
- 3 tablespoons butter, melted
- 2 tablespoons brown sugar
- ¼ cup chopped pecans
- 2 tablespoons rolled oats*
- 1 tablespoon flour*
- vanilla ice cream

- caramel sauce

Directions:
1. Place the apples cut side down on a cutting board. Slicing from stem end to blossom end, make 8 to 10 slits down the apple halves but only slice three quarters of the way through the apple, not all the way through to the cutting board.
2. Preheat the air fryer to 330°F/165°C and pour a little water into the bottom of the air fryer drawer. (This will help prevent the grease that drips into the bottom drawer from burning and smoking.)
3. Transfer the apples to the air fryer basket, flat side down. Combine ¼ cup of melted butter, cinnamon and sugar in a small bowl. Brush this butter mixture onto the apples and air-fry at 330°F/165°C for 15 minutes. Baste the apples several times with the butter mixture during the cooking process.
4. While the apples are air-frying, make the filling. Combine 3 tablespoons of melted butter with the brown sugar, pecans, rolled oats and flour in a bowl. Stir with a fork until the mixture resembles small crumbles.
5. When the timer on the air fryer is up, spoon the topping down the center of the apples. Air-fry at 330°F/165°C for an additional 5 minutes.
6. Transfer the apples to a serving plate and serve with vanilla ice cream and caramel sauce.

S'mores Pockets

Servings: 6
Cooking Time: 5 Minutes
Ingredients:
- 12 sheets phyllo dough, thawed
- 1½ cups butter, melted
- ¾ cup graham cracker crumbs
- 1 (7-ounce) Giant Hershey's® milk chocolate bar
- 12 marshmallows, cut in half

Directions:
1. Place one sheet of the phyllo on a large cutting board. Keep the rest of the phyllo sheets covered with a slightly damp, clean kitchen towel. Brush the phyllo sheet generously with some melted butter. Place a second phyllo sheet on top of the first and brush it with more butter. Repeat with one more phyllo sheet until you have a stack of 3 phyllo sheets with butter brushed between the layers. Cover the phyllo sheets with one quarter of the graham cracker crumbs leaving a 1-inch border on one of the short ends of the rectangle. Cut the phyllo sheets lengthwise into 3 strips.
2. Take 2 of the strips and crisscross them to form a cross with the empty borders at the top and to the left. Place 2 of the chocolate rectangles in the center of the cross. Place 4 of the marshmallow halves on top of the chocolate. Now fold the pocket together by folding the bottom phyllo strip up over the chocolate and marshmallows. Then fold the right side over, then the top strip down and finally the left side over. Brush all the edges generously with melted butter to seal shut. Repeat with the next three sheets of phyllo, until all the sheets have been used. You will be able to make 2 pockets with every second batch because you will have an extra graham cracker crumb strip from the previous set of sheets.
3. Preheat the air fryer to 350°F/175°C.
4. Transfer 3 pockets at a time to the air fryer basket. Air-fry at 350°F/175°C for 4 to 5 minutes, until the phyllo dough is light brown in color. Flip the pockets over halfway through the cooking process. Repeat with the remaining 3 pockets.
5. Serve warm.

Giant Buttery Oatmeal Cookie

Servings: 4
Cooking Time: 16 Minutes
Ingredients:
- 1 cup Rolled oats (not quick-cooking or steel-cut oats)
- ½ cup All-purpose flour
- ½ teaspoon Baking soda
- ½ teaspoon Ground cinnamon
- ½ teaspoon Table salt
- 3½ tablespoons Butter, at room temperature
- ⅓ cup Packed dark brown sugar
- 1½ tablespoons Granulated white sugar
- 3 tablespoons (or 1 medium egg, well beaten) Pasteurized egg substitute, such as Egg Beaters
- ¾ teaspoon Vanilla extract
- ⅓ cup Chopped pecans
- Baking spray

Directions:
1. Preheat the air fryer to 350°F/175°C .
2. Stir the oats, flour, baking soda, cinnamon, and salt in a bowl until well combined.
3. Using an electric hand mixer at medium speed , beat the butter, brown sugar, and granulated white sugar until creamy and thick, about 3 minutes, scraping down the inside of the bowl occasionally. Beat in the egg substitute or egg (as applicable) and vanilla until uniform.
4. Scrape down and remove the beaters. Fold in the flour mixture and pecans with a rubber spatula just until all the flour is moistened and the nuts are even throughout the dough.
5. For a small air fryer, coat the inside of a 6-inch round cake pan with baking spray. For a medium air fryer, coat the inside of a 7-inch round cake pan with baking spray. And for a large air fryer, coat the inside of an 8-inch round cake pan with baking spray. Scrape and gently press the dough into the prepared pan, spreading it into an even layer to the perimeter.
6. Set the pan in the basket and air-fry undisturbed for 16 minutes, or until puffed and browned.
7. Transfer the pan to a wire rack and cool for 10 minutes. Loosen the cookie from the perimeter with a spatula, then invert the pan onto a cutting board and let the cookie come free. Remove the pan and reinvert the cookie onto the wire rack. Cool for 5 minutes more before slicing into wedges to serve.

Date Oat Cookies

Servings: 6
Cooking Time: 20 Minutes
Ingredients:
- ¼ cup butter, softened
- 2 ½ tbsp milk
- ½ cup sugar
- ½ tsp vanilla extract
- ½ tsp lemon zest
- ½ tsp ground cinnamon
- 3/4 cup flour
- ¼ tsp salt
- ¾ cup rolled oats
- ¼ tsp baking soda
- ¼ tsp baking powder
- 2 tbsp dates, chopped

Directions:
1. Use an electric beater to whip the butter until fluffy. Add the milk, sugar, lemon zest, and vanilla. Stir until well combined. Add the cinnamon, flour, salt, oats, baking soda, and baking powder in a separate bowl and stir. Add the dry mix to the wet mix and stir with a wooden spoon. Pour in the dates.
2. Preheat air fryer to 350°F/175°C. Drop tablespoonfuls of the batter onto a greased baking pan, leaving room in between each. Bake for 6 minutes or until light brown. Make all the cookies at once, or save the batter in the fridge for later. Let them cool and enjoy!

Coconut Crusted Bananas With Pineapple Sauce

Servings: 4
Cooking Time: 5 Minutes
Ingredients:
- Pineapple Sauce
- 1½ cups puréed fresh pineapple
- 2 tablespoons sugar
- juice of 1 lemon
- ¼ teaspoon ground cinnamon
- 3 firm bananas
- ¼ cup sweetened condensed milk
- 1¼ cups shredded coconut
- ⅓ cup crushed graham crackers (crumbs)*
- vegetable or canola oil, in a spray bottle
- vanilla frozen yogurt or ice cream

Directions:
1. Make the pineapple sauce by combining the pineapple, sugar, lemon juice and cinnamon in a saucepan. Simmer the mixture on the stovetop for 20 minutes, and then set it aside.
2. Slice the bananas diagonally into ½-inch thick slices and place them in a bowl. Pour the sweetened condensed milk into the bowl and toss the bananas gently to coat. Combine the coconut and graham cracker crumbs together in a shallow dish. Remove the banana slices from the condensed milk and let any excess milk drip off. Dip the banana slices in the coconut and crumb mixture to coat both sides. Spray the coated slices with oil.
3. Preheat the air fryer to 400°F/205°C.
4. Grease the bottom of the air fryer basket with a little oil. Air-fry the bananas in batches at 400°F/205°C for 5 minutes, turning them over halfway through the cooking time. Air-fry until the bananas are golden brown on both sides.
5. Serve warm over vanilla frozen yogurt with some of the pineapple sauce spooned over top.

Choco-granola Bars With Cranberries

Servings: 6
Cooking Time: 20 Minutes
Ingredients:
- 2 tbsp dark chocolate chunks
- 2 cups quick oats
- 2 tbsp dried cranberries
- 3 tbsp shredded coconut
- ½ cup maple syrup
- 1 tsp ground cinnamon
- ⅛ tsp salt
- 2 tbsp smooth peanut butter

Directions:
1. Preheat air fryer to 360°F/180°C. Stir together all the ingredients in a bowl until well combined. Press the oat mixture into a parchment-lined baking pan in a single layer. Put the pan into the frying basket and Bake for 15 minutes. Remove the pan from the fryer, and lift the granola cake out of the pan using the edges of the parchment paper. Leave to cool for 5 minutes. Serve sliced and enjoy!.

Brown Sugar Baked Apples

Servings: 4
Cooking Time: 15 Minutes
Ingredients:
- 3 Small tart apples, preferably McIntosh
- 4 tablespoons (¼ cup/½ stick) Butter
- 6 tablespoons Light brown sugar
- Ground cinnamon
- Table salt

Directions:
1. Preheat the air fryer to 400°F/205°C.
2. Stem the apples, then cut them in half through their "equators" (that is, not the stem ends). Use a melon baller to core the apples, taking care not to break through the flesh and skin at any point but creating a little well in the center of each half.
3. When the machine is at temperature, remove the basket and set it on a heat-safe work surface. Set the apple halves cut side up in the basket with as much air space between them as possible. Even a fraction of an inch will work. Drop 2 teaspoons of butter into the well in the center of each apple half. Sprinkle each half with 1 tablespoon brown sugar and a pinch each ground cinnamon and table salt.
4. Return the basket to the machine. Air-fry undisturbed for 15 minutes, or until the apple halves have softened and the brown sugar has caramelized.
5. Use a nonstick-safe spatula to transfer the apple halves cut side up to a wire rack. Cool for at least 10 minutes before serving, or serve at room temperature.

Cheese & Honey Stuffed Figs

Servings: 4
Cooking Time: 15 Minutes
Ingredients:
- 8 figs, stem off
- 2 oz cottage cheese
- ¼ tsp ground cinnamon
- ¼ tsp orange zest
- ¼ tsp vanilla extract
- 2 tbsp honey
- 1 tbsp olive oil

Directions:
1. Preheat air fryer to 360°F/180°C. Cut an "X" in the top of each fig 1/3 way through, leaving intact the base. Mix together the cottage cheese, cinnamon, orange zest, vanilla extract and 1 tbsp of honey in a bowl. Spoon the cheese mixture into the cavity of each fig. Put the figs in a single layer in the frying basket. Drizzle the olive oil over the top of the figs and Roast for 10 minutes. Drizzle with the remaining honey. Serve and enjoy!

Fried Pineapple Chunks

Servings: 3
Cooking Time: 10 Minutes
Ingredients:
- 3 tablespoons Cornstarch
- 1 Large egg white, beaten until foamy
- 1 cup (4 ounces) Ground vanilla wafer cookies (not low-fat cookies)
- ¼ teaspoon Ground dried ginger
- 18 (about 2¼ cups) Fresh 1-inch chunks peeled and cored pineapple

Directions:
1. Preheat the air fryer to 400°F/205°C.
2. Put the cornstarch in a medium or large bowl. Put the beaten egg white in a small bowl. Pour the cookie crumbs and ground dried ginger into a large zip-closed plastic bag, shaking it a bit to combine them.
3. Dump the pineapple chunks into the bowl with the cornstarch. Toss and stir until well coated. Use your cleaned fingers or a large fork like a shovel to pick up a few pineapple chunks, shake off any excess cornstarch, and put them in the bowl with the egg white. Stir gently, then pick them up and let any excess egg white slip back into the rest. Put them in the bag with the crumb mixture. Repeat the cornstarch-then-egg process until all the pineapple chunks are in the bag. Seal the bag and shake gently, turning the bag this way and that, to coat the pieces well.
4. Set the coated pineapple chunks in the basket with as much air space between them as possible. Even a fraction of an inch will work, but they should not touch. Air-fry undisturbed for 10 minutes, or until golden brown and crisp.
5. Gently dump the contents of the basket onto a wire rack. Cool for at least 5 minutes or up to 15 minutes before serving.

Fall Pumpkin Cake

Servings: 6
Cooking Time: 50 Minutes
Ingredients:
- 1/3 cup pecan pieces
- 5 gingersnap cookies
- 1/3 cup light brown sugar
- 6 tbsp butter, melted
- 3 eggs
- ½ tsp vanilla extract
- 1 cup pumpkin purée
- 2 tbsp sour cream
- ½ cup flour
- ¼ cup tapioca flour
- ½ tsp cornstarch
- ½ cup granulated sugar
- ½ tsp baking soda
- 1 tsp baking powder
- 1 tsp pumpkin pie spice
- 6 oz mascarpone cheese
- 1 1/3 cups powdered sugar
- 1 tsp cinnamon
- 2 tbsp butter, softened
- 1 tbsp milk
- 1 tbsp flaked almonds

Directions:
1. Blitz the pecans, gingersnap cookies, brown sugar, and 3 tbsp of melted butter in a food processor until combined. Press mixture into the bottom of a lightly greased cake pan. Preheat air fryer at 350ºF. In a bowl, whisk the eggs, remaining melted butter, ½ tsp of vanilla extract, pumpkin purée, and sour cream. In another bowl, combine the flour, tapioca flour, cornstarch, granulated sugar, baking soda, baking powder, and pumpkin pie spice. Add wet ingredients to dry ingredients and combine. Do not overmix. Pour the batter into a cake pan and cover it with aluminum foil. Place cake pan in the frying basket and Bake for 30 minutes. Remove the foil and cook for another 5 minutes. Let cool onto a cooling rack for 10 minutes. Then, turn cake onto a large serving platter. In a small bowl, whisk the mascarpone cheese, powdered sugar, remaining vanilla extract, cinnamon, softened butter, and milk. Spread over cooled cake and cut into slices. Serve sprinkled with almonds and enjoy!

Air-fried Beignets

Servings: 24
Cooking Time: 5 Minutes
Ingredients:
- ¾ cup lukewarm water (about 90°F)
- ¼ cup sugar
- 1 generous teaspoon active dry yeast (½ envelope)
- 3½ to 4 cups all-purpose flour
- ½ teaspoon salt
- 2 tablespoons unsalted butter, room temperature and cut into small pieces
- 1 egg, lightly beaten
- ½ cup evaporated milk
- ¼ cup melted butter
- 1 cup confectioners' sugar
- chocolate sauce or raspberry sauce, to dip

Directions:
1. Combine the lukewarm water, a pinch of the sugar and the yeast in a bowl and let it proof for 5 minutes. It should froth a little. If it doesn't froth, your yeast is not active and you should start again with new yeast.
2. Combine 3½ cups of the flour, salt, 2 tablespoons of butter and the remaining sugar in a large bowl, or in the bowl of a stand mixer. Add the egg, evaporated milk and yeast mixture to the bowl and mix with a wooden spoon (or the paddle attachment of the stand mixer) until the dough comes together in a sticky ball. Add a little more flour if necessary to get the dough to form. Transfer the dough to an oiled bowl, cover with plastic wrap or a clean kitchen towel and let it rise in a warm place for at least 2 hours or until it has doubled in size. Longer is better for flavor development and you can even let the dough rest in the refrigerator overnight (just remember to bring it to room temperature before proceeding with the recipe).
3. Roll the dough out to ½-inch thickness. Cut the dough into rectangular or diamond-shaped pieces. You can make the beignets any size you like, but this recipe will give you 24 (2-inch x 3-inch) rectangles.
4. Preheat the air fryer to 350°F/175°C.
5. Brush the beignets on both sides with some of the melted butter and air-fry in batches at 350°F /175°C for 5 minutes, turning them over halfway through if desired. (They will brown on all sides without being flipped, but flipping them will brown them more evenly.)
6. As soon as the beignets are finished, transfer them to a plate or baking sheet and dust with the confectioners' sugar. Serve warm with a chocolate or raspberry sauce.

Holiday Pear Crumble

Servings: 4
Cooking Time: 40 Minutes
Ingredients:
- 2 tbsp coconut oil
- ¼ cup flour
- ¼ cup demerara sugar
- ⅛ tsp salt
- 2 cups finely chopped pears
- ½ tbsp lemon juice
- ¾ tsp cinnamon

Directions:
1. Combine the coconut oil, flour, sugar, and salt in a bowl and mix well. Preheat air fryer to 320°F/160°C. Stir the pears with 3 tbsp of water, lemon juice, and cinnamon into a baking pan until combined. Sprinkle the chilled topping over the pears. Bake for 30 minutes or until they are softened and the topping is crispy and golden. Serve.

Tortilla Fried Pies

Servings: 12
Cooking Time: 5 Minutes
Ingredients:
- 12 small flour tortillas (4-inch diameter)
- ½ cup fig preserves
- ¼ cup sliced almonds
- 2 tablespoons shredded, unsweetened coconut
- oil for misting or cooking spray

Directions:
1. Wrap refrigerated tortillas in damp paper towels and heat in microwave 30 seconds to warm.
2. Working with one tortilla at a time, place 2 teaspoons fig preserves, 1 teaspoon sliced almonds, and ½ teaspoon coconut in the center of each.
3. Moisten outer edges of tortilla all around.
4. Fold one side of tortilla over filling to make a half-moon shape and press down lightly on center. Using the tines of a fork, press down firmly on edges of tortilla to seal in filling.
5. Mist both sides with oil or cooking spray.
6. Place hand pies in air fryer basket close but not overlapping. It's fine to lean some against the sides and corners of the basket. You may need to cook in 2 batches.
7. Cook at 390°F/200°C for 5minutes or until lightly browned. Serve hot.
8. Refrigerate any leftover pies in a closed container. To serve later, toss them back in the air fryer basket and cook for 2 or 3minutes to reheat.

Sea-salted Caramel Cookie Cups

Servings: 12
Cooking Time: 12 Minutes
Ingredients:
- ⅓ cup butter
- ¼ cup brown sugar
- 1 teaspoon vanilla extract
- 1 large egg
- 1 cup all-purpose flour
- ½ cup old-fashioned oats
- ½ teaspoon baking soda
- ¼ teaspoon salt
- ⅓ cup sea-salted caramel chips

Directions:
1. Preheat the air fryer to 300°F/150°C.
2. In a large bowl, cream the butter with the brown sugar and vanilla. Whisk in the egg and set aside.
3. In a separate bowl, mix the flour, oats, baking soda, and salt. Then gently mix the dry ingredients into the wet. Fold in the caramel chips.
4. Divide the batter into 12 silicon muffin liners. Place the cookie cups into the air fryer basket and cook for 12 minutes or until a toothpick inserted in the center comes out clean.
5. Remove and let cool 5 minutes before serving.

Magic Giant Chocolate Cookies

Servings: 2
Cooking Time: 30 Minutes
Ingredients:
- 2 tbsp white chocolate chips
- ½ cup flour
- 1/8 tsp baking soda
- ¼ cup butter, melted
- ¼ cup light brown sugar
- 2 tbsp granulated sugar
- 2 eggs
- 2 tbsp milk chocolate chips

- ¼ cup chopped pecans
- ¼ cup chopped hazelnuts
- ½ tsp vanilla extract
- Salt to taste

Directions:
1. Preheat air fryer at 350ºF/175°C. In a bowl, combine the flour, baking soda, butter, brown sugar, granulated sugar, eggs, milk chocolate chips, white chocolate chips, pecans, hazelnuts, vanilla extract, and salt. Press cookie mixture onto a greased pizza pan. Place pizza pan in the frying basket and Bake for 10 minutes. Let cool completely for 10 minutes. Turn over on a plate and serve.

Oreo-coated Peanut Butter Cups

Servings:8
Cooking Time: 4 Minutes

Ingredients:
- 8 Standard ¾-ounce peanut butter cups, frozen
- ⅓ cup All-purpose flour
- 2 Large egg white(s), beaten until foamy
- 16 Oreos or other creme-filled chocolate sandwich cookies, ground to crumbs in a food processor
- Vegetable oil spray

Directions:
1. Set up and fill three shallow soup plates or small pie plates on your counter: one for the flour, one for the beaten egg white(s), and one for the cookie crumbs.
2. Dip a frozen peanut butter cup in the flour, turning it to coat all sides. Shake off any excess, then set it in the beaten egg white(s). Turn it to coat all sides, then let any excess egg white slip back into the rest. Set the candy bar in the cookie crumbs. Turn to coat on all parts, even the sides. Dip the peanut butter cup back in the egg white(s) as before, then into the cookie crumbs as before, making sure you have a solid, even coating all around the cup. Set aside while you dip and coat the remaining cups.
3. When all the peanut butter cups are dipped and coated, lightly coat them on all sides with the vegetable oil spray. Set them on a plate and freeze while the air fryer heats.
4. Preheat the air fryer to 400°F/205°C.
5. Set the dipped cups wider side up in the basket with as much air space between them as possible. Air-fry undisturbed for 4 minutes, or until they feel soft but the coating is set.
6. Turn off the machine and remove the basket from it. Set aside the basket with the fried cups for 10 minutes. Use a nonstick-safe spatula to transfer the fried cups to a wire rack. Cool for at least another 5 minutes before serving.

Fried Oreos

Servings: 12
Cooking Time: 6 Minutes Per Batch

Ingredients:
- oil for misting or nonstick spray
- 1 cup complete pancake and waffle mix
- 1 teaspoon vanilla extract
- ½ cup water, plus 2 tablespoons
- 12 Oreos or other chocolate sandwich cookies
- 1 tablespoon confectioners' sugar

Directions:
1. Spray baking pan with oil or nonstick spray and place in basket.
2. Preheat air fryer to 390°F/200°C.
3. In a medium bowl, mix together the pancake mix, vanilla, and water.
4. Dip 4 cookies in batter and place in baking pan.
5. Cook for 6minutes, until browned.
6. Repeat steps 4 and 5 for the remaining cookies.

7. Sift sugar over warm cookies.

Peanut Butter-banana Roll-ups

Servings: 4
Cooking Time: 20 Minutes

Ingredients:
- 2 ripe bananas, halved crosswise
- 4 spring roll wrappers
- ¼ cup molasses
- ¼ cup peanut butter
- 1 tsp ground cinnamon
- 1 tsp lemon zest

Directions:
1. Preheat air fryer to 375°F/190°C. Place the roll wrappers on a flat surface with one corner facing up. Spread 1 tbsp of molasses on each, then 1 tbsp of peanut butter, and finally top with lemon zest and 1 banana half. Sprinkle with cinnamon all over. For the wontons, fold the bottom over the banana, then fold the sides, and roll-up. Place them seam-side down and Roast for 10 minutes until golden brown and crispy. Serve warm.

Greek Pumpkin Cheesecake

Servings: 4
Cooking Time: 35 Minutes + Chilling Time

Ingredients:
- 2 tbsp peanut butter
- ¼ cup oat flour
- ½ cup Greek yogurt
- 2 tbsp sugar
- ¼ cup ricotta cheese
- ¼ cup canned pumpkin
- 1 tbsp vanilla extract
- 2 tbsp cornstarch
- ¼ tsp ground cinnamon

Directions:
1. Preheat air fryer to 320°F/160°C. For the crust: Whisk the peanut butter, oat flour, 1 tbsp of Greek yogurt, and 1 tsp of sugar until you get a dough. Remove the dough onto a small cake pan and press down to get a ½-inch thick crust. Set aside. Mix the ricotta cheese, pumpkin, vanilla extract, cornstarch, cinnamon, ½ cup of Greek yogurt, and 1 tbsp of sugar until smooth. Pour over the crust and Bake for 20 minutes until golden brown. Let cool completely and refrigerate for 1 hour before serving.

Blueberry Cheesecake Tartlets

Servings: 9
Cooking Time: 6 Minutes

Ingredients:
- 8 ounces cream cheese, softened
- ¼ cup sugar
- 1 egg
- ½ teaspoon vanilla extract
- zest of 2 lemons, divided
- 9 mini graham cracker tartlet shells*
- 2 cups blueberries
- ½ teaspoon ground cinnamon
- juice of ½ lemon
- ¼ cup apricot preserves

Directions:
1. Preheat the air fryer to 330°F/165°C.
2. Combine the cream cheese, sugar, egg, vanilla and the zest of one lemon in a medium bowl and blend until smooth by hand or with an electric hand mixer. Pour the cream cheese mixture into the tartlet shells.

3. Air-fry 3 tartlets at a time at 330°F/165°C for 6 minutes, rotating them in the air fryer basket halfway through the cooking time.

4. Combine the blueberries, cinnamon, zest of one lemon and juice of half a lemon in a bowl. Melt the apricot preserves in the microwave or over low heat in a saucepan. Pour the apricot preserves over the blueberries and gently toss to coat.

5. Allow the cheesecakes to cool completely and then top each one with some of the blueberry mixture. Garnish the tartlets with a little sugared lemon peel and refrigerate until you are ready to serve.

Fried Banana S'mores

Servings: 4
Cooking Time: 6 Minutes
Ingredients:
- 4 bananas
- 3 tablespoons mini semi-sweet chocolate chips
- 3 tablespoons mini peanut butter chips
- 3 tablespoons mini marshmallows
- 3 tablespoons graham cracker cereal

Directions:
1. Preheat the air fryer to 400°F/205°C.
2. Slice into the un-peeled bananas lengthwise along the inside of the curve, but do not slice through the bottom of the peel. Open the banana slightly to form a pocket.
3. Fill each pocket with chocolate chips, peanut butter chips and marshmallows. Poke the graham cracker cereal into the filling.
4. Place the bananas in the air fryer basket, resting them on the side of the basket and each other to keep them upright with the filling facing up. Air-fry for 6 minutes, or until the bananas are soft to the touch, the peels have blackened and the chocolate and marshmallows have melted and toasted.
5. Let them cool for a couple of minutes and then simply serve with a spoon to scoop out the filling.

Easy Churros

Servings: 12
Cooking Time: 10 Minutes
Ingredients:
- ½ cup Water
- 4 tablespoons (¼ cup/½ stick) Butter
- ¼ teaspoon Table salt
- ½ cup All-purpose flour
- 2 Large egg(s)
- ¼ cup Granulated white sugar
- 2 teaspoons Ground cinnamon

Directions:
1. Bring the water, butter, and salt to a boil in a small saucepan set over high heat, stirring occasionally.
2. When the butter has fully melted, reduce the heat to medium and stir in the flour to form a dough. Continue cooking, stirring constantly, to dry out the dough until it coats the bottom and sides of the pan with a film, even a crust. Remove the pan from the heat, scrape the dough into a bowl, and cool for 15 minutes.
3. Using an electric hand mixer at medium speed, beat in the egg, or eggs one at a time, until the dough is smooth and firm enough to hold its shape.
4. Mix the sugar and cinnamon in a small bowl. Scoop up 1 tablespoon of the dough and roll it in the sugar mixture to form a small, coated tube about ½ inch in diameter and 2 inches long. Set it aside and make 5 more tubes for the small batch or 11 more for the large one.

5. Set the tubes on a plate and freeze for 20 minutes. Meanwhile, Preheat the air fryer to 375°F/190°C .
6. Set 3 frozen tubes in the basket for a small batch or 6 for a large one with as much air space between them as possible. Air-fry undisturbed for 10 minutes, or until puffed, brown, and set.
7. Use kitchen tongs to transfer the churros to a wire rack to cool for at least 5 minutes. Meanwhile, air-fry and cool the second batch of churros in the same way.

Fried Twinkies

Servings:6
Cooking Time: 5 Minutes
Ingredients:
- 2 Large egg white(s)
- 2 tablespoons Water
- 1½ cups (about 9 ounces) Ground gingersnap cookie crumbs
- 6 Twinkies
- Vegetable oil spray

Directions:
1. Preheat the air fryer to 400°F/205°C.
2. Set up and fill two shallow soup plates or small pie plates on your counter: one for the egg white(s), whisked with the water until foamy; and one for the gingersnap crumbs.
3. Dip a Twinkie in the egg white(s), turning it to coat on all sides, even the ends. Let the excess egg white mixture slip back into the rest, then set the Twinkie in the crumbs. Roll it to coat on all sides, even the ends, pressing gently to get an even coating. Then repeat this process: egg white(s), followed by crumbs. Lightly coat the prepared Twinkie on all sides with vegetable oil spray. Set aside and coat each of the remaining Twinkies with the same double-dipping technique, followed by spraying.
4. Set the Twinkies flat side up in the basket with as much air space between them as possible. Air-fry for 5 minutes, or until browned and crunchy.
5. Use a nonstick-safe spatula to gently transfer the Twinkies to a wire rack. Cool for at least 10 minutes before serving.

Baked Stuffed Pears

Servings: 4
Cooking Time: 15 Minutes + Cooling Time
Ingredients:
- 4 cored pears, halved
- ½ cup chopped cashews
- ½ cup dried cranberries
- ¼ cup agave nectar
- ½ stick butter, softened
- ½ tsp ground cinnamon
- ½ cup apple juice

Directions:
1. Preheat the air fryer to 350°F/175°C. Combine the cashews, cranberries, agave nectar, butter, and cinnamon and mix well. Stuff this mixture into the pears, heaping it up on top. Set the pears in a baking pan and pour the apple juice into the bottom of the pan. Put the pan in the fryer and Bake for 10-12 minutes or until the pears are tender. Let cool before serving.

Dark Chocolate Cream Galette

Servings: 4
Cooking Time: 55 Minutes + Cooling Time
Ingredients:
- 16 oz cream cheese, softened
- 1 cup crumbled graham crackers
- 1 cup dark cocoa powder
- ½ cup white sugar
- 1 tsp peppermint extract
- 1 tsp ground cinnamon
- 1 egg
- 1 cup condensed milk
- 2 tbsp muscovado sugar
- 1 ½ tsp butter, melted

Directions:
1. Preheat air fryer to 350°F/175°C. Place the crumbled graham crackers in a large bowl and stir in the muscovado sugar and melted butter. Spread the mixture into a greased pie pan, pressing down to form the galette base. Place the pan into the air fryer and Bake for 5 minutes. Remove the pan and set aside.
2. Place the cocoa powder, cream cheese, peppermint extract, white sugar, cinnamon, condensed milk, and egg in a large bowl and whip thoroughly to combine. Spoon the chocolate mixture over the graham cracker crust and level the top with a spatula. Put in the air fryer and Bake for 40 minutes until firm. Transfer the cookies to a wire rack to cool. Serve and enjoy!

Mango Cobbler With Raspberries

Servings: 4
Cooking Time: 30 Minutes
Ingredients:
- 1 ½ cups chopped mango
- 1 cup raspberries
- 1 tbsp brown sugar
- 2 tsp cornstarch
- 1 tsp lemon juice
- 2 tbsp sunflower oil
- 1 tbsp maple syrup
- 1 tsp vanilla
- ½ cup rolled oats
- 1/3 cup flour
- 3 tbsp coconut sugar
- 1 tsp cinnamon
- ¼ tsp nutmeg
- ⅛ tsp salt

Directions:
1. Place the mango, raspberries, brown sugar, cornstarch, and lemon juice in a baking pan. Stir with a rubber spatula until combined. Set aside.
2. In a separate bowl, add the oil, maple syrup, and vanilla and stir well. Toss in the oats, flour, coconut sugar, cinnamon, nutmeg, and salt. Stir until combined. Sprinkle evenly over the mango-raspberry filling. Preheat air fryer to 320°F/160°C. Bake for 20 minutes or until the topping is crispy and golden. Enjoy warm.

Coconut Macaroons

Servings: 12
Cooking Time: 8 Minutes
Ingredients:
- 1⅓ cups shredded, sweetened coconut
- 4½ teaspoons flour
- 2 tablespoons sugar
- 1 egg white
- ½ teaspoon almond extract

Directions:
1. Preheat air fryer to 330°F/165°C.
2. Mix all ingredients together.
3. Shape coconut mixture into 12 balls.
4. Place all 12 macaroons in air fryer basket. They won't expand, so you can place them close together, but they shouldn't touch.
5. Cook at 330°F/165°C for 8 minutes, until golden.

Orange-chocolate Cake

Servings: 6
Cooking Time: 35 Minutes
Ingredients:
- ¾ cup flour
- ½ cup sugar
- 7 tbsp cocoa powder
- ½ tsp baking soda
- ½ cup milk
- 2 ½ tbsp sunflower oil
- ½ tbsp orange juice
- 2 tsp vanilla
- 2 tsp orange zest
- 3 tbsp butter, softened
- 1 ¼ cups powdered sugar

Directions:
1. Use a whisk to combine the flour, sugar, 2 tbsp of cocoa powder, baking soda, and a pinch of salt in a bowl. Once combined, add milk, sunflower oil, orange juice, and orange zest. Stir until combined. Preheat the air fryer to 350°F/175°C. Pour the batter into a greased cake pan and Bake for 25 minutes or until a knife inserted in the center comes out clean.
2. Use an electric beater to beat the butter and powdered sugar together in a bowl. Add the remaining cocoa powder and vanilla and whip until fluffy. Scrape the sides occasionally. Refrigerate until ready to use. Allow the cake to cool completely, then run a knife around the edges of the baking pan. Turn it upside-down on a plate so it can be frosted on the sides and top. When the frosting is no longer cold, use a butter knife or small spatula to frost the sides and top. Cut into slices and enjoy!

Rustic Berry Layer Cake

Servings: 6
Cooking Time: 45 Minutes
Ingredients:
- 2 eggs, beaten
- ½ cup milk
- 2 tbsp Greek yogurt
- ¼ cup maple syrup
- 1 tbsp apple cider vinegar
- 1 tbsp vanilla extract
- ¾ cup all-purpose flour
- 1 tsp baking powder
- ½ tsp baking soda
- ¼ cup dark chocolate chips
- 1/3 cup raspberry jam

Directions:
1. Preheat air fryer to 350°F/175°C. Combine the eggs, milk, Greek yogurt, maple syrup, apple vinegar, and vanilla extract in a bowl. Toss in flour, baking powder, and baking soda until combined. Pour the batter into a 6-inch round cake pan, distributing well, and Bake for 20-25 minutes until a toothpick comes out clean. Let cool completely.

2. Turn the cake onto a plate, cut lengthwise to make 2 equal layers. Set aside. Add chocolate chips to a heat-proof bowl and Bake for 3 minutes until fully melted. In the meantime, spread raspberry jam on top of the bottom layer, distributing well, and top with the remaining layer. Once the chocolate is ready, stir in 1 tbsp of milk. Pour over the layer cake and spread well. Cut into 6 wedges and serve immediately.

One-bowl Chocolate Buttermilk Cake

Servings: 6
Cooking Time: 16-20 Minutes
Ingredients:
- ¾ cup All-purpose flour
- ½ cup Granulated white sugar
- 3 tablespoons Unsweetened cocoa powder
- ½ teaspoon Baking soda
- ¼ teaspoon Table salt
- ½ cup Buttermilk
- 2 tablespoons Vegetable oil
- ¾ teaspoon Vanilla extract
- Baking spray (see here)

Directions:
1. Preheat the air fryer to 325°F/160°C (or 330°F/165°C, if that's the closest setting).
2. Stir the flour, sugar, cocoa powder, baking soda, and salt in a large bowl until well combined. Add the buttermilk, oil, and vanilla. Stir just until a thick, grainy batter forms.
3. Use the baking spray to generously coat the inside of a 6-inch round cake pan for a small batch, a 7-inch round cake pan for a medium batch, or an 8-inch round cake pan for a large batch. Scrape and spread the chocolate batter into this pan, smoothing the batter out to an even layer.
4. Set the pan in the basket and air-fry undisturbed for 16 minutes for a 6-inch layer, 18 minutes for a 7-inch layer, or 20 minutes for an 8-inch layer, or until a toothpick or cake tester inserted into the center of the cake comes out clean. Start checking it at the 14-minute mark to know where you are.
5. Use hot pads or silicone baking mitts to transfer the cake pan to a wire rack. Cool for 5 minutes. To unmold, set a cutting board over the baking pan and invert both the board and the pan. Lift the still-warm pan off the cake layer. Set the wire rack on top of the cake layer and invert all of it with the cutting board so that the cake layer is now right side up on the wire rack. Remove the cutting board and continue cooling the cake for at least 10 minutes or to room temperature, about 30 minutes, before slicing into wedges.

Homemade Chips Ahoy

Servings: 4
Cooking Time: 20 Minutes
Ingredients:
- 1 tbsp coconut oil, melted
- 1 tbsp honey
- 1 tbsp milk
- ½ tsp vanilla extract
- ¼ cup oat flour
- 2 tbsp coconut sugar
- ¼ tsp salt
- ¼ tsp baking powder
- 2 tbsp chocolate chips

Directions:
1. Combine the coconut oil, honey, milk, and vanilla in a bowl. Add the oat flour, coconut sugar, salt, and baking powder. Stir until combined. Add the chocolate chips and stir. Preheat air fryer to 350°F/175°C. Pour the batter into a

greased baking pan, leaving a little room in between. Bake for 7 minutes or until golden. Do not overcook. Move to a cooling rack and serve chilled.

Bananas Foster Bread Pudding

Servings: 4
Cooking Time: 25 Minutes
Ingredients:
- ½ cup brown sugar
- 3 eggs
- ¾ cup half and half
- 1 teaspoon pure vanilla extract
- 6 cups cubed Kings Hawaiian bread (½-inch cubes), ½ pound
- 2 bananas, sliced
- 1 cup caramel sauce, plus more for serving

Directions:
1. Preheat the air fryer to 350°F/175°C.
2. Combine the brown sugar, eggs, half and half and vanilla extract in a large bowl, whisking until the sugar has dissolved and the mixture is smooth. Stir in the cubed bread and toss to coat all the cubes evenly. Let the bread sit for 10 minutes to absorb the liquid.
3. Mix the sliced bananas and caramel sauce together in a separate bowl.
4. Fill the bottom of 4 (8-ounce) greased ramekins with half the bread cubes. Divide the caramel and bananas between the ramekins, spooning them on top of the bread cubes. Top with the remaining bread cubes and wrap each ramekin with aluminum foil, tenting the foil at the top to leave some room for the bread to puff up during the cooking process.
5. Air-fry two bread puddings at a time for 25 minutes. Let the puddings cool a little and serve warm with additional caramel sauce drizzled on top. A scoop of vanilla ice cream would be nice too and in keeping with our Bananas Foster theme!

Caramel Apple Crumble

Servings: 6
Cooking Time: 50 Minutes
Ingredients:
- 4 apples, peeled and thinly sliced
- 2 tablespoons sugar
- 1 tablespoon flour
- 1 teaspoon ground cinnamon
- ¼ teaspoon ground allspice
- healthy pinch ground nutmeg
- 10 caramel squares, cut into small pieces
- Crumble Topping:
- ¾ cup rolled oats
- ¼ cup sugar
- ⅓ cup flour
- ¼ teaspoon ground cinnamon
- 6 tablespoons butter, melted

Directions:
1. Preheat the air fryer to 330°F/165°C.
2. Combine the apples, sugar, flour, and spices in a large bowl and toss to coat. Add the caramel pieces and mix well. Pour the apple mixture into a 1-quart round baking dish that will fit in your air fryer basket (6-inch diameter).
3. To make the crumble topping, combine the rolled oats, sugar, flour and cinnamon in a small bowl. Add the melted butter and mix well. Top the apples with the crumble mixture. Cover the entire dish with aluminum foil and transfer the dish to the air fryer basket, lowering the dish into the basket using a sling made of aluminum foil (fold a piece of aluminum foil

into a strip about 2-inches wide by 24-inches long). Fold the ends of the aluminum foil over the top of the dish before returning the basket to the air fryer.

4. Air-fry at 330°F/165°C for 25 minutes. Remove the aluminum foil and continue to air-fry for another 25 minutes. Serve the crumble warm with whipped cream or vanilla ice cream, if desired.

Vanilla-strawberry Muffins

Servings: 4
Cooking Time: 25 Minutes
Ingredients:
- ¼ cup diced strawberries
- 2 tbsp powdered sugar
- 1 cup flour
- ½ tsp baking soda
- 1/3 cup granulated sugar
- ¼ tsp salt
- 1 tsp vanilla extract
- 1 egg
- 1 tbsp butter, melted
- ½ cup diced strawberries
- 2 tbsp chopped walnuts
- 6 tbsp butter, softened
- 1 ½ cups powdered sugar
- 1/8 tsp peppermint extract

Directions:
1. Preheat air fryer at 375ºF/190°C. Combine flour, baking soda, granulated sugar, and salt in a bowl. In another bowl, combine the vanilla, egg, walnuts and melted butter. Pour wet ingredients into dry ingredients and toss to combine. Fold in half of the strawberries and spoon mixture into 8 greased silicone cupcake liners.

2. Place cupcakes in the frying basket and Bake for 6-8 minutes. Let cool onto a cooling rack for 10 minutes. Blend the remaining strawberries in a food processor until smooth. Slowly add powdered sugar to softened butter while beating in a bowl. Stir in peppermint extract and puréed strawberries until blended. Spread over cooled cupcakes. Serve sprinkled with powdered sugar

Nutty Cookies

Servings: 6
Cooking Time: 25 Minutes
Ingredients:
- ¼ cup pistachios
- ¼ cup evaporated cane sugar
- ¼ cup raw almonds
- ½ cup almond flour
- 1 tsp pure vanilla extract
- 1 egg white

Directions:
1. Preheat air fryer to 375°F/190°C. Add ¼ cup of pistachios and almonds into a food processor. Pulse until they resemble crumbles. Roughly chop the rest of the pistachios with a sharp knife. Combine all ingredients in a large bowl until completely incorporated. Form 6 equally-sized balls and transfer to the parchment-lined frying basket. Allow for 1 inch between each portion. Bake for 7 minutes. Cool on a wire rack for 5 minutes. Serve and enjoy.

Mini Carrot Cakes

Servings: 6
Cooking Time: 25 Minutes
Ingredients:
- 1 cup grated carrots

- ¼ cup raw honey
- ¼ cup olive oil
- ½ tsp vanilla extract
- ½ tsp lemon zest
- 1 egg
- ¼ cup applesauce
- 1 1/3 cups flour
- ¾ tsp baking powder
- ½ tsp baking soda
- ½ tsp ground cinnamon
- ¼ tsp ground nutmeg
- ⅛ tsp ground ginger
- ⅛ tsp salt
- ¼ cup chopped hazelnuts
- 2 tbsp chopped sultanas

Directions:
1. Preheat air fryer to 380°F/195°C. Combine the carrots, honey, olive oil, vanilla extract, lemon zest, egg, and applesauce in a bowl. Sift the flour, baking powder, baking soda, cinnamon, nutmeg, ginger, and salt in a separate bowl. Add the wet ingredients to the dry ingredients, mixing until just combined. Fold in the hazelnuts and sultanas. Fill greased muffin cups three-quarters full with the batter, and place them in the frying basket. Bake for 10-12 minutes until a toothpick inserted in the center of a cupcake comes out clean. Serve and enjoy!

Coconut-carrot Cupcakes

Servings: 4
Cooking Time: 25 Minutes
Ingredients:
- 1 cup flour
- ½ tsp baking soda
- 1/3 cup light brown sugar
- ¼ tsp salt
- ¼ tsp ground cinnamon
- 1 ½ tsp vanilla extract
- 1 egg
- 1 tbsp buttermilk
- 1 tbsp vegetable oil
- ¼ cup grated carrots
- 2 tbsp coconut shreds
- 6 oz cream cheese
- 1 1/3 cups powdered sugar
- 2 tbsp butter, softened
- 1 tbsp milk
- 1 tbsp coconut flakes

Directions:
1. Preheat air fryer at 375ºF/190°C. Combine flour, baking soda, brown sugar, salt, and cinnamon in a bowl. In another bowl, combine egg, 1 tsp of vanilla, buttermilk, and vegetable oil. Pour wet ingredients into dry ingredients and toss to combine. Do not overmix. Fold in carrots and coconut shreds. Spoon mixture into 8 greased silicone cupcake liners. Place cupcakes in the frying basket and Bake for 6-8 minutes. Let cool onto a cooling rack for 15 minutes. Whisk cream cheese, powdered sugar, remaining vanilla, softened butter, and milk in a bowl until smooth. Spread over cooled cupcakes. Garnish with coconut flakes and serve.

Molten Chocolate Almond Cakes

Servings: 3
Cooking Time: 13 Minutes
Ingredients:
- butter and flour for the ramekins
- 4 ounces bittersweet chocolate, chopped
- ½ cup (1 stick) unsalted butter
- 2 eggs
- 2 egg yolks
- ¼ cup sugar
- ½ teaspoon pure vanilla extract, or almond extract
- 1 tablespoon all-purpose flour
- 3 tablespoons ground almonds
- 8 to 12 semisweet chocolate discs (or 4 chunks of chocolate)
- cocoa powder or powdered sugar, for dusting
- toasted almonds, coarsely chopped

Directions:
1. Butter and flour three (6-ounce) ramekins. (Butter the ramekins and then coat the butter with flour by shaking it around in the ramekin and dumping out any excess.)
2. Melt the chocolate and butter together, either in the microwave or in a double boiler. In a separate bowl, beat the eggs, egg yolks and sugar together until light and smooth. Add the vanilla extract. Whisk the chocolate mixture into the egg mixture. Stir in the flour and ground almonds.
3. Preheat the air fryer to 330°F/165°C.
4. Transfer the batter carefully to the buttered ramekins, filling halfway. Place two or three chocolate discs in the center of the batter and then fill the ramekins to ½-inch below the top with the remaining batter. Place the ramekins into the air fryer basket and air-fry at 330°F for 13 minutes. The sides of the cake should be set, but the centers should be slightly soft. Remove the ramekins from the air fryer and let the cakes sit for 5 minutes. (If you'd like the cake a little less molten, air-fry for 14 minutes and let the cakes sit for 4 minutes.)
5. Run a butter knife around the edge of the ramekins and invert the cakes onto a plate. Lift the ramekin off the plate slowly and carefully so that the cake doesn't break. Dust with cocoa powder or powdered sugar and serve with a scoop of ice cream and some coarsely chopped toasted almonds.

Banana Fritters

Servings: 6
Cooking Time: 20 Minutes
Ingredients:
- 1 egg
- ¼ cup cornstarch
- ¼ cup bread crumbs
- 3 bananas, halved crosswise
- ¼ cup caramel sauce

Directions:
1. Preheat air fryer to 350°F/175°C. Set up three small bowls. In the first bowl, add cornstarch. In the second bowl, beat the egg. In the third bowl, add bread crumbs. Dip the bananas in the cornstarch first, then the egg, and then dredge in bread crumbs. Put the bananas in the greased frying basket and spray with oil. Air Fry for 8 minutes, flipping once around minute 5. Remove to a serving plate and drizzle with caramel sauce. Serve warm and enjoy.

Brownies After Dark

Servings: 4
Cooking Time: 13 Minutes
Ingredients:
- 1 egg
- ½ cup granulated sugar
- ¼ teaspoon salt
- ½ teaspoon vanilla
- ¼ cup butter, melted
- ¼ cup flour, plus 2 tablespoons
- ¼ cup cocoa
- cooking spray
- Optional
- vanilla ice cream
- caramel sauce
- whipped cream

Directions:
1. Beat together egg, sugar, salt, and vanilla until light.
2. Add melted butter and mix well.
3. Stir in flour and cocoa.
4. Spray 6 x 6-inch baking pan lightly with cooking spray.
5. Spread batter in pan and cook at 330°F/165°C for 13 minutes. Cool and cut into 4 large squares or 16 small brownie bites.

Mixed Berry Pie

Servings: 4
Cooking Time: 25 Minutes
Ingredients:
- 2/3 cup blackberries, cut into thirds
- ¼ cup sugar
- 2 tbsp cornstarch
- ¼ tsp vanilla extract
- ¼ tsp peppermint extract
- ½ tsp lemon zest
- 1 cup sliced strawberries
- 1 cup raspberries
- 1 refrigerated piecrust
- 1 large egg

Directions:
1. Mix the sugar, cornstarch, vanilla, peppermint extract, and lemon zest in a bowl. Toss in all berries gently until combined. Pour into a greased dish. On a clean workspace, lay out the dough and cut into a 7-inch diameter round. Cover the baking dish with the round and crimp the edges. With a knife, cut 4 slits in the top to vent.
2. Beat 1 egg and 1 tbsp of water to make an egg wash. Brush the egg wash over the crust. Preheat air fryer to 350°F/175°C. Put the baking dish into the frying basket. Bake for 15 minutes or until the crust is golden and the berries are bubbling through the vents. Remove from the air fryer and let cool for 15 minutes. Serve warm.

Cheesecake Wontons

Servings:16
Cooking Time: 6 Minutes
Ingredients:
- ¼ cup Regular or low-fat cream cheese (not fat-free)
- 2 tablespoons Granulated white sugar
- 1½ tablespoons Egg yolk
- ¼ teaspoon Vanilla extract
- ⅛ teaspoon Table salt
- 1½ tablespoons All-purpose flour
- 16 Wonton wrappers (vegetarian, if a concern)
- Vegetable oil spray

Directions:
1. Preheat the air fryer to 400°F/205°C.
2. Using a flatware fork, mash the cream cheese, sugar, egg yolk, and vanilla in a small bowl until smooth. Add the salt and flour and continue mashing until evenly combined.

3. Set a wonton wrapper on a clean, dry work surface so that one corner faces you (so that it looks like a diamond on your work surface). Set 1 teaspoon of the cream cheese mixture in the middle of the wrapper but just above a horizontal line that would divide the wrapper in half. Dip your clean finger in water and run it along the edges of the wrapper. Fold the corner closest to you up and over the filling, lining it up with the corner farthest from you, thereby making a stuffed triangle. Press gently to seal. Wet the two triangle tips nearest you, then fold them up and together over the filling. Gently press together to seal and fuse. Set aside and continue making more stuffed wontons, 11 more for the small batch, 15 more for the medium batch, or 23 more for the large one.

4. Lightly coat the stuffed wrappers on all sides with vegetable oil spray. Set them with the fused corners up in the basket with as much air space between them as possible. Air-fry undisturbed for 6 minutes, or until golden brown and crisp.

5. Gently dump the contents of the basket onto a wire rack. Cool for at least 5 minutes before serving.

Sweet Potato Pie Rolls

Servings:3
Cooking Time: 8 Minutes
Ingredients:
- 6 Spring roll wrappers
- 1½ cups Canned yams in syrup, drained
- 2 tablespoons Light brown sugar
- ¼ teaspoon Ground cinnamon
- 1 Large egg(s), well beaten
- Vegetable oil spray

Directions:
1. Preheat the air fryer to 400°F/205°C.
2. Set a spring roll wrapper on a clean, dry work surface. Scoop up ¼ cup of the pulpy yams and set along one edge of the wrapper, leaving 2 inches on each side of the yams. Top the yams with about 1 teaspoon brown sugar and a pinch of ground cinnamon. Fold the sides of the wrapper perpendicular to the yam filling up and over the filling, partially covering it. Brush beaten egg(s) over the side of the wrapper farthest from the yam. Starting with the yam end, roll the wrapper closed, ending at the part with the beaten egg that you can press gently to seal. Lightly coat the roll on all sides with vegetable oil spray. Set it aside seam side down and continue filling, rolling, and spraying the remaining wrappers in the same way.
3. Set the rolls seam side down in the basket with as much air space between them as possible. Air-fry undisturbed for 8 minutes, or until crisp and golden brown.
4. Use a nonstick-safe spatula and perhaps kitchen tongs for balance to gently transfer the rolls to a wire rack. Cool for at least 5 minutes or up to 30 minutes before serving.

Chocolate Cake

Servings: 8
Cooking Time: 20 Minutes
Ingredients:
- ½ cup sugar
- ¼ cup flour, plus 3 tablespoons
- 3 tablespoons cocoa
- ½ teaspoon baking powder
- ½ teaspoon baking soda
- ¼ teaspoon salt
- 1 egg
- 2 tablespoons oil
- ½ cup milk

- ½ teaspoon vanilla extract

Directions:
1. Preheat air fryer to 330°F/165°C.
2. Grease and flour a 6 x 6-inch baking pan.
3. In a medium bowl, stir together the sugar, flour, cocoa, baking powder, baking soda, and salt.
4. Add all other ingredients and beat with a wire whisk until smooth.
5. Pour batter into prepared pan and bake at 330°F/165°C for 20 minutes, until toothpick inserted in center comes out clean or with crumbs clinging to it.

Orange Gooey Butter Cake

Servings: 6
Cooking Time: 85 Minutes
Ingredients:
- Crust Layer:
- ½ cup flour
- ¼ cup sugar
- ½ teaspoon baking powder
- ⅛ teaspoon salt
- 2 ounces (½ stick) unsalted European style butter, melted
- 1 egg
- 1 teaspoon orange extract
- 2 tablespoons orange zest
- Gooey Butter Layer:
- 8 ounces cream cheese, softened
- 4 ounces (1 stick) unsalted European style butter, melted
- 2 eggs
- 2 teaspoons orange extract
- 2 tablespoons orange zest
- 4 cups powdered sugar
- Garnish:
- powdered sugar
- orange slices

Directions:
1. Preheat the air fryer to 350°F/175°C.
2. Grease a 7-inch cake pan and line the bottom with parchment paper. Combine the flour, sugar, baking powder and salt in a bowl. Add the melted butter, egg, orange extract and orange zest. Mix well and press this mixture into the bottom of the greased cake pan. Lower the pan into the basket using an aluminum foil sling (fold a piece of aluminum foil into a strip about 2-inches wide by 24-inches long). Fold the ends of the aluminum foil over the top of the dish before returning the basket to the air fryer. Air-fry uncovered for 8 minutes.
3. To make the gooey butter layer, beat the cream cheese, melted butter, eggs, orange extract and orange zest in a large bowl using an electric hand mixer. Add the powdered sugar in stages, beat until smooth with each addition. Pour this mixture on top of the baked crust in the cake pan. Wrap the pan with a piece of greased aluminum foil, tenting the top of the foil to leave a little room for the cake to rise.
4. Air-fry for 60 minutes at 350°F/175°C. Remove the aluminum foil and air-fry for an additional 17 minutes.
5. Let the cake cool inside the pan for at least 10 minutes. Then, run a butter knife around the cake and let the cake cool completely in the pan. When cooled, run the butter knife around the edges of the cake again and invert it onto a plate and then back onto a serving platter. Sprinkle the powdered sugar over the top of the cake and garnish with orange slices.

Rich Blueberry Biscuit Shortcakes

Servings: 4
Cooking Time: 35 Minutes
Ingredients:
- 1 lb blueberries, halved
- ¼ cup granulated sugar
- 1 tsp orange zest
- 1 cup heavy cream
- 1 tbsp orange juice
- 2 tbsp powdered sugar
- ¼ tsp cinnamon
- ¼ tsp nutmeg
- 2 cups flour
- 1 egg yolk
- 1 tbsp baking powder
- ½ tsp baking soda
- ½ tsp cornstarch
- ½ tsp salt
- ½ tsp vanilla extract
- ½ tsp honey
- 4 tbsp cold butter, cubed
- 1 ¼ cups buttermilk

Directions:
1. Combine blueberries, granulated sugar, and orange zest in a bowl. Let chill the topping covered in the fridge until ready to use. Beat heavy cream, orange juice, egg yolk, vanilla extract and powdered sugar in a metal bowl until peaks form. Let chill the whipped cream covered in the fridge until ready to use.
2. Preheat air fryer at 350ºF/175°C. Combine flour, cinnamon, nutmeg, baking powder, baking soda, cornstarch, honey, butter cubes, and buttermilk in a bowl until a sticky dough forms. Flour your hands and form dough into 8 balls. Place them on a lightly greased pizza pan. Place pizza pan in the frying basket and Air Fry for 8 minutes. Transfer biscuits to serving plates and cut them in half. Spread blueberry mixture to each biscuit bottom and place tops of biscuits. Garnish with whipped cream and serve.

Fast Brownies

Servings: 4
Cooking Time: 25 Minutes
Ingredients:
- ½ cup flour
- 2 tbsp cocoa
- 1/3 cup granulated sugar
- ¼ tsp baking soda
- 3 tbsp butter, melted
- 1 egg
- ¼ tsp salt
- ½ cup chocolate chips
- ¼ cup chopped hazelnuts
- 1 tbsp powdered sugar
- 1 tsp vanilla extract

Directions:
1. Preheat air fryer at 350ºF/175°C. Combine all ingredients, except chocolate chips, hazelnuts, and powdered sugar, in a bowl. Fold in chocolate chips and pecans. Press mixture into a greased cake pan. Place cake pan in the frying basket and Bake for 12 minutes. Let cool for 10 minutes before slicing into 9 brownies. Scatter with powdered sugar and serve.

Giant Vegan Chocolate Chip Cookie

Servings: 4
Cooking Time: 16 Minutes
Ingredients:
- ⅔ cup All-purpose flour
- 5 tablespoons Rolled oats (not quick-cooking or steel-cut oats)
- ¼ teaspoon Baking soda
- ¼ teaspoon Table salt
- 5 tablespoons Granulated white sugar
- ¼ cup Vegetable oil
- 2½ tablespoons Tahini (see here)
- 2½ tablespoons Maple syrup
- 2 teaspoons Vanilla extract
- ⅔ cup Vegan semisweet or bittersweet chocolate chips
- Baking spray

Directions:
1. Preheat the air fryer to 325°F/160°C (or 330°F/165°C, if that's the closest setting).
2. Whisk the flour, oats, baking soda, and salt in a bowl until well combined.
3. Using an electric hand mixer at medium speed, beat the sugar, oil, tahini, maple syrup, and vanilla until rich and creamy, about 3 minutes, scraping down the inside of the bowl occasionally.
4. Scrape down and remove the beaters. Fold in the flour mixture and chocolate chips with a rubber spatula just until all the flour is moistened and the chocolate chips are even throughout the dough.
5. For a small air fryer, coat the inside of a 6-inch round cake pan with baking spray. For a medium air fryer, coat the inside of a 7-inch round cake pan with baking spray. And for a large air fryer, coat the inside of an 8-inch round cake pan with baking spray. Scrape and gently press the dough into the prepared pan, spreading it into an even layer to the perimeter.
6. Set the pan in the basket and air-fry undisturbed for 16 minutes, or until puffed, browned, and firm to the touch.
7. Transfer the pan to a wire rack and cool for 10 minutes. Loosen the cookie from the perimeter with a spatula, then invert the pan onto a cutting board and let the cookie come free. Remove the pan and reinvert the cookie onto the wire rack. Cool for 5 minutes more before slicing into wedges to serve.

Carrot-oat Cake Muffins

Servings: 4
Cooking Time: 20 Minutes
Ingredients:
- 3 tbsp butter, softened
- ¼ cup brown sugar
- 1 tbsp maple syrup
- 1 egg white
- ½ tsp vanilla extract
- 1/3 cup finely grated carrots
- ½ cup oatmeal
- 1/3 cup flour
- ½ tsp baking soda
- ¼ cup raisins

Directions:
1. Preheat air fryer to 350°F/175°C. Mix the butter, brown sugar, and maple syrup until smooth, then toss in the egg white, vanilla, and carrots. Whisk well and add the oatmeal, flour, baking soda, and raisins. Divide the mixture between muffin cups. Bake in the fryer for 8-10 minutes.

Banana-lemon Bars

Servings: 6
Cooking Time: 40 Minutes
Ingredients:
- ¾ cup flour
- 2 tbsp powdered sugar
- ¼ cup coconut oil, melted
- ½ cup brown sugar
- 1 tbsp lemon zest
- ¼ cup lemon juice
- ⅛ tsp salt
- ¼ cup mashed bananas
- 1¾ tsp cornstarch
- ¾ tsp baking powder

Directions:
1. Combine the flour, powdered sugar, and coconut oil in a bowl. Place in the fridge. Mix the brown sugar, lemon zest and juice, salt, bananas, cornstarch, and baking powder in a bowl. Stir well. Preheat air fryer to 350°F/175°C. Spray a baking pan with oil. Remove the crust from the fridge and press it into the bottom of the pan to form a crust. Place in the air fryer and Bake for 5 minutes or until firm. Remove and spread the lemon filling over the crust. Bake for 18-20 minutes or until the top is golden. Cool for an hour in the fridge. Once firm and cooled, cut into pieces and serve.

Blueberry Crisp

Servings: 6
Cooking Time: 13 Minutes
Ingredients:
- 3 cups Fresh or thawed frozen blueberries
- ⅓ cup Granulated white sugar
- 1 tablespoon Instant tapioca
- ⅓ cup All-purpose flour
- ⅓ cup Rolled oats (not quick-cooking or steel-cut)
- ⅓ cup Chopped walnuts or pecans
- ⅓ cup Packed light brown sugar
- 5 tablespoons plus 1 teaspoon (⅔ stick) Butter, melted and cooled
- ¾ teaspoon Ground cinnamon
- ¼ teaspoon Table salt

Directions:
1. Preheat the air fryer to 400°F/205°C.
2. Mix the blueberries, granulated white sugar, and instant tapioca in a 6-inch round cake pan for a small batch, a 7-inch round cake pan for a medium batch, or an 8-inch round cake pan for a large batch.
3. When the machine is at temperature, set the cake pan in the basket and air-fry undisturbed for 5 minutes, or just until the blueberries begin to bubble.
4. Meanwhile, mix the flour, oats, nuts, brown sugar, butter, cinnamon, and salt in a medium bowl until well combined.
5. When the blueberries have begun to bubble, crumble this flour mixture evenly on top. Continue air-frying undisturbed for 8 minutes, or until the topping has browned a bit and the filling is bubbling.
6. Use two hot pads or silicone baking mitts to transfer the cake pan to a wire rack. Cool for at least 10 minutes or to room temperature before serving.

Oatmeal Blackberry Crisp

Servings: 6
Cooking Time: 20 Minutes
Ingredients:
- 1 cup rolled oats
- ½ cup flour

- ¼ cup olive oil
- ¼ tsp salt
- 1 tsp cinnamon
- 1/3 cup honey
- 4 cups blackberries

Directions:
1. Preheat air fryer to 350°F/175°C. Combine rolled oats, flour, olive oil, salt, cinnamon, and honey in a large bowl. Mix well. Spread blackberries on the bottom of a greased cooking pan. Cover them with the oat mixture. Place pan in air fryer and Bake for 15 minutes. Cool for a few minutes. Serve and enjoy.

Fried Cannoli Wontons

Servings: 10
Cooking Time: 8 Minutes
Ingredients:
- 8 ounces Neufchâtel cream cheese
- ¼ cup powdered sugar
- 1 teaspoon vanilla extract
- ¼ teaspoon salt
- ¼ cup mini chocolate chips
- 2 tablespoons chopped pecans (optional)
- 20 wonton wrappers
- ¼ cup filtered water

Directions:
1. Preheat the air fryer to 370°F/185°C.
2. In a large bowl, use a hand mixer to combine the cream cheese with the powdered sugar, vanilla, and salt. Fold in the chocolate chips and pecans. Set aside.
3. Lay the wonton wrappers out on a flat, smooth surface and place a bowl with the filtered water next to them.
4. Use a teaspoon to evenly divide the cream cheese mixture among the 20 wonton wrappers, placing the batter in the center of the wontons.
5. Wet the tip of your index finger, and gently moisten the outer edges of the wrapper. Then fold each wrapper until it creates a secure pocket.
6. Liberally spray the air fryer basket with olive oil mist.
7. Place the wontons into the basket, and cook for 5 to 8 minutes. When the outer edges begin to brown, remove the wontons from the air fryer basket. Repeat cooking with remaining wontons.
8. Serve warm.

Honey Apple-pear Crisp

Servings: 4
Cooking Time: 25 Minutes
Ingredients:
- 1 peeled apple, chopped
- 2 peeled pears, chopped
- 2 tbsp honey
- ½ cup oatmeal
- 1/3 cup flour
- 3 tbsp sugar
- 2 tbsp butter, softened
- ½ tsp ground cinnamon

Directions:
1. Preheat air fryer to 380°F/195°C. Combine the apple, pears, and honey in a baking pan. Mix the oatmeal, flour, sugar, butter, and cinnamon in a bowl. Note that this mix won't be smooth. Dust the mix over the fruit, then Bake for 10-12 minutes. Serve hot.

Cinnamon Canned Biscuit Donuts

Servings: 4
Cooking Time: 25 Minutes
Ingredients:
- 1 can jumbo biscuits
- 1 cup cinnamon sugar

Directions:
1. Preheat air fryer to 360°F/180°C. Divide biscuit dough into 8 biscuits and place on a flat work surface. Cut a small circle in the center of the biscuit with a small cookie cutter. Place a batch of 4 donuts in the air fryer. Spray with oil and Bake for 8 minutes, flipping once. Drizzle the cinnamon sugar over the donuts and serve.

Cheese Blintzes

Servings: 6
Cooking Time: 10 Minutes
Ingredients:
- 1½ 7½-ounce package(s) farmer cheese
- 3 tablespoons Regular or low-fat cream cheese (not fat-free)
- 3 tablespoons Granulated white sugar
- ¼ teaspoon Vanilla extract
- 6 Egg roll wrappers
- 3 tablespoons Butter, melted and cooled

Directions:
1. Preheat the air fryer to 375°F/190°C .
2. Use a flatware fork to mash the farmer cheese, cream cheese, sugar, and vanilla in a small bowl until smooth.
3. Set one egg roll wrapper on a clean, dry work surface. Place ¼ cup of the filling at the edge closest to you, leaving a ½-inch gap before the edge of the wrapper. Dip your clean finger in water and wet the edges of the wrapper. Fold the perpendicular sides over the filling, then roll the wrapper closed with the filling inside. Set it aside seam side down and continue filling the remainder of the wrappers.
4. Brush the wrappers on all sides with the melted butter. Be generous. Set them seam side down in the basket with as much space between them as possible. Air-fry undisturbed for 10 minutes, or until lightly browned.
5. Use a nonstick-safe spatula to transfer the blintzes to a wire rack. Cool for at least 5 minutes or up to 20 minutes before serving.

Struffoli

Servings: X
Cooking Time: 20 Minutes
Ingredients:
- ¼ cup butter, softened
- ⅔ cup sugar
- 5 eggs
- 2 teaspoons vanilla extract
- zest of 1 lemon
- 4 cups all-purpose flour
- 2 teaspoons baking soda
- ¼ teaspoon salt
- 16 ounces honey
- 1 teaspoon ground cinnamon
- zest of 1 orange
- 2 tablespoons water
- nonpareils candy sprinkles

Directions:
1. Cream the butter and sugar together in a bowl until light and fluffy using a hand mixer (or a stand mixer). Add the eggs, vanilla and lemon zest and mix. In a separate bowl, combine the flour, baking soda and salt. Add the dry ingredients to the wet ingredients and mix until you have a soft dough. Shape the dough into a ball, wrap it in plastic and let it rest for 30 minutes.

2. Divide the dough ball into four pieces. Roll each piece into a long rope. Cut each rope into about 25 (½-inch) pieces. Roll each piece into a tight ball. You should have 100 little balls when finished.
3. Preheat the air fryer to 370°F/185°C.
4. In batches of about 20, transfer the dough balls to the air fryer basket, leaving a small space in between them. Air-fry the dough balls at 370°F/185°C for 3 to 4 minutes, shaking the basket when one minute of cooking time remains.
5. After all the dough balls are air-fried, make the honey topping. Melt the honey in a small saucepan on the stovetop. Add the cinnamon, orange zest, and water. Simmer for one minute. Place the air-fried dough balls in a large bowl and drizzle the honey mixture over top. Gently toss to coat all the dough balls evenly. Transfer the coated struffoli to a platter and sprinkle the nonpareil candy sprinkles over top. You can dress the presentation up by piling the balls into the shape of a wreath or pile them high in a cone shape to resemble a Christmas tree.
6. Struffoli can be made ahead. Store covered tightly.

Strawberry Donuts

Servings: 4
Cooking Time: 55 Minutes
Ingredients:
- ¾ cup Greek yogurt
- 2 tbsp maple syrup
- 1 tbsp vanilla extract
- 2 tsp active dry yeast
- 1 ½ cups all-purpose flour
- 3 tbsp milk
- ½ cup strawberry jam

Directions:
1. Preheat air fryer to 350°F/175°C. Whisk the Greek yogurt, maple syrup, vanilla extract, and yeast until well combined. Then toss in flour until you get a sticky dough. Let rest covered for 10 minutes. Flour a parchment paper on a flat surface, lay the dough, sprinkle with some flour, and flatten to ½-inch thick with a rolling pin.
2. Using a 3-inch cookie cutter, cut the donuts. Repeat the process until no dough is left. Place the donuts in the basket and let rise for 15-20 minutes. Spread some milk on top of each donut and Air Fry for 4 minutes. Turn the donuts, spread more milk, and Air Fry for 4 more minutes until golden brown. Let cool for 15 minutes. Using a knife, cut the donuts 3/4 lengthwise, brush 1 tbsp of strawberry jam on each and close them. Serve.

Honeyed Tortilla Fritters

Servings: 8
Cooking Time: 10 Minutes
Ingredients:
- 2 tbsp granulated sugar
- ½ tsp ground cinnamon
- 1 tsp vanilla powder
- Salt to taste
- 8 flour tortillas, quartered
- 2 tbsp butter, melted
- 4 tsp honey
- 1 tbsp almond flakes

Directions:
1. Preheat air fryer at 400ºF/205°C. Combine the sugar, cinnamon, vanilla powder, and salt in a bowl. Set aside. Brush tortilla quarters with melted butter and sprinkle with sugar mixture. Place tortilla quarters in the frying basket and Air Fry for 4 minutes, turning once. Let cool on a large plate for 5 minutes until hardened. Drizzle with honey and scatter with almond flakes to serve.

Almond-roasted Pears

Servings: 4
Cooking Time: 15 Minutes
Ingredients:
- Yogurt Topping
- 1 container vanilla Greek yogurt (5–6 ounces)
- ¼ teaspoon almond flavoring
- 2 whole pears
- ¼ cup crushed Biscoff cookies (approx. 4 cookies)
- 1 tablespoon sliced almonds
- 1 tablespoon butter

Directions:
1. Stir almond flavoring into yogurt and set aside while preparing pears.
2. Halve each pear and spoon out the core.
3. Place pear halves in air fryer basket.
4. Stir together the cookie crumbs and almonds. Place a quarter of this mixture into the hollow of each pear half.
5. Cut butter into 4 pieces and place one piece on top of crumb mixture in each pear.
6. Cook at 360°F/180°C for 15 minutes or until pears have cooked through but are still slightly firm.
7. Serve pears warm with a dollop of yogurt topping.

Vanilla Cupcakes With Chocolate Chips

Servings: 2
Cooking Time: 25 Minutes + Cooling Time
Ingredients:
- ½ cup white sugar
- 1 ½ cups flour
- 2 tsp baking powder
- ½ tsp salt
- 2/3 cup sunflower oil
- 1 egg
- 2 tsp maple extract
- ¼ cup vanilla yogurt
- 1 cup chocolate chips

Directions:
1. Preheat air fryer to 350°F/175°C. Combine the sugar, flour, baking powder, and salt in a bowl and stir to combine. Whisk the egg in a separate bowl. Pour in the sunflower oil, yogurt, and maple extract, and continue whisking until light and fluffy. Spoon the wet mixture into the dry ingredients and stir to combine. Gently fold in the chocolate chips with a spatula. Divide the batter between cupcake cups and Bake in the air fryer for 12-15 minutes or until a toothpick comes out dry. Remove the cupcakes let them cool. Serve.

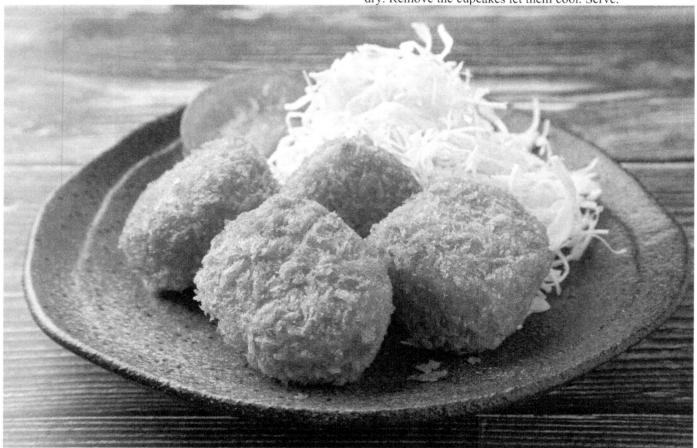

RECIPE INDEX

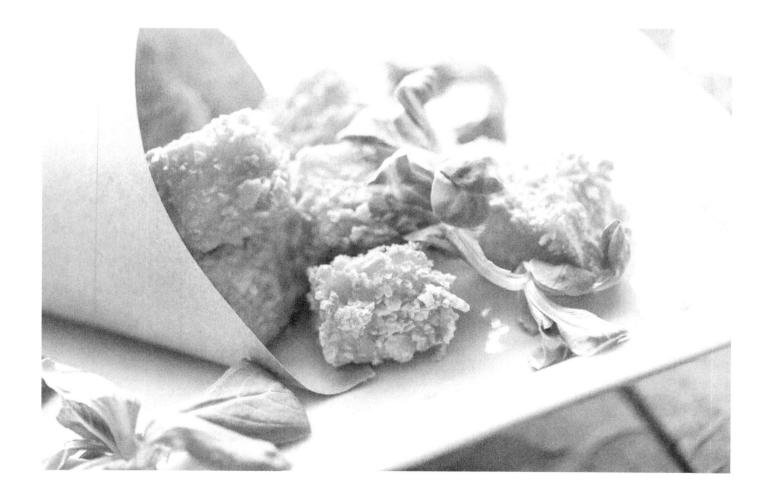

Printed in Great Britain
by Amazon